Santiago Canyon College
Library

Assistive Technology for the Hearing-impaired, Deaf and Deafblind

Springer
*London
Berlin
Heidelberg
New York
Hong Kong
Milan
Paris
Tokyo*

Marion A. Hersh, Michael A. Johnson (Eds.)
with Conny Andersson, Douglas Campbell, Alistair
Farquharson, Stephen Furner, John Gill, Alan Jackson,
Jay Lucker, Keith Nolde, Erhard Werner and Mike Whybray

Assistive Technology for the Hearing-impaired, Deaf and Deafblind

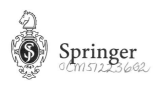

Springer

Marion A. Hersh, MSc, PhD
Department of Electronic and Electrical Engineering, University of Glasgow, Glasgow, G12 8LT, UK

Michael A. Johnson, MSc, PhD
Department of Electronic and Electrical Engineering, University of Strathclyde, Glasgow, G1 1QE, UK

British Library Cataloguing in Publication Data
Assistive technology for the hearing-impaired, deaf and deafblind
  1.Self-help devices for people with disabilities 2.Hearing impaired 3.Hearing aids – Design and construction
  I.Hersh, Marion A. II.Johnson, Michael A. (Michael Arthur), 1948-
  617.8'9
  ISBN 1852333820

Library of Congress Cataloging-in-Publication Data
Assistive technology for the hearing-impaired, deaf and deafblind / Marion A. Hersh, Michael A. Johnson (eds), with Conny Andersson ... [et al.].
  p. cm.
  Includes bibliographical references and index.
  ISBN 1-85233-382-0 (alk. paper)
  1. Deaf--Means of communication. 2. Communication devices for people with disabilities. 3. Deaf--Means of communication--Technological innovations. 4. Communication devices for people with disabilities--Technological innovations. I. Hersh, Marion A., 1956- II. Johnson, Michael A., 1948-

HV2502.A875 2003
362.4'283--dc21
                                        2002044538

Apart from any fair dealing for the purposes of research or private study, or criticism or review, as permitted under the Copyright, Designs and Patents Act 1988, this publication may only be reproduced, stored or transmitted, in any form or by any means, with the prior permission in writing of the publishers, or in the case of reprographic reproduction in accordance with the terms of licences issued by the Copyright Licensing Agency. Enquiries concerning reproduction outside those terms should be sent to the publishers.

ISBN 1-85233-382-0 Springer-Verlag London Berlin Heidelberg
a member of BertelsmannSpringer Science+Business Media GmbH

© Springer-Verlag London Limited 2003

The use of registered names, trademarks, etc. in this publication does not imply, even in the absence of a specific statement, that such names are exempt from the relevant laws and regulations and therefore free for general use.

Product liability: The publisher can give no guarantee for information about drug dosage and application thereof contained in this book. In every individual case the respective user must check its accuracy by consulting other pharmaceutical literature.

Typeset by Ian Kingston Editorial Services, Nottingham, UK
Printed and bound in the United States of America
28/3830-543210 Printed on acid-free paper SPIN 10781975

For my mother and father
Marion A. Hersh

That this book might inspire my two young friends, Holly and Joe
Michael A. Johnson

Preface

Affirmative legislative action in many countries now requires public spaces to be accessible and service providers to change or introduce practices, policies, or procedures that allow equal accessibility by disabled people. Although this is often interpreted as access for wheelchair users, such legislation also covers people with vision or hearing impairments. In these cases it is often the provision of advanced technological devices that enable people with sensory impairments to enjoy the theatre, cinema, a political meeting or a religious meeting to the full. Hearing-impaired and deaf people have been especial beneficiaries of this slow, but growing, technological provision, and this book is about this particular branch of assistive technology.

The field of assistive technology has steadily grown, driven by the desire to provide disabled people with equal access to the facilities and products of society and to provide an enhanced quality of life for this community group. Many different engineering ideas and disciplines have been used to produce the technological solutions required. However, there have been few, if any, systematic attempts to draw together the themes of assistive technology and create a coherent technological and engineering discipline. It is true that organisations like the Rehabilitation Engineering Society of North America (RESNA) and the Association for the Advancement of Assistive Technology in Europe (AAATE) try to present a cohesive programme for assistive technology, but our experience has been that, although many engineers are active in these organisations, assistive technology has not yet become part of mainstream engineering.

Part of the problem is simply the lack of a coherent educational framework for involving *engineers* in the assistive technology field. This is not to say that engineers do not wish to study the subject, since our experience is that young undergraduate and postgraduate engineers relish the idea of trying to solve problems in assistive engineering. Indeed, there are some really challenging technical problems still to be tackled. What is missing are books that demonstrate that it is possible to bring together the themes of human physiology, fundamental engineering principles, design principles, engineering technology, and human end-user issues (such as ethics) to make a coherent course that can contribute to the higher education of electrical and mechanical engineers. This particular collaborative book is an attempt to demonstrate just how this might be accomplished for the assistive technology needed by the hearing impaired and deaf community. The book is envisaged as the first of a series of three texts dealing, in turn, with assistive technologies and devices for people with hearing, vision and mobility impairments.

In parallel with developing this textbook, we have been pioneering the introduction of a course module on Assistive Technology in the Electronic and Electrical Engineering degrees at our respective universities. The experience gained in developing the educational framework has also been fed into the book as it progressed. The consequence has been a strong editorial steer on the various chapters to give the type of information required in degree courses and the strong engineering approach in the book. This particular book is about the application of electrical technology to all aspects of communication and daily living for those people with hearing impairments. The first chapter, on physiological aspects of hearing, sets the background for the various technological areas, namely hearing-aid development, induction and infrared communications for public spaces, and accessibility. The book then continues with facilitating technologies and devices for telephony and daily living. The penultimate chapter takes a look at assistive technology for deafblind people, a really challenging area with a number of unsolved research questions. The final chapter of the book presents a basic introduction to human end-user issues and ethics, as well as the distribution of devices to end users. This is not a long chapter, but it deals with topics that are often omitted from existing engineering courses.

We believe we set ourselves ambitious objectives in writing this book, which could not have been accomplished without the cooperation and enthusiasm of our collaborating authors. We would like to thank them all for their help and patience in seeing the project come to fruition. We have been lucky to meet many of our collaborators at the Conference and Workshop on Assistive Technologies for Vision and Hearing Impairment, which we organise with invaluable European Union support (from the High Level Scientific Conference Programme), and this has given us the opportunity to discuss and debate together many of the engineering ideas and techniques reported in the book. Needless to say, we have made many new friends in the process and gained many useful insights into assistive technology for people with hearing and vision impairments. We hope this book will inspire many new projects, new courses and new ways to assist people with sensory impairments.

Marion Hersh and Michael Johnson
Glasgow, Scotland, UK

Who Should Read This Book

This book is designed to inform a wide range of current and future professionals about basic engineering principles and the way these principles are turned into assistive technology devices, the possible future technology developments, and the human end-user aspects in assistive technology for hearing-impaired and deaf people. As far as we have been able to ascertain, there are no other textbooks for electrical engineering, mechanical engineering and scientific professionals on this technological area at this depth or with this higher educational approach. This is expected to change as legislative pressures drive the need for more engineering and social professionals to become aware of these technologies. Similarly, we have not been able to find any undergraduate course texts of adequate detail and depth for the discipline of assistive technology. Thus, we hope this book will be well placed to meet this need, as it has been designed to be read by electrical engineering undergraduates as a course book or to supplement existing courses. The authors have been encouraged to see many engineering undergraduates enjoy this type of material, and it is hoped that this enjoyment will fire the ingenuity of engineering students to find new and innovative ways to develop technology to support hearing-impaired and deaf people.

An Overview of the Book

This book provides detailed coverage of the full range of assistive technologies used to support deaf and hearing-impaired people, including state-of-the-art techniques. Division into chapters is based on either the type of technology or the field of application. The following applications are discussed: audiology and assessment of hearing loss, hearing aids, telecommunications, devices for daily living and devices for deafblind people. Systems and devices based on the induction-loop technology and infrared technology are presented. To provide a background to the technologies, particularly the hearing assessment and hearing-aid technologies, the first chapter discusses the physiology of the ear and causes of deafness.

The book is designed so that each chapter is self-contained and can be read on its own, though familiarity with the material in Chapter 1 will be assumed in some of the other chapters. Each chapter is motivated by specific learning objectives and contains an introduction to the subject, such as the basic principles of the underlying technology or the application area. This is usually followed by a full discussion of the applications of the technology to support the hearing impaired. The chapters close with suggestions for projects and reference to further reading sources, books, journal and conference papers and Web sites. There may be many professionals for whom this is a new area and who may not be familiar with the underpinning pedagogical engineering topics covered in the various chapters, so Table 1 is given to provide an outline plan of the book and the disciplines involved.

Editorial Responsibilities

The concept of this book originated with Marion Hersh and Michael Johnson, who were also responsible for the overall task of collating and integrating the various contributions. The book is more a close collaboration between editors and chapter contributors than the usual book of edited chapters and papers. This was necessary to try and obtain the style of a textbook on assistive technology for hearing-impaired and deaf people.

Table 1 An outline plan of book and pedagogical fundamentals.

Chapter		Key fundamentals in the chapter
1	Anatomy and Physiology of Hearing, Hearing Impairment and Treatment	Human physiology (of the ear) Acoustics, speech and sound Hearing-loss categories
2	Audiology: The Measurement of Hearing	Measurement principles Frequency response and decibels Instrumentation – medical Calibration and standards
3	Hearing-aid Principles and Technology	Signal-processing principles Human body as an engineering environment Electronics – analogue and digital
4	Induction-loop Systems	Electromagnetic principles Electrical circuit equivalents Calibration and standards
5	Infrared Communication Systems	Electromagnetic spectrum Basic communication system principles Diodes – LEDs and IREDs System design, construction and standards
6	Telephone Technology	Basic telephony principles Electromagnetic induction Textphone principles Videophone principles Ergonomics
7	Alarm and Alerting Systems for Hearing-impaired and Deaf People	Unifying generic system structures Sensors, transmission modules and actuators Amplifier types and principles Interface design and ergonomics
8	Dual Sensory Impairment: Devices for Deafblind People	Sensory impairment demography and classes Braille principles Sensors and actuators Difficult interface design and ergonomics Information technology
9	The Final Product: Issues in the Design and Distribution of Assistive Technology Devices	Human issues Working with end users Social research methods Ethics for engineers and other professionals

Chapter Contributions

Chapter 1 on, Anatomy and Physiology of Hearing, Hearing Impairment and Treatment, was the work of Jay Lucker with input from Marion Hersh. Marion Hersh and Michael Johnson contributed Chapter 2, on Audiology: The Measurement of Hearing, in which an engineering perspective to the measurement aspect of audiology is taken. Douglas Campbell, who was a Leverhulme Fellow in Hearing Aid Technology, contributed Chapter 3, Hearing-aid Principles and Technology. Bo-Edin is a Swedish company specialising in induction-loop technology, and Conny Andersson drew on his wide applications experience to write Chapter 4 on Induction-loop Systems. Similarly, Erhard Werner used his deep technical expertise garnered from a long career with the Sennheiser

Company to write Chapter 5 on Infrared Communications Systems. British Telecommunications research laboratories, located within BTexact at Adastral Park in Suffolk, have a world renowned reputation in assistive technology for telecommunications. Stephen Furner and his colleagues from BT at Adastral Park wrote Chapter 6 on Telephone Technology for hearing-impaired people. Chapter 7, on Alarm and Alerting Systems for Hearing-impaired and Deaf People, was written by Marion Hersh with input from Jay Lucker. The presentation of a common and generic engineering framework in which to discuss the various devices was an important component of this chapter. John Gill used his long association with the RNIB to write Chapter 8, Dual Sensory Impairment: Devices for Deafblind People; this material was augmented by contributions from Marion Hersh. Finally, Chapter 9, The Final Product: Issues in the Design and Distribution of Assistive Technology Devices, was contributed by Marion Hersh.

The Contributors and Their Affiliations

Marion Hersh, Department of Electronics and Electrical Engineering, University of Glasgow, Glasgow G12 8LT, Scotland, UK.

Michael A. Johnson, Department of Electronic and Electrical Engineering, University of Strathclyde, Glasgow G1 1QE, Scotland, UK.

Jay R. Lucker, formerly with Department of Audiology & Speech–Language Pathology, Gallaudet University, Washington, DC 20002-3695, USA. Now in private practice: PO Box 4177, Silver Spring, MD 20914-4177, USA.

Douglas R. Campbell, School of Information and Communication Technologies, University of Paisley, High Street, Paisley, PA1 2BE, Scotland, UK.

Conny Andersson, Bo-Edin, S-18175 Lidingo, Sweden.

Erhard Werner, formerly with Sennheiser, Germany.

Stephen Furner, Alan Jackson, Keith Nolde, Mike Whybray and Alistair Farquharson, British Telecommunications, Adastral Park, Martlesham Heath, Suffolk IP5 3RE, UK.

John Gill, Royal National Institute for the Blind, Falcon Park, Neasden Lane, London NW10 1RN, England, UK.

More detailed biographical sketches of the individual contributors can be found at the end of the book.

Contents

1 **Anatomy and Physiology of Hearing, Hearing Impairment and Treatment** 1
   1.1 Introduction 1
       1.1.1 Learning Objectives 1
       1.1.2 Overview of Hearing 2
       1.1.3 The Auditory System in Engineering Terms 3
   1.2 Acoustics of Hearing 4
       1.2.1 Amplitude 6
       1.2.2 Phase 7
       1.2.3 Frequency and Period 8
       1.2.4 Sound Intensity and the Decibel Scale 8
       1.2.5 Simple and Complex Sounds 9
       1.2.6 Spectral Analysis of Complex Sounds 10
       1.2.7 Filtering Sound 10
   1.3 Anatomy and Physiology of the Auditory System 14
       1.3.1 Some Terminology Used in Describing Anatomical Structures 14
   1.4 The Anatomy and Functions of the Outer-ear Structures 15
       1.4.1 The Pinna 16
       1.4.2 External Auditory Meatus 16
       1.4.3 Functions of the Outer-ear Structures 17
   1.5 The Anatomy and Functions of the Middle-ear Structures 18
       1.5.1 The Tympanic Membrane 18
       1.5.2 Middle-ear Ossicles 19
       1.5.3 The Middle-ear Cavity 20
       1.5.4 The Functions of the Middle-ear Structures 22
   1.6 The Anatomy and Functions of the Inner-ear Structures 23
       1.6.1 Vestibule 24
       1.6.2 The Cochlea 24
       1.6.3 Sound Processing in the Cochlea 27
   1.7 The Central Auditory Nervous System 27
   1.8 Classification of Hearing Loss 29
       1.8.1 Degrees of Hearing Loss 31
       1.8.2 Hearing Loss Due to Problems in the Outer Ear 31
       1.8.3 Hearing Loss Due to Problems in Middle Ear 32
       1.8.4 Hearing Loss Due to Problems in the Cochlea 32

		1.8.5 Problems in the Auditory (Eighth) Nerve and Central Auditory Pathways	33

- 1.9 Medical and Non-medical Treatments ... 36
  - 1.9.1 Medical and Surgical Treatment of Problems in the Auditory System ... 36
  - 1.9.2 Non-medical or Non-surgical Interventions ... 36
- 1.10 Learning Highlights of the Chapter ... 37
- Projects and Investigations ... 38
- References and Further Reading ... 39

2 Audiology: The Measurement of Hearing ... 41
- 2.1 Introduction: The Measurement of Hearing ... 41
  - 2.1.1 Learning Objectives ... 41
- 2.2 Measurement Systems ... 42
  - 2.2.1 Definitions ... 42
  - 2.2.2 Frequency-response Curves ... 43
  - 2.2.3 Gain in Decibels ... 43
  - 2.2.4 Amplifiers ... 44
- 2.3 Measurement of Biological Variables and Sources of Error ... 44
  - 2.3.1 Types of Error ... 44
  - 2.3.2 Physiological and Environmental Sources of Error ... 45
- 2.4 The Test Decision Process ... 46
- 2.5 Pure-tone Audiometry ... 47
  - 2.5.1 Audiograms ... 47
  - 2.5.2 Noise ... 48
  - 2.5.3 The Test ... 48
  - 2.5.4 Masking ... 51
  - 2.5.5 Instrumentation ... 52
  - 2.5.6 Technical Description of an Audiometer ... 53
  - 2.5.7 Technical Specifications ... 55
- 2.6 Immittance Audiometry ... 56
  - 2.6.1 Definitions ... 56
  - 2.6.2 Measurement ... 57
  - 2.6.3 Static Acoustic Immittance ... 58
  - 2.6.4 Tympanometry ... 58
  - 2.6.5 Acoustic Reflex Threshold ... 59
- 2.7 Electric Response Audiometry (ERA) ... 59
  - 2.7.1 Electrocochleography ... 60
  - 2.7.2 Brain-stem Response Audiometry ... 61
- 2.8 Standards ... 61
- 2.9 Audiometric Equipment Design and Calibration ... 62
  - 2.9.1 Earphone Calibration ... 63
  - 2.9.2 Calibration of Pure-tone Audiometers ... 64
  - 2.9.3 Calibration of Couplers and Sound-level Meters ... 64
  - 2.9.4 Calibration of Bone Vibrators ... 65
  - 2.9.5 Calibration of Acoustic Immittance Devices ... 65
- 2.10 Artificial Ears ... 65
  - 2.10.1 The 2cc Coupler ... 66
  - 2.10.2 Zwislocki Coupler ... 67
  - 2.10.3 KEMAR ... 67

	2.11	Learning Highlights of the Chapter	68

Acknowledgements ... 68
Projects and Investigations ... 68
References and Further Reading ... 69

3 Hearing-aid Principles and Technology ... 71
3.1 Learning Objectives ... 71
3.2 Introduction ... 71
3.2.1 Review of Technical Terms ... 73
3.2.2 Human Hearing Viewed from an Engineering Perspective ... 73
3.2.3 Hearing-aid Prescription (in Brief) ... 77
3.3 Categories of Electronic Aids ... 80
3.3.1 Body-worn Aid ... 81
3.3.2 Behind-the-ear Aid ... 81
3.3.3 Spectacles Aid ... 83
3.3.4 In-the-ear Aid ... 83
3.3.5 Bone-conduction Aid ... 84
3.3.6 Middle-ear Implant Aid ... 85
3.3.7 Cochlear Implant Aid ... 85
3.3.8 Auditory Brain-stem Implant Aid ... 86
3.4 Historical Background ... 87
3.5 The Ear as an Environment ... 88
3.5.1 Aid-on-body Considerations ... 88
3.5.2 Body-on-aid Considerations ... 90
3.6 Processing Strategies ... 91
3.6.1 Single-channel Processing Schemes ... 91
3.6.2 Multiple-channel Processing Schemes ... 103
3.7 Modern Hearing-aid Technology ... 106
3.7.1 Analogue Hearing Aids ... 106
3.7.2 Digital Hearing Aids ... 106
3.7.3 Portable Speech Processors ... 108
3.8 Conclusion and Learning Highlights of the Chapter ... 109
3.8.1 Current Research ... 110
3.8.2 A Future Possibility? ... 110
3.8.3 Learning Highlights of the Chapter ... 110

Acknowledgements ... 111
Projects and Investigations ... 111
References and Further Reading ... 113

4 Induction-loop Systems ... 117
4.1 Learning Objectives ... 117
4.2 Audio-frequency Induction-loop Systems ... 117
4.3 The Electromagnetic Principles of a Loop System ... 118
4.4 Induction-loop Systems ... 121
4.4.1 Hearing-aid Receiver or Telecoil ... 121
4.4.2 The Effect of Different Materials and Loop Shapes ... 122
4.4.3 Magnetic Field Strength ... 123
4.4.4 Magnetic Field Direction ... 124
4.4.5 Magnetic Field Distribution ... 124

		4.4.6 Overspill	128
	4.5	Loop Installation	132
		4.5.1 Multi-combination Loop System	136
	4.6	The Electrical Equivalent of a Loop System	136
		4.6.1 Loop Inductance	137
		4.6.2 Loop Resistance	137
		4.6.3 Loop Impedance	137
		4.6.4 Two-turn Loop	141
	4.7	Automatic Gain Control	143
	4.8	Loop System Measurements	146
		4.8.1 The Dynamic Range of a Loop System	146
		4.8.2 Magnetic Field Strength as a Function of Level and Frequency	147
		4.8.3 Measurement of the Loop Amplifier	147
		4.8.4 Field-strength Meters	148
	4.9	Standards for Loop Systems	149
	4.10	Learning Highlights for the Chapter	150
	Projects and Investigations		151
	References and Further Reading		152
5	**Infrared Communication Systems**		**153**
	5.1	Learning Objectives and Introduction	153
		5.1.1 Learning Objectives	153
	5.2	Basic Principles	153
		5.2.1 General Technical Requirements for Audio Applications	154
		5.2.2 Applications	155
		5.2.3 Technical Features and Application Requirements	157
	5.3	System Components	158
		5.3.1 Audio Sources and Signal Processing in the Transmitter	159
		5.3.2 Radiators	160
		5.3.3 Receivers	164
	5.4	Compatibility and Use with Hearing Aids	169
	5.5	Design Issues	169
		5.5.1 System Placement	170
		5.5.2 Interference Issues	170
		5.5.3 Ergonomic and Operational Issues	170
	5.6	Technical Standards and Regulations	172
	5.7	Advantages and Disadvantages of Infrared Systems	172
	5.8	Conclusions and Learning Highlights	173
		5.8.1 Learning Highlights of the Chapter	173
	Acknowledgements		173
	Projects and Investigations		174
	References and Further Reading		175
6	**Telephone Technology**		**177**
	6.1	Introducing Telephony and Learning Objectives	177
	6.2	User-centred Telephone Design	178
		6.2.1 Designing for Hearing Impairment	178

	6.2.2	Putting It All Together	180
6.3	Design of an Electronic Telephone		180
	6.3.1	Introducing the Modern Telephone	182
	6.3.2	Indication of the Start of the Call	184
	6.3.3	Transmission of Signalling Information	184
	6.3.4	Design of the Transmission Circuit	187
	6.3.5	Call Arrival Indication (Ringing)	190
	6.3.6	Telephone Design Enhancements to Provide Additional Accessibility Features	192
6.4	The Text Telephone		195
	6.4.1	Introduction	195
	6.4.2	Basic Principles	196
6.5	The Videophone		203
	6.5.1	Basic Principles	203
	6.5.2	Application Aspects	206
	6.5.3	Systems and Standards	208
	6.5.4	Future Systems	210
6.6	Conclusions and Learning Highlights		210
	6.6.1	Learning Highlights of the Chapter	210
	Projects and Investigations		211
References and Further Reading			212

7 Alarm and Alerting Systems for Hearing-impaired and Deaf People — 215

7.1	Learning Objectives		215
7.2	The Engineering Principles of Alarm and Alerting Devices		215
	7.2.1	Design Issues	216
	7.2.2	Categorisation of Alarm and Alerting Systems	218
7.3	Sensors, Transducers and Actuators		220
	7.3.1	The Sensors in Fire Alarms	221
	7.3.2	Carbon Monoxide Sensors	223
	7.3.3	Intruder Detectors	225
	7.3.4	Piezoelectric Sensors: Sound and Pressure	226
	7.3.5	Microphones: Sound Sensors	228
7.4	Signal Conditioning		229
	7.4.1	Voltage and Power Amplifiers	230
	7.4.2	Transistor	231
	7.4.3	Voltage Amplifiers	233
	7.4.4	Small-signal Tuned Amplifiers	234
	7.4.5	Class C Power Amplifiers	235
	7.4.6	Class AB Power Amplifiers	237
7.5	Radio Frequency Transmission		237
	7.5.1	Transmitter	238
	7.5.2	Superheterodyne Receiver	239
	7.5.3	Modulation	241
	7.5.4	Modulator	242
	7.5.5	Demodulator	244
7.6	Actuators		246
	7.6.1	Auditory Signals: Loud Bells and Buzzers	246
	7.6.2	Lights	247

	7.6.3	Light-emitting Diodes	248
	7.6.4	Television	248
	7.6.5	Vibro-tactile Devices	249
	7.6.6	Electro-tactile Devices	250
	7.6.7	Paging Systems	250
7.7	Learning Highlights of the Chapter		253
Projects and Investigations			253
References and Further Reading			254

8 Dual Sensory Impairment: Devices for Deafblind People 257

- 8.1 Learning Objectives 257
- 8.2 Definitions and Demographics of Deafblindness 257
- 8.3 Communication for Deafblind People 258
  - 8.3.1 Assistive Technology for Deafblind Communication .. 261
- 8.4 Braille Devices 262
  - 8.4.1 Braille Displays 262
  - 8.4.2 Multifunction Braille Notetakers 263
  - 8.4.3 Text–Braille Conversion and Braille Embossers 264
- 8.5 Automating Fingerspelling for Deafblind Communication 266
  - 8.5.1 Developing Mechanical Fingerspelling Hands for Deafblind People 266
  - 8.5.2 Dexter I 267
  - 8.5.3 Dexter II and III 268
  - 8.5.4 Fingerspelling Hand for Gallaudet 268
  - 8.5.5 Ralph 270
  - 8.5.6 The Handtapper – a UK Development 271
  - 8.5.7 Speaking Hands and Talking Gloves 272
  - 8.5.8 Comparison and Availability 273
- 8.6 Other Communication Aids 274
  - 8.6.1 The Optacon and Optical Character Recognition (OCR) 274
  - 8.6.2 Tactile Sound-recognition Devices 275
- 8.7 Low-technology Devices and Domestic Appliances 276
- 8.8 Bluetooth 278
- 8.9 Alerting Devices for Deafblind People 279
  - 8.9.1 Vibrating Alarm Clocks 280
  - 8.9.2 A Multifunction Domestic Alert System 282
  - 8.9.3 Tactiwatch 284
  - 8.9.4 Tam 284
- 8.10 Access to Information Technology 284
  - 8.10.1 The Universal Communications Text Browser (Ucon) 286
- 8.11 Provision of Telecommunications Equipment and Services .. 286
  - 8.11.1 Hardware 287
  - 8.11.2 Software and Access to Telecommunications 289
- 8.12 Future Research Directions 290
- Projects and Investigations 292
- References and Further Reading 293

9 The Final Product: Issues in the Design and Distribution of Assistive Technology Devices **297**
   9.1   Development and Distribution of Devices 297
   9.2   Working with End Users 299
         9.2.1   Methods for Involving End Users 300
         9.2.2   FORTUNE Concept of User Participation in Projects . 300
   9.3   Communication Issues 301
   9.4   Other Important Issues 302
         9.4.1   Deaf Culture and Deaf Awareness 302
         9.4.2   Ethical Issues 303
         9.4.3   Data Protection Legislation 304
   Acknowledgements 304
   References and Further Reading 305

Biographies of the Contributors (in Alphabetical Order of Family Name) **307**

Index **313**

1 Anatomy and Physiology of Hearing, Hearing Impairment and Treatment

1.1 Introduction

The auditory system is a complex network that transduces pressure gradients caused by sound vibrations into neuroelectrical energy in the central nervous system. These neuroelectrical signals are then interpreted in the brain as, for instance, speech or music. Problems in the auditory system can lead to hearing difficulties or deafness.

Sound is an important source of information. Most face-to-face communication is by sound signals in the form of speech. However, persons who are deaf or hard-of-hearing may not be able to make use of sound signals for communicating effectively. Technology plays an important role in supporting the communication and information needs of deaf people and people who are hard-of-hearing. This includes hearing aids (Chapter 3), induction loop and infrared listening devices (Chapters 4 and 5), text and video telephones (Chapter 6), and visual or vibrating alarms and alerting devices (Chapter 7). Further research and development is still required in many of these technological areas, but especially those of the electro-vibratory and electro-tactile transmission of speech signals and speech–sign language text–signal language translation.

Understanding the basic principles of the auditory system and the basic causes of some of the main types of hearing loss can help engineers and technology experts to develop appropriate assistive devices, as well as to decide when assisted auditory, visual or tactile access to communication is more appropriate. This chapter aims to provide this basic understanding of hearing and hearing loss in order to serve as a foundation for understanding how to approach the development of assistive technology devices for deaf people and those who are hard-of-hearing.

1.1.1 Learning Objectives

The basic aim of this chapter is to give readers an understanding of the acoustics of sound and the functioning of the auditory system. Specific learning objectives include the following:

- basic understanding of the acoustics of sound, including how sound is propagated and how the propagation of sound relates to hearing;
- basic knowledge of the anatomy of the auditory system;
- some understanding of the functioning of each part of the ear;
- understanding how hearing loss is measured and various degrees and types of hearing loss;
- basic knowledge of the causes of the main types of hearing loss;
- basic knowledge of some primary medical and non-medical treatments for different types of hearing loss.

1.1.2 Overview of Hearing

Hearing is one of the five senses, along with vision, taste, smell, and touch. The ears receive sound and transmits it to the brain, where it is interpreted, so that speech, music, and other signals can be heard. Therefore, the auditory system requires a source of sound, a mechanism for receiving this sound, mechanisms for relaying sounds to the central nervous system, and pathways in the central nervous systems to deliver this sensory information to the brain where it can be interpreted, integrated, and stored. A cross-section of the ear, including the outer, the middle, and the inner ear with cochlea and auditory nerve, can be seen in Figure 1.1.

Most sounds are produced by vibration of air molecules from an oscillating source. In the case of speech, the vibrating source is the *vocal folds* or voice box in the throat or *larynx*. The ear can be divided into three main components: the outer, middle, and inner ear. The outer ear consists of the *pinna* or *auricle* and

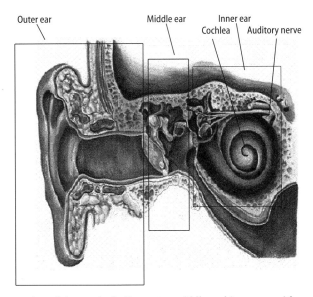

Figure 1.1 Cross-section of the ear, including outer, middle and inner ear with cochlea and auditory nerve (based on illustration courtesy of http://www.earaces.com/).

the ear canal or *external auditory meatus* (EAM). The eardrum or *tympanic membrane* is sometimes considered as part of the outer ear and sometimes as part of the middle ear.

The pinna generally protrudes to make it easier to capture sound waves. These captured waves are then funnelled by the pinna down the ear canal and strike the eardrum. The sound wave vibrations striking the eardrum make the membrane vibrate. The middle ear consists of three small bones or *ossicles*, the *malleus* (hammer), *incus* (anvil) and *stapes* (stirrup). Vibrations of the eardrum make the malleus, which is attached to it, move. This motion is transmitted to the other two ossicles. The three ossicles, or *ossicular chain*, transmit the eardrum vibrations to the end portion of the stapes, called the *footplate*, as it resembles the part of a stirrup into which the foot is placed when mounting a horse.

The middle ear is separated from the inner ear by a bony wall. The footplate fits into the *oval window*, an oval hole in this wall. The inner ear is divided into two sensory parts. The first part is called the *vestibular system* and is the sensory system of the inner ear involved with balance, motion, and feedback related to the body's position in space. It is *not* involved in hearing or auditory sensitivity. The auditory portion of the inner ear is called the *cochlea*. It is a fluid-filled portion of the temporal bone that houses the sensory receptor structures of the auditory system in its central portion, or *cochlear duct*. This duct can be thought of as a membranous canal in the fluid-filled cochlea. The auditory receptor cells are in the cochlear duct. They are called *hair cells*, as they have hair-like protrusions (*cilia*).

Motion of the footplate causes waves in the fluids of the cochlea. As the waves travel down the cochlea, the cochlear duct moves up and down. This movement leads to a bending of the cilia, causing the hair cells to release neurochemicals from their bases. The fibres or *neurons* of the auditory nerve, known as the eighth cranial nerve or the eighth nerve, are below the hair cells. These neurons receive the neurochemicals, giving rise to a neural impulse that travels along the fibres or *axons* of the eighth nerve. The cochlea, its internal structures, and the eighth nerve make up the auditory portion of the inner ear.

The auditory nerve connects the cochlea with the *brainstem*, a portion of the central nervous system above the spinal cord, but below the *cortex* or brain. In the brainstem, the auditory sensory information from the stimulation of the cochlea is transmitted as neuroelectrochemical activity through a succession of neurons to the auditory reception areas of the cortex. In the cortex, the nerve connections transmit the sound sensations to various parts of the brain, where they are interpreted, form mental images, and are stored for later use. The brainstem and cortical auditory pathways are known as the *central auditory nervous system* (CANS) or more simply as the auditory pathways.

1.1.3 The Auditory System in Engineering Terms

The signals of interest originate as sound pressure waves and are transformed into electrochemical nerve signals that are processed by the auditory brainstem and in the auditory cortex of the brain.

The ear can be considered as a signal-processing device that performs the following functions (Figure 1.2):

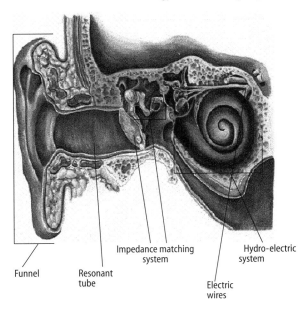

Figure 1.2 The auditory system in engineering terms (based on illustration courtesy of http://www.earaces.com/).

- transduction
- filtering
- amplification
- non-linear compression
- impedance matching
- spectral analysis.

Although this type of engineering system is useful, it is also important to recognise the difference between human and electromechanical systems. Other factors, including processing in the brain, individual perceptions, and emotions, also affect hearing.

1.2 Acoustics of Hearing

Hearing begins with the propagation of a sound wave. Therefore, to understand hearing and hearing loss, it is necessary to understand how sound is generated and how it travels from its source to the ear. Sound is produced by a vibrating or oscillating body. It then travels as *longitudinal waves* through a medium, usually air, to the ear. It can also travel through other mediums, such as liquids and solids.

The vibrating body transmits the vibration to the molecules of air in contact with it, making them vibrate. This motion is resisted by the *frictional resistance* of air, which converts some of the kinetic energy of motion into heat and

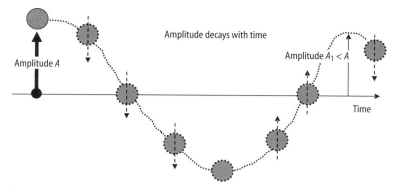

Figure 1.3 Oscillatory motion of air molecule and the effect of frictional resistance.

reduces the amplitude of the oscillation until the air molecules stop moving. However, the vibration is communicated to other molecules and will travel through the air until it encounters an object that acts as an opposing force. Objects that are elastic, such as the eardrum, will start oscillating due to the force of the air molecules striking them.

The graph in Figure 1.3 shows displacement from the rest position against time. The *amplitude* of a particular wave is the distance between any wave peak (*e.g.* amplitudes A and A_1 in Figure 1.3) and the position of rest on the horizontal axis. The effect of frictional resistance is to reduce the amplitude as time progresses.

The longitudinal sound wave resulting from the vibration of an object being communicated to and travelling through the air molecules is illustrated in Figure 1.4. The difference between the vibration of each air molecule about a point of rest and the wave that moves through the air molecules should be noted. The figure illustrates points of *compression*, where the air molecules are clumped together due to the motion, and points of *rarefaction*, where the molecules are spread out.

Figure 1.5 shows the sound wave travelling from its source as a series of concentric circles. Each circle represents points of compression and the spaces between the circles represent points of rarefaction.

Important features of a sound wave include amplitude, frequency and phase.

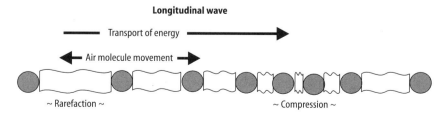

Figure 1.4 Longitudinal sound wave.

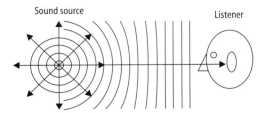

Figure 1.5 Sound spreading out from a source (by kind courtesy of http://interface.cipic.ucdavis.edu/CIL_tutorial/3D_phys/sines.htm).

1.2.1 Amplitude

The amplitude of a sound wave is the maximum displacement of an air molecule from its rest position. Since it is produced by a vibrating body making contact with air molecules and applying a force to them, sound amplitude is measured as the *sound pressure level* (SPL), as pressure is equal to force divided by area, in this case the force from the vibrating body over the area into which it comes in contact with or the area of the eardrum when this vibration is transmitted to the eardrum.

The smallest SPL at which sound can be perceived is taken as 20 μPa (micropascals). This gives the first point (zero) of the amplitude scale. The amplitude of sound measured is generally measured relative to the *peak amplitude*, *i.e.* the SPL measured in micropascals at the peak (see root-mean-square below). Sound pressure can also be measured at other points than peaks on a sound wave.

It can also be shown that the sound wave moves with *simple harmonic motion* with distance from rest or amplitude given by

$$y = A\sin 2\pi ft = A\sin \omega t$$

where A is the peak amplitude and ω is a measure of angular velocity, given by $\omega = 2\pi f$ with f the frequency of the wave. Since the amplitude of the signal y is measured as a sine function, the sound wave can be considered as a *sine wave*. The above sine wave equation can be obtained by considering the wave motion of the sound wave as *uniform circular motion*, in which the motion of any point P on the sound wave can be seen to be analogous to motion around the circumference of a circle, as shown in Figure 1.6.

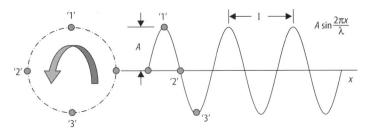

Figure 1.6 Circular motion.

On this circle, the points at rest are the two points on the circle circumference on the *x* axis and the points of maximum displacement are the two points on the circle circumference on the *y* axis.

Sound amplitude is generally measured using the *root-mean-square* (r.m.s.) amplitude, which is denoted by A_{rms}. In the case of a sine wave, the r.m.s. value is 0.707 times the peak amplitude or 70.7% of the peak amplitude. Thus, $A_{rms} = 0.707A$, where A is the peak amplitude.

1.2.2 Phase

As already seen above, sound waves can be represented by sine waves. The *phase* of a sine or sound wave indicates at what point in the cycle the sound wave starts. For instance, a sound wave with phase of 90° starts with its maximum amplitude rather than at rest and, therefore, is equivalent to a cosine wave (see Figure 1.7(a) and (b)). Phase angle varies from 0 to 360°. It is also useful to compare the phase angles of different sine waves to obtain the relative phase, as shown in Figure 1.7, where the three sine waves shown have relative phases of 0°, 90° and 180°. This factor becomes important when considering that sound in the environment is made from various sine waves that may have differing phases. The interaction of phase becomes important when, for

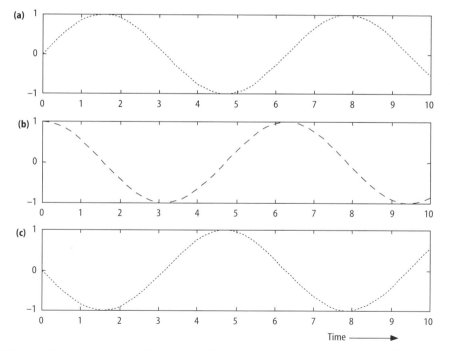

Figure 1.7 The relative phase of three sinusoidal waves: (a) sine wave with no phase shift; (b) sine wave with 90° phase shift; (c) sine wave with 180° phase shift.

example, two sounds of the same frequency and intensity are 180° out of phase. In such a case, the sounds cancel each other out, leading to no sound being perceived (consider adding the two sine waves in Figure 1.7(a) and (c) together). This is one method for eliminating unwanted sound.

1.2.3 Frequency and Period

Frequency is the number of cycles or complete oscillations per second. A cycle is an oscillation of an air molecule from rest through the points of maximum displacement (A and B) and back to the initial point of rest. Frequency is generally measured in hertz or cycles per second. In terms of circular motion, a cycle is equivalent to moving round the circle once or going through 360° or 2π radians. Therefore, frequency is also sometimes measured as angular frequency in radians per second.

Period is the length of time taken to complete one cycle. Therefore, it is the inverse of the frequency. Thus, a sound with a frequency of 1000 Hz has a period of 1/1000 s or 1 ms.

1.2.4 Sound Intensity and the Decibel Scale

The amplitude or SPL of a sound is also related to the *intensity* of a sound. Intensity is the measure of energy used per unit of time per unit of area. Since the area of molecular movement for sound waves is fairly small, it is usually measured in centimetres squared (cm^2) and time is measured in units of seconds. Thus, intensity is measured as joules/second/cm^2 or equivalently as watts/cm^2. Sound intensity is used in acoustics, for example, when measuring sound from a loudspeaker. However, in hearing it is the pressure of sound striking the eardrum rather than the sound intensity that is significant.

Studies of sound perception have shown that sound intensity is related to the ratio of the measured pressure P_m for the sound under investigation to the pressure P_r for the softest sound that can be heard (called the reference pressure). This reference pressure is $P_r = 20$ µPa. Thus, sound intensity is perceived as the ratio $(P_m/P_r)^2$. It has also been shown experimentally that multiplying the sound pressure in micropascals by a factor of ten is required to give a perceived doubling of loudness. For instance, a sound of 200 µPa is twice as loud as one of 20 µPa, and a sound of 2000 µPa is four times as loud as one of 20 µPa.

This finding suggests the use of a scale based on logarithms to the base ten would be convenient. Such a scale, called the bel (B) scale, is used in sound and acoustics and is named after the pioneering engineer in this field, Alexander Graham Bell. However, when measurements of sound are made, using bels gives a rather small range and also gives many sound pressures with values of one decimal place, such as 3.5 or 6.4 B. This is not so convenient, so the decibel (dB) is generally used. A bel is equal to 10 dB, and 6.4 B would become 64 dB.

The SPL can be obtained from measurements of the sound pressure P_m of a particular sound as

$$\text{Sound Pressure Level} = 10\log_{10}\left(\frac{P_m}{P_r}\right)^2 \text{ dB SPL}$$

$$= 20\log_{10}\left(\frac{P_m}{P_r}\right) \text{ dB SPL}$$

In decibels, the softest sound has a value of

$$20\log_{10}\left(\frac{P_r}{P_r}\right) = 20\log_{10} 1 = 0 \text{ dB SPL}$$

and the loudest sound that can be experienced at the threshold of pain is 140 dB SPL. Thus dB SPL is measured with respect to the sound reference pressure, $P_r = 20\ \mu\text{Pa}$ and this is a very useful measure of sound range.

1.2.5 Simple and Complex Sounds

A *simple sound* has a single frequency regardless of amplitude or SPL. Thus, 1000 Hz, 250 Hz, and 12,500 Hz are all simple sounds. The term *pure tone* is sometimes used to denote a sound at a single frequency. Pure tones are used in measuring hearing and hearing loss (see Chapter 2). A simple sound is produced by a single vibrating mass (sound source) producing an audible sound (of 0 dB SPL or greater); the sound is of a single frequency. However, most vibrating sources are more than just a single mass. For example, the vocal folds that produce voice are housed in a structure (the throat or *pharynx*) that is itself able to vibrate. The initial sound from the vocal folds then causes oscillation in the vocal tract of the pharynx. The oscillation of other masses or structures due to an original sound is called *resonance* and the structure is said to *resonate*. Therefore, most complex sounds, such as speech, are due to an initial sound mixed with resonated sounds.

A *complex sound* consists of a base or *fundamental* frequency plus *harmonics*, i.e. multiples of the fundamental frequency. For example, a complex sound with fundamental frequency of 100 Hz could also have harmonics at 200, 300, 400, and 500 Hz. The harmonics are often denoted f_0, f_1, f_2 and so on, with f_0 the first harmonic or fundamental frequency, f_1 the first *overtone* or second harmonic, and so on. However, a complex sound does not always have its entire harmonics. For instance, a complex sound with five harmonics could consist of the first five harmonics or the fundamental plus odd harmonics, e.g. 100, 300, 500, and 700 Hz. Speech is produced by this fundamental plus odd harmonics resonance pattern and, therefore, the ability to hear complex sounds rather than only pure tones is important for understanding speech.

In the case of speech, the vocal tract is a tube that can be thought of as a resonant tube. The initial sound produced by the vocal folds is called the *fundamental frequency of voice* (for the given person). The resonance characteristics of the vocal tract determine the fundamental plus odd harmonics characteristics of speech.

Resonance is an important factor in speech and hearing. In addition to speech resulting from sound resonating within the vocal tract, the ear, itself, is a resonator. This resonance affects the ability to hear. Damage to the ear or using a hearing aid can change the resonant characteristics of the auditory system.

1.2.6 Spectral Analysis of Complex Sounds

Resonating systems produce sounds at two or more different frequencies. Complex sounds can be analysed using *spectral analysers* or *spectrograms* that carry out Fourier analyses of the sound. In the case of speech, and many other sounds that change rapidly over time, *fast Fourier transformation* (FFT) analysis is used.

When a spectral analyser completes an FFT, it provides a display of the results in numeric or data format or in graphical form. In hearing measurement, a graphical representation called a spectrogram is generally used. The spectrogram displays graphs of the amplitude (generally in dB SPL) along the y-axis against frequency (in hertz) on the x-axis. This information can be represented in two ways.

One type of spectrogram shows discrete frequency and amplitude information as a series of lines or bars, like a bar graph. A line is drawn for each frequency for which the intensity is greater than 0 dB SPL. This type of graph is sometimes called a *line display*. Figure 1.8 shows the line display for four harmonics of complex sound with a fundamental frequency of 50 Hz.

The most commonly used spectrogram in the field of hearing is called a *wave envelope*, as an envelope is produced by drawing lines to connect the peaks or tops of each line in the line display. There may also be, but are not always, lines below the envelope. Figure 1.9 shows the wave envelope for the complex sound in Figure 1.8.

1.2.7 Filtering Sound

Another important function that takes place in the auditory system is *filtering*. The inner ear can be considered, in part, as a series of band-pass filters that

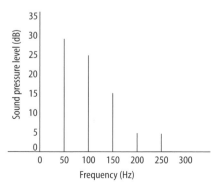

Figure 1.8 Line display spectrogram.

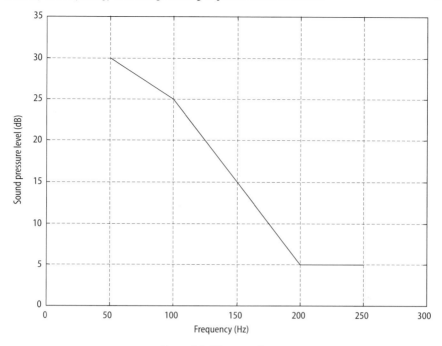

Figure 1.9 Wave envelope.

extract information from complex sounds. Filtering affects the spectral composition of a signal by reducing some frequencies in intensity and filtering out other frequencies. For instance, if an input sound having harmonics at the frequencies 50, 100, 150, 200, 250, and 300 Hz is passed through a system and the output sound has frequency components at 100, 150, 200, and 250 Hz, then the system has filtered out the harmonics at 50 and 300 Hz.

The filter *transfer function* describes the effect of a filter on an input signal, such as a sound signal. It is generally expressed as a rational function of frequency, as it determines the effect of the filter on frequency in the input signal. A typical filter transfer function could have the formula

$$G(j\omega) = \frac{K}{j\tau\omega + 1} = \frac{Y(j\omega)}{U(j\omega)}$$

The transfer function gives the ratio of the system output $Y(j\omega)$, as a function of frequency, to the input $U(j\omega)$, as a function of frequency. Evaluating the transfer function at a particular frequency gives a *multiplicative* effect on that frequency component. For instance, if the transfer function has an absolute gain of 0.7 at the frequency of 1000 Hz, then any signal passing through the filter will have its component at that frequency multiplied by the gain factor of 0.7, or its input dB amplitude reduced by $20\log_{10} 0.7 \approx -3\,\text{dB}$. The signal amplitude reduction or attenuation occurs because the absolute gain factor is less than unity. Similarly, if the transfer function has an absolute gain of 0.3 at the frequency of 2000 Hz, then the frequency component at 2000 Hz in the incoming signal will leave the filter with its 2000 Hz component multiplied by the gain factor of 0.3, or its dB amplitude reduced by $20\log_{10} 0.3 \approx -10.5\,\text{dB}$. Again, the signal amplitude reduction or attenuation occurs because the gain factor is less than unity. The formula applied is given by

Output amplitude = [Gain value] × Input amplitude

In dB or logarithmic form this is

[Output amplitude] dB = $20\log_{10}$ [Gain value] dB + [Input amplitude] dB

Thus if the absolute gain value is less than unity, then $20\log_{10}$ [Gain value] dB will be a negative dB value and a dB reduction in dB input signal amplitude occurs. If the absolute gain value had been greater than unity, then the output amplitude would be greater than the input amplitude and signal *amplification* will occur. In this case, the quantity $20\log_{10}$ [Gain value] dB will be a *positive* dB value and a dB addition to the dB input signal amplitude occurs.

In some cases the filter transfer function will be defined by the effect on different frequencies, *i.e.* a table of the filter reductions in dB at different frequencies, rather than as a mathematical expression. The system transfer function can be plotted on a graph, called a *filter curve*.

Example

Consider a complex sound consisting of the frequencies 100, 200, 300, 400, 500, 600, and 700 Hz, all at 40 dB SPL. The sound enters the system with each of the frequencies at 40 dB SPL. The output sound levels for the different harmonics are as follows:

100 Hz: 10.4 dB SPL
200 Hz: 14.0 dB SPL
300 Hz: 20.0 dB SPL
400 Hz: 40 dB SPL
500 Hz: 20.0 dB SPL
600 Hz: 14.0 dB SPL
700 Hz: 10.4 dB SPL

The amount of filtering at each frequency can be calculated to give the transfer function as follows:

100 Hz: 40 −10.4 = 29.6 dB SPL of filtering
200 Hz: 40 −14.0 = 26.0 dB SPL of filtering
300 Hz: 40 − 20.0 = 20.0 dB SPL of filtering
400 Hz: 40 −40 = 0 dB SPL of filtering
500 Hz: 40 − 20.0 = 20.0 dB SPL of filtering
600 Hz: 40 −14.0 = 26.0 dB SPL of filtering
700 Hz: 40 −10.4 = 29.6 dB SPL of filtering

The filter curve for this system is shown in Figure 1.10. It is a curve that is symmetric about the frequency 400 Hz, at which no filtering occurs.

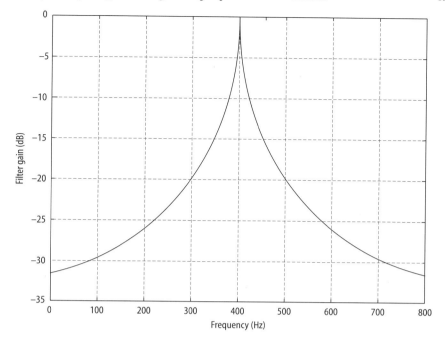

Figure 1.10 Filter curve.

Important filter characteristics include the upper and lower cut-off frequencies, the centre frequency, and the filter range, bandwidth or filter band. The *centre frequency* of a filter is the frequency in the middle of the range of frequencies for which no, or minimal, filtering occurs. It is generally assumed that a filter lets through frequencies where the amplitude is reduced by less than or equal to 3 dB and filters out frequencies that are reduced by more than 3 dB. This is known as the *3 dB down* point on the filter characteristic.

The *cut-off frequencies* are the frequencies at which filtering of –3 dB occurs, *i.e.* the outer limits of the frequencies let through. Some filters have both *upper* f_U and *lower* f_L cut-off frequencies, and others have either upper or lower cut-off frequencies but not both. The bandwidth or filter range is the difference between the upper and lower cut-off frequencies, namely, $f_U - f_L$ and the *frequency response* the range between the upper and lower cut-off frequencies. A filter can be specified in terms of its centre frequency f_c, and the cut-off frequencies that provide the limits of the frequency range of the filter.

Example

Consider a system with input 10 dB SPL at all frequencies and the following output levels:

100 Hz: 6 dB SPL
200 Hz: 7 dB SPL
300 Hz: 8 dB SPL
400 Hz: 9 dB SPL
500 Hz: 10 dB SPL
600 Hz: 9 dB SPL
700 Hz: 8 dB SPL
800 Hz: 7 dB SPL
900 Hz: 6 dB SPL

The centre frequency is 500 Hz with 10 dB SPL. Therefore, a reduction of 3 dB is 7 dB and the upper and lower cut-off frequencies are 200 Hz and 800 Hz.

Filters can also be described by their filter *band*, which is generally given by the number of octaves within the $f_L - f_U$ range. Harmonics are multiples of the fundamental and octaves involve doubling of the previous frequency. For example, for a fundamental frequency of 200 Hz, the harmonics are 200, 400, 600, 800, 1000, 1200, 1400, 1600, 1800, 2000 Hz, *etc.* and the octaves are: 200, 400, 800, 1600, 3200, 6400 Hz, *etc.*

For a filter with f_L = 500 Hz and f_U = 2000 Hz, the number of octaves from 500 to 2000 Hz is two. Thus, this filter has a *two-octave bandwidth*.

Sound is reduced or *attenuated* by a filter. The filter attenuation rate can be given in decibels per octave. A two-octave filter with 12 dB attenuation at one octave above or below the centre frequency has a 12 dB/octave attenuation rate.

Most filters can be categorised as low pass, band pass or high pass. *Band-pass filters* allow a particular band of frequencies to pass through the filter and have both upper and lower cut-off frequencies. *Low-pass filters* pass through all frequencies less than a certain frequency and, therefore, have only an upper cut-off frequency. *High-pass filters* pass through all frequencies above a certain frequency and have only a lower cut-off frequency.

1.3 Anatomy and Physiology of the Auditory System

1.3.1 Some Terminology Used in Describing Anatomical Structures

Before considering the specifics of the anatomical structures that receive and transmit sound and deliver it to the brain for processing, some of the terminology used in describing anatomical structures will be presented.

The term *frontal view* is used to describe a structure as seen from the front, whereas *dorsal view* refers to a back or rear perspective. *Lateral view* describes a perspective towards the side and *medial view* a perspective from the inside looking out; see Figure 1.11.

In addition to these four perspectives, anatomical structures are sometimes described in relation to each other. Structures on top are referred to as *superior*, whereas those underneath are referred to as *inferior*. Structures in back are *posterior* and those in front are *anterior*.

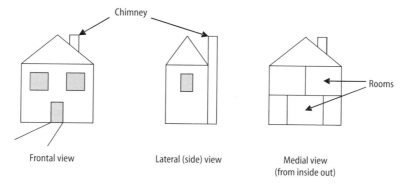

Figure 1.11 Anatomical perspectives.

The ear can be divided into three main parts: the outer, middle and inner ear (Figure 1.12). The anatomy and functions of these three parts will be discussed in the following sections.

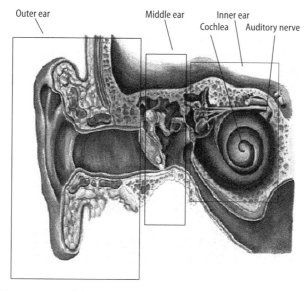

Figure 1.12 The structure of the ear (based on illustration courtesy of http://www.earaces.com/).

1.4 The Anatomy and Functions of the Outer-ear Structures

The outer ear consists of the pinna or the auricle and the ear canal or EAM that ends in the eardrum or tympanic membrane. The eardrum is sometimes considered as an outer-ear structure and sometimes as a middle-ear structure. It will be discussed here as part of the middle ear, as its functioning primarily involves the total physiology of the middle ear. The main function of the outer

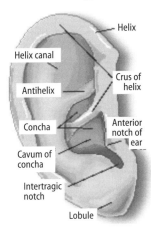

Figure 1.13 The pinna (based on an illustration courtesy of http://www.orlions.org/).

ear is to receive sound and funnel it down to the eardrum. Both the pinna and the EAM also act as a resonator of sound, and the EAM additionally filters out low-frequency sounds.

1.4.1 The Pinna

The *pinna* or the *auricle* receives sound from the environment and channels it into the auditory system. It is made of cartilage covered with skin and has a small inferior portion consisting of fatty tissue covered with skin.

Some animals, such as rabbits and dogs, can move their pinnae using the muscles attached to their pinnae to allow the structure to provide a directional factor and allow the pinna to pick up sounds from different directions. In humans, these muscles are dormant and do not function, although some people can "wiggle" their ears. Instead, movements of the neck twist the head, allowing the pinna to pick up sound from different directions.

Some of the main features of the pinna are shown in Figure 1.13. The superior portion is called the *helix*, which somewhat flaps over the *antihelix*. The helix comes down the posterior portion of the pinna to a soft part of the ear that consists of fatty tissue covered with skin having no cartilage. This is actually the *ear lobe* or *lobule*. In many animals, and in some people, the lobule is attached to the head and is not easily identifiable.

Superior and somewhat anterior to the lobule is a notch called the *tragal notch*. Superior to this is a part of the ear that often sticks out a bit, called the *tragus*. Opposite to this is the *antitragus*.

1.4.2 External Auditory Meatus

Between the tragus and antitragus is a recess that leads to the opening of the ear into the head. This recess is called the *concha* and it is the part of the pinna

Anatomy and Physiology of Hearing, Hearing Impairment and Treatment

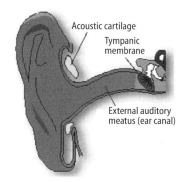

Figure 1.14 EAM (based on an illustration courtesy of http://www.orlions.org/).

that channels sound to the *ear canal* or *EAM*. The outermost portion of the EAM consists of cartilage covered with skin. As the EAM moves medially, the cartilage changes to bone, although it is still covered with skin, as shown in Figure 1.14.

The EAM ends, medially, at the eardrum or *tympanic membrane*, which, as noted above, some people refer to as a structure of the outer ear rather than the middle ear. Cells in the walls and floor of the EAM produce *cerumen* or earwax. Additionally, there are hairs in the lateral part of the EAM. Both the hairs and cerumen serve to trap foreign matter and objects that may enter the ear canal, helping to prevent them from getting down to the tympanic membrane, where they could possibly cause serious problems.

1.4.3 Functions of the Outer-ear Structures

The major function of the outer ear is to capture sound and funnel that sound down to the eardrum. The pinna sticks out to allow people to pick up sounds better from the front than from the back. This can be demonstrated by listening carefully to two sound sources from in front and behind, noting the volume or loudness of both sounds. When cupped hands are put around the pinna on both sides, the sound from in front should seem much louder than it was previously and the sound at the back quieter.

It is important to remember that sounds from in front are louder than those behind when considering a person wearing a hearing aid. With a behind-the-ear (BTE) or body-worn hearing aid, the sound is picked up from a microphone that is placed outside the region of the pinna. Thus, the localisation effects of the pinna are not available in these types of hearing aid and people often complain of interfering background sounds more when using BTE and body-worn hearing aids. A more complete discussion of hearing aids will be given in Chapter 3.

In addition to picking up sound, the pinna acts as a slight resonator of sound. The concha is recessed and forms a small cave-like structure, called the *cavum concha*. The cavum concha makes sound resonate slightly, but enough to enhance the loudness of sound entering the ear, especially from the front.

The final auditory function of the pinna, especially the concha, is to funnel the sound to the opening to the EAM, where the sound travels to the tympanic membrane. The EAM is a tube closed medially and open laterally. As tubes cause resonance, the EAM acts as an acoustic resonator. In humans, the resonant characteristics of the EAM are around 10 dB in the frequency range from 2500 to 5000 Hz. The peak is usually around 3000 Hz. Thus, higher frequencies of sound enter the EAM and are resonated by a factor of about +10 dB.

This EAM resonance is important for understanding speech. Consonants carry important linguistic information. For instance, consider the words "hat" and "cat". There is a considerable difference in meaning, but the only acoustic difference is the slight, high-frequency energy difference in the consonant sounds of "h" and "c" (represented as the speech sound or *phoneme*s /h/ and /k/). Vowels contain a great deal of acoustic energy; this contrasts with the consonants, which have significantly less, especially the high-frequency consonants. Thus, the EAM helps to increase the energy in these high-frequency sounds by resonating these frequencies when they travel through the outer ear.

The other important concept to understand about the EAM tube is that it is open at its lateral end. This allows low-frequency sounds to be filtered out of the EAM. Again, this serves to enhance the energy for the higher frequencies. Therefore, the EAM functions as a high-pass filter.

This filtering factor becomes important in considering the effects of fitting a hearing aid. For most hearing-aid users, the hearing aid is fitted into the ear with an earmould, whether part of the hearing aid (as with in-the-ear and in-the-canal models) or separate from the hearing aid (as with BTE and body-aid models). Placing an earmould into the opening of the EAM removes the open-tube filtering effects of the ear canal and changes its resonant characteristics. Chapter 3 has a more detailed discussion of hearing aids and earmould effects.

1.5 The Anatomy and Functions of the Middle-ear Structures

The middle ear consists of three ossicles and the tympanic membrane, which can be considered as either part of the outer or middle ears. It will be discussed here as part of the middle ear, as its function has been shown to be integrally related to the middle-ear impedance matching.

1.5.1 The Tympanic Membrane

As its name implies, the tympanic membrane (Figure 1.15) is a membrane. The acoustic energy from the sound travelling down the EAM is translated into motion of the tympanic membrane. This motion is directly related to the compression and rarefaction motion of the air molecules travelling as the sound wave. Thus, when compression occurs, the tympanic membrane moves medially; and when rarefaction occurs, the tympanic membrane moves laterally. Thus, the tympanic membrane moves in-and-out or back-and-forth.

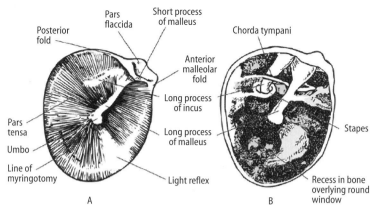

Figure 1.15 Tympanic membrane (by kind courtesy of http://www.merck.com/pubs/mmanual/figures/).

1.5.2 Middle-ear Ossicles

There are three small bones, or ossicles, in the middle ear, called the *malleus* (hammer), *incus* (anvil) and *stapes* (stirrup); see Figure 1.16. The malleus, or hammer, is attached to the tympanic membrane. Like the hammer from which it derives its name, the malleus has two parts, the head and the arm, called the *manubrium*.

The lateral end of the manubrium is attached to the centre, or *umbo*, of the tympanic membrane. Thus, movement or oscillation of the tympanic membrane is transmitted directly to the malleus. The malleus is also suspended from the bony walls of the middle ear at several points, so that it can move as the vibrations of the tympanic membrane are transmitted to it. Thus, as the tympanic membrane moves medially, the malleus does the same because of this direct vibration.

The head of the malleus is rounded like a mallet and is attached to the head of the incus, the next middle-ear ossicle, via ligaments (see Figure 1.16). The head of the incus is indented to form a *ball-in-socket* attachment. This type of

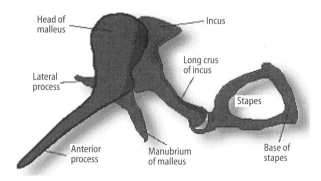

Figure 1.16 Malleus, incus and stapes (based on an illustration courtesy of http://www.orlions.org/).

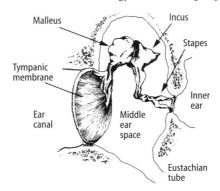

Figure 1.17 Tympanic membrane and the three ossicles (by kind courtesy of http://depts.washington.edu/otoweb/).

attachment allows free motion of the malleus and incus. The movements of the incus are in opposition to those of the malleus, *i.e.* as the malleus moves medially the incus moves laterally. This causes a lever-type action between these two ossicles. This lever is one of the important mechanical devices involved in the functioning of the middle ear.

The head of the incus leads to the body and the *long process* of the incus (see Figure 1.16). The next ossicle, called the stapes or stirrup, is attached to the end of this process. The attachment between the incus and the stapes is such that any movement of the incus leads to movement of the stapes in the same direction. Therefore, as the incus moves in, the stapes moves in as well. The stapes is the third and last ossicle, making up what is called the *ossicular chain*.

The stapes bone has four main parts: the head, neck, arms or *crura*, and the *footplate*. The footplate is the end part of the stapes and resembles the part of a stirrup into which the foot is put when mounting a horse. This footplate is oval in shape and fits in an oval-shaped opening in the medial bony wall, separating the middle ear from the inner ear, called the *oval window*. In anatomical terminology, a window is an open space in a bony wall. The ligaments that hold the footplate in the oval window allow this part of the stapes to rock in and out of the inner ear. This rocking motion sets up waves in the fluid of the inner ear.

Figure 1.17 shows how the middle-ear structures fit together. It also shows that the tympanic membrane is significantly larger in area than the footplate. This area difference is important and is discussed below in the section on middle-ear functioning.

1.5.3 The Middle-ear Cavity

The structures of the middle ear are situated in a part of the *temporal bone* of the skull known as the *mastoid process*. The tympanic membrane is attached to an opening in the bony walls making up the outer-ear canal leading to the middle ear. The bony middle-ear walls form a cavity known as the *middle ear* or *tympanic cavity*. In contrast to the bony ear canal, which is covered by skin, the walls of the middle-ear cavity are covered with *mucous membrane* (Figure 1.18).

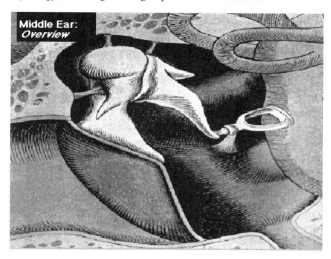

Figure 1.18 The middle-ear cavity (by kind courtesy of http://www.neurophys.wisc.edu/~ychen/auditory/anatomy/).

Attached to the walls of the middle ear are ligaments and other attachments that hold the ossicles in place. The *tympanic ring* is a cartilaginous ring in the most lateral part of the middle ear that holds the tympanic membrane in place. The superior portion of the middle-ear cavity is called the *attic*. The attic is a bony shelf, above which is the brain. Therefore, the middle ear is separated from the brain only by this bone. The bony walls of the attic are filled with holes or cells, known as the *mastoid cells*.

The medial wall of the middle-ear cavity contains the oval window, as described above, and has two other prominent features. The first is another window or hole in the bony wall; this is round and is called the *round window*. This window is covered with a membrane called the *round window membrane* and it functions to relieve pressure from the fluid of the inner ear when the footplate of the stapes sets up waves in this fluid. This will be discussed further below in the section on inner-ear functioning. The other prominent structure is called the *promontory*, a part of the medial bony wall that sticks into the middle ear. The promontory is a portion of one of the channels of the inner ear called the *scala media*, which is discussed further below in the section on inner-ear structures.

The most prominent feature of the floor of the middle-ear cavity is an opening that leads to a long tube connecting the middle ear with the back of the throat near the adenoids. This tube is called the *auditory* or *Eustachian tube* and is a critical part of the middle-ear cavity.

As a cavity, there is no normal opening between the middle ear and the outer world. However the middle-ear cavity is full of air and the mucous membrane cellular structures lining the middle ear require oxygen. Thus, the cells of this mucous membrane use up air in the middle-ear space and this would eventually cause a vacuum if the air were not replaced. The Eustachian tube is the structure that allows replacement of the air that has been exhausted. It is normally closed in children, from toddler age to adult. Movement of the muscles attached to the lateral part of the Eustachian tube in the area of the throat makes the tube open and allows air to rush into the middle-ear cavity. This effect is often noticed when there is a change in air pressure such as when going up high into the mountains or flying in an aeroplane. Passengers in cars and planes usually swallow, yawn or do something else to cause the muscles to open their Eustachian tubes allowing an equalisation of pressure between the middle ear and the outer world.

1.5.4 The Functions of the Middle-ear Structures

The middle ear converts the acoustic energy of the sound received by the pinna and funnelled down to the eardrum into mechanical energy by the motions of the eardrum and the bones in the middle ear. In order to facilitate understanding of the reasons for this conversion of acoustic to mechanical energy and the purposes of the middle ear, the anatomy of the inner ear will be discussed briefly.

The inner ear is the portion of the ear beyond the medial bony wall of the middle ear. Its structures are housed completely in fluids. Thus, energy travelling through the inner ear is in the form of hydraulic energy. Since the inner ear is fluid filled, sound received by the outer ear must be transmitted to this fluid. Sound waves will lose energy in going from air to fluid, as there is an impedance differential between the thinner medium of air and that of the fluid. In essence, the fluids of the inner ear have the basic characteristics of seawater contained in a closed tube. The change from acoustic energy travelling in air to acoustic energy travelling in seawater would lead to a loss of about 99% of the transmitted sound. Thus, to make up for this energy loss, the middle ear acts as an impedance-matching device by allowing the signal at the end of the middle ear (the footplate of the stapes) to have a greater energy than the acoustic energy striking the tympanic membrane at the start of the middle ear.

The impedance matching function of the middle ear has two components: the size differential of the tympanic membrane and stapes and the length differential between the manubrium of the malleus and the long process of the incus. Since pressure is force per unit area, the reduced area of the stapes compared with the tympanic membrane means that the same force striking it will give increased pressure. Sound pressure striking the tympanic membrane makes only 70% of the membrane oscillate, *i.e.* an area of about 0.594 cm^2. As the footplate of the stapes is rigid, this oscillation causes all of it to oscillate, *i.e.* an area of 0.032 cm^2.

Thus, the ratio of the tympanic membrane to the stapes footplate is 0.594/0.032 = 18.6. Therefore, the area reduction from the tympanic membrane to the footplate is a factor of 18.6. This leads to an *area size ratio increase* in pressure between the tympanic membrane and footplate of 18.6, therefore, providing an increase is energy between the sound striking the tympanic membrane and the energy transmitted to the footplate.

However, this is not the only change that occurs. Between the tympanic membrane and stapes are two other middle-ear ossicles, the malleus and incus. These ossicles function as a lever that further increases the energy transmitted along their path. The energy increase due to the lever action is related to the difference in the length of the handle or manubrium of the malleus and the long process of the incus. The difference is a factor of 1.3 in humans. Thus, energy is increased by a factor of 1.3 due to this lever action.

Combining the energy increase due to the area size ratio with that due to lever action gives a total energy increase of $18.6 \times 1.3 = 24.2$.

Therefore, the middle-ear mechanical transformation of sound energy leads to an increase of about 24 times. This can be converted into SPL in dB to give $20 \log_{10} 24.2 \approx 28$ dB. Therefore, middle-ear impedance matching adds 28 dB to the sound pressure of the acoustic energy striking the tympanic membrane. The energy loss when going from air to fluid is about 30 dB. Therefore, the middle-ear impedance matching approximately cancels out this energy loss, so there is very little overall energy loss when sound enters the inner ear.

1.6 The Anatomy and Functions of the Inner-ear Structures

The entire inner ear is actually a hole in part of the skull known as the temporal bone. This hole contains a labyrinth of membranous structures that house the sensory cells of hearing and balance. Therefore, the inner ear has a *bony labyrinth* and a *membranous labyrinth* (Figure 1.19). The inner ear carries out two sensory functions, *viz.* hearing and balance, which are localised in the cochlea and the vestibular system respectively. The two sensory systems interconnect within both of these labyrinthine systems, but have unique sensory cells that react differently, to allow neural information about sound (hearing) and balance to be transmitted. The auditory part of the inner ear has two main components: the cochlea and the auditory nerve, *i.e.* the eighth cranial nerve, sometimes referred to as just the eighth nerve.

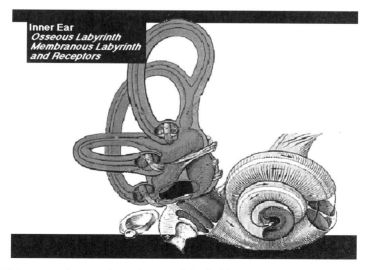

Figure 1.19 Inner-ear bony and membranous labyrinthine systems (by kind courtesy of http://www.neurophys.wisc.edu/~ychen/auditory/anatomy/).

The movements of the footplate of the stapes in the oval window set up waves in the fluids of the inner ear. It is at this point that the mechanical motions of the middle-ear structures are converted to hydraulic energy in the inner ear.

1.6.1 Vestibule

Beyond the footplate of the stapes is a fluid-filled area called the *vestibule*. Superior to the vestibule is a membranous structure consisting of two parts with three half-rings protruding from the superior part. The two parts are known as the *saccule* and *utricle*, and these are involved in providing information about body motion and movement in space. The three rings or canals protruding from the utricle are called the *semicircular canals*. Each of the three semicircular canals is oriented to one of the three dimensions of space: up-and-down, back-and-forth, and side-to-side (Figure 1.20). Thus, sensory information gathered from these canals provides information about our motion and movement in three-dimensional space.

Attached to one end of the utricle are a sac and duct known as the *endolymphatic sac* and *endolymphatic duct*. The sac produces endolymph, an inner-ear fluid that is found in the membranous parts of the inner ear. At the inferior end of the saccule there is a very narrow membranous duct that leads from the structures of the vestibular system to the membranous structures of the auditory system in the *cochlea*.

1.6.2 The Cochlea

The cochlear membrane differs from the vestibular membrane in many ways. One of the most important differences is that the membranous structures of

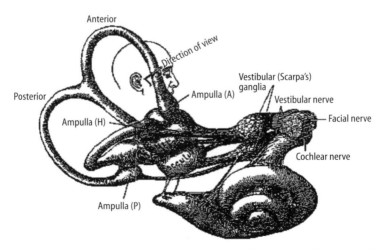

Figure 1.20 The balance system with the utricle, saccule and the three semicircular canals (by kind courtesy of http://www.anatomy.wisc.edu/Bs97/text/).

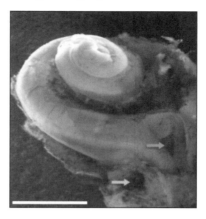

Figure 1.21 The cochlea (by kind courtesy of http://www.iurc.montp.inserm.fr/cric/audition/english/cochlea/).

the saccule, utricle and semicircular canals are floating in the fluids found in the bony labyrinth, whereas the cochlear membrane or *cochlear duct* is attached at the sides to the bony wall of the cochlea, and is only free to move on the top and bottom. This attachment leads to the formation of three chambers or canals called scalae (singular scala): one in the centre made of membranous walls, and the other two above and below this membranous cochlear duct.

The membranous duct is too long to fit into the small space of the bony cochlea section of the inner ear without folding and, therefore, curls like the shell of a snail. As shown in Figure 1.21, the cochlea has two and one-half turns.

The upper scala is mainly bone, with a membranous floor made from the superior membrane of the middle channel. It is called the *scala vestibuli*, since it comes from the vestibule. The bottom canal is also mainly bone, with a membranous ceiling from the inferior membrane or base of the cochlear duct. It is called the *scala tympani*, since it runs towards the middle ear or *tympanic cavity*. The middle cochlear duct is called the scala media and its floor and ceiling are entirely membranous (Figure 1.22).

The bony canals, scala vestibuli and scala tympani, are filled with perilymph, a fluid similar to cerebral spinal fluid and similar in viscosity to seawater. Perilymph flows throughout the bony labyrinth in both the cochlea and the vestibular system. The membranous canal or scala media, which is continuous from the duct connecting it to the saccule, is filled with endolymph.

The upper membrane of the scala media, called *Reisner's membrane*, is slanted. The floor or base of the scala media is made of the *basilar membrane*. It is on this membrane that the sensory cells of hearing are situated.

The sensory organ of hearing, known as the *organ of Corti*, is easy to see in Figure 1.23. It sits on the basilar membrane and consists of a series of cells, known as *supporting cells*, because they support the important sensory cells that transmit auditory stimulation to the central nervous system. The sensory cells are called *hair cells*, as they have *cilia* or hair-like structures protruding from them. It is damage, dysfunction, deterioration, or developmental problems with these hair cells that lead to the majority of permanent hearing loss often called *nerve deafness* or *sensorineural hearing loss*.

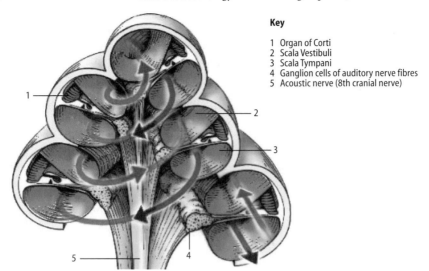

Figure 1.22 Cross-sectional view of the cochlea (by kind courtesy of http://www.iurc.montp.inserm.fr/cric/audition/english/cochlea/).

Figure 1.23 also shows that there are three hair cells followed by a structure looking like and inverted "V" followed by a fourth hair cell. The upside down structure is a supporting structure known as the *pillars of Corti*. The pillars of Corti support the *tectorial membrane* that sits on top of the hair cells. There are hair cells throughout the entire length of the scala media and they form rows of inner and outer hair cells. The *inner hair cells* are situated between the pillars of Corti and the innermost wall of the scala media. The remaining rows of hair cells are called *outer hair cells*.

At the base of each of the hair cells there is a small junction (space) in which are the neural endings of the *auditory nerve*. Stimulation of the cilia causes changes in these hair cells, leading to a release of neurochemicals into this junction called a *synapse*. The neurochemicals are picked up by the ends or *dendrites* of the auditory nerve and the neural transmission of sound sensation to the brain begins.

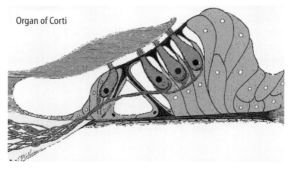

Figure 1.23 Organ of Corti (by kind courtesy of http://www9.biostr.washington.edu/cgi-bin/).

1.6.3 Sound Processing in the Cochlea

The movements of the footplate of the stapes are the final mechanical motion of the middle-ear structures. These movements cause waves in the perilymph fluid. The waves in the perilymph move from the oval window along the scala vestibuli to the helicotrema, which is the end where the scala vestibuli meets the scala tympani. The waves continue to flow along the scala tympani to the end of this canal. Since the perilymph is housed in a closed structure, the cochlea, there needs to be some release of the pressure that builds up as the footplate pushes into the fluid. This release is provided by the *membrane of the round window*, which covers a round opening in the bone at the lateral end of the scala tympani. Thus, as the footplate moves in, the round window membrane moves out, and *vice versa*.

As the wave moves along the scala vestibuli, its downward motion depresses Reisner's membrane, causing it to move down. Since the scala media is also enclosed and filled with endolymph fluid, the downward movement of Reisner's membrane compresses the endolymph, causing a downward displacement of the basilar member. Additionally, the tectorial membrane floating within the endolymph moves. While this is occurring, the basilar membrane is also moving down as the endolymph pushes the structures attached to this membrane. The motion of the tectorial and basilar membranes leads to a back-and-forth *shearing* action in the cilia attached to the hair cells. This shearing action leads to a change in the hair cells, thus causing the cell membrane at the base to allow neurochemicals to be released into the synaptic junction between the hair cells and the neurons of the auditory nerve (or eighth nerve) seated beneath.

The neural endings, or dendrites, pick up these neurochemicals and transmit them to the cell body, where they are stored until a sufficient quantity of neurochemicals has built up in the cell body, leading to a rapid and sudden discharge of the nerve cell called a *nerve impulse*. The nerve impulse flows down a long structure of the nerve called the *axon* and ends at the axon ending or foot. There, the permeability of the walls of the axon foot change. This allows a release of other neurochemicals into another synaptic junction, where awaiting dendrites from the next higher level neurons pick them up, move the neurochemicals to their respective cell bodies, leading to a neural discharge along their respective axons, releasing more neurochemicals into the synapses at their axonal endings. This neural transmission continues until the nerve impulses have brought the information to the brain for interpretation and comprehension of the message.

1.7 The Central Auditory Nervous System

As described above, the neurochemicals released by the hair cells are picked up by the neurons of the eighth or auditory nerve. The nerve impulses flow along the eighth nerve into the brainstem and eventually to the brain or *cortex*. The pathways from the eighth nerve to the brain are known as the *central auditory pathways* or the CANS. Transmission of information in the CANS is electrochemical, in the form of neurochemicals released into the synaptic junctions picked up by the next-level neurons causing a neural discharge.

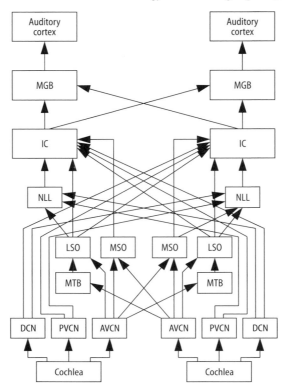

Figure 1.24 Block diagram of the pathways of the CANS (by kind courtesy of http://earlab.bu.edu/intro/).

The central auditory pathways are a complexity of neurons interconnected in intricate ways. Neurons function rather like capacitors, since they store neural energy until a level is reached at which they discharge totally, sending a DC voltage down the axon. Thus, neural activity is like direct current flow, in one direction, all-or-none, on-or-off.

The central auditory pathways, as with electric junction boxes, allow for multiple connections at each junction or synapse. That is, if one neuron leads to a synapse, there can be multiple neural connections at that junction. In this manner, neural information can flow to many different places from one source. Various junctions along the auditory pathways can be seen in Figure 1.24. The various blocks in the diagram have not been given in a key table since the figure is included only to provide an appreciation of the complexity of the pathways.

The first level in the system is at the eighth nerve, whose neurons begin at the base of the cochlear hair cells. The auditory nerve travels from the inner ear via a bony channel called the *internal auditory meatus* and enters the central nervous system below the brain or *cortex* at a level known as the *low brainstem*. Specifically, the auditory nerve projects to the *cerebellar–pontine angle* at the level of the *cerebellum* and *pons* within the upper end of the *medulla*. From there, these nerve endings meet with the next-level neurons at a region in the lower brainstem called the pons. This junction is known as the *cochlear neucleus*. Leaving the cochlear neucleus, fibres travel to either the next level in the system or bypass that level and jump to higher levels.

The next level above the cochlear neucleus is called the *superior olivary complex*. It is a complex of neural synaptic junctions. From the low brainstem, the pathway travels into the upper brainstem leaving the superior olivary complex, travelling along the *lateral lemniscus* to the *inferior colliculus* in the *mid-brain*. Here, the pathways project into a region of the brain called the *thalamus*. The auditory portion of the thalamus is called the *medial geniculate bodies*, since there are two: one on the right side and one on the left side. From here, neural fibres radiate out into the higher levels of the brain known as the *cortex*. Most nerve fibres project to the auditory receiving areas of the cortex known as *Heschl's gyrus*. From here, there are intricate connections to other parts of the cortex, between the right and left parts or *hemispheres* of the cortex, and, eventually, to areas of memory, visual regions, language regions, *etc*. Thus, the auditory pathways can be viewed as a complex system of "wires" with multiple connections and multiple routes through which neural discharges flow. This all-or-none discharging provides sufficient activity in the brain to make sense of sound, so long as all of the structures are functioning properly, coordinated in their functioning, and sound energy striking the tympanic membrane is transmitted to the inner ear and travels to the brain.

1.8 Classification of Hearing Loss

In order to determine whether there is a hearing loss, and, if so, the type and extent of hearing loss, hearing measurement is required. This will be discussed in more detail in Chapter 2. Measurement of hearing generally includes measurement of both air- and bone-conduction thresholds. The *hearing threshold* at a particular frequency is the minimum sound pressure given in dB HL required to perceive that frequency. *Air conduction* refers to sound travelling through air and then through the whole auditory system, whereas *bone conduction* refers to sound travelling through the bones of the skull, thereby avoiding the outer and middle ears (Figure 1.25). Hearing loss is generally indicated by raised thresholds. There is an *air–bone gap* when there is a difference between the air conduction and bone conduction thresholds.

The main types of hearing loss are categorised as:

- conductive
- sensorineural
- mixed
- central.

Conductive hearing loss results when there is a problem in the outer and/or middle ears. In this case, there will be an air–bone gap, as sound travelling through the bone conduction pathway would be heard better than sound travelling through the air conduction pathway that includes the outer and middle ear. Consequently, air conduction thresholds will be raised, but bone conduction thresholds will be "normal".

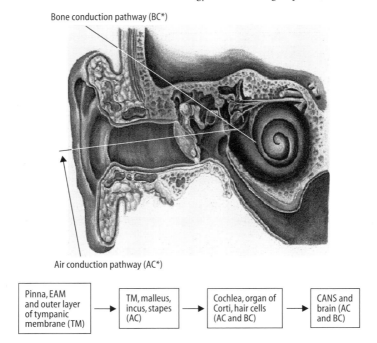

Figure 1.25 Air- and bone-conduction pathways (based on illustration courtesy of http://www.earaces.com/).

Sensorineural hearing loss results when there is a problem in the cochlea or inner ear. This can be further divided into *sensory hearing loss*, due to problems in the cochlea, and neural hearing loss, due to problems in the auditory nerve. Neural hearing loss is often referred to as *retrocochlear* hearing loss. In retrocochlear hearing loss, there is a lesion in the auditory nerve. It is relatively uncommon.

In the case of sensorineural hearing loss, both the air conduction and bone conduction thresholds are raised and there is no air–bone gap.

Mixed hearing loss occurs when there are problems in both the inner ear or auditory nerve and the middle or outer ears. This results in raised air- and bone-conduction thresholds, as well as an air–bone gap.

The last type of hearing loss is called a *central hearing loss*. Central losses are due to lesions, disorders, or dysfunctioning within the pathways of the CANS. In cases of pure central hearing loss, those without associated sensorineural loss, hearing thresholds are normal and there are no air–bone gaps. Central hearing losses lead to distortions in the processing of auditory messages rather than the loss of hearing sensitivity that is accompanied by the other three types of hearing loss.

This information is summarised in Table 1.1.

Measurement of the degree and type of hearing loss can be used to help diagnose problems in the auditory system. In most cases, it is the type of hearing loss that helps identify possible auditory disorders and ear "pathologies". The initial concern may be with the hearing loss, and there is a range of different

Table 1.1 Types of hearing loss and air- and bone-conduction thresholds.

Disorder of part of the ear	Air conduction threshold	Bone conduction threshold	Air–bone gap	Type of hearing loss
Outer ear	Raised	Normal	Yes	Conductive
Middle ear	Raised	Normal	Yes	Conductive
Outer + middle	Raised	Normal	Yes	Conductive
Cochlea	Raised	Raised	No	Sensorineural
Cochlea + outer	Raised	Raised	Yes	Mixed
Cochlea + middle	Raised	Raised	Yes	Mixed
Auditory nerve	Raised	Raised	No	Sensorineural
CANS	Normal	Normal	No	Central

causes. The majority of causes of hearing loss do not have any other consequences, but occasionally they are symptomatic of another problem, such as tumours.

1.8.1 Degrees of Hearing Loss

In addition to the type of hearing loss, the *degree of hearing* loss can also be categorised, using the hearing threshold. Slightly different categories are used in different countries. Table 1.2 presents the categories of degree of hearing loss defined by the American Speech–Language–Hearing Association (ASHA) and accepted in normal use by audiologists and hearing professionals in the USA.

Table 1.2 Degree of hearing loss.

Degree of hearing loss	Hearing loss range (dB HL)
Normal	–10 to 15
Slight	16 to 25
Mild	26 to 40
Moderate	41 to 55
Moderately severe	56 to 70
Severe	71 to 90
Profound	>90

1.8.2 Hearing Loss Due to Problems in the Outer Ear

Disorders of the outer ear generally cause conductive hearing loss, for instance due to blockage of the air conduction pathway. One common problem in the outer ear is the build up of cerumen (earwax), which can completely block the ear canal or EAM. In some cases, the build up of cerumen is so bad that the wax becomes impacted in the EAM and has to be syringed out by a nurse or doctor. Some of the other common outer-ear causes of hearing loss are outlined in Table 1.3. It should be noted that conductive hearing loss only results from problems of the outer ear if they result in total blockage of the air conduction

Table 1.3 Common problems of the outer ear that cause conductive hearing loss.

Problem	Structure involved	Causes and treatments
Cerumen	EAM	Cerumen softeners, ear washing (irrigation) or removal by doctor
Foreign objects in EAM	EAM	Irrigation or removal by doctor
Congenital atresia	EAM	Birth defect in which the ear canal does not form. Surgery is done for cosmetic purposes only
Otitis externa, outer ear infection (sometimes referred to as swimmer's ear)	EAM	Antibiotics and sometime anti-inflammatory medication to reduce swelling of EAM

pathway. For example, cerumen in the ear does not generally cause hearing difficulties until the wax totally blocks the EAM. This is also true of foreign objects and swelling of the ear canal. The conductive hearing loss lasts only as long as the outer ear is totally blocked and prevents sound reaching the tympanic membrane. Thus, most outer-ear problems cause temporary rather than permanent hearing loss.

1.8.3 Hearing Loss Due to Problems in Middle Ear

In contrast to the outer ear, there are a number of structures that can malfunction leading to problems with middle-ear transmission of sound to the inner ear. As with the outer ear, disorders of the middle ear lead to conductive hearing losses. The most common problems of the middle ear are infections and build up of fluid that may lead to infections, called *otitis media*. Otitis media can occur with effusion (fluid), with infection (acute), or as just a swelling of the middle ear with no fluid or infection present (just otitis media). In many cases, the middle-ear problems persist, leading to *chronic otitis media*. Otitis media with effusion is one of the most common causes of ear problems and temporary hearing loss in children. As with outer-ear disorders, many middle-ear problems are temporary and only cause hearing loss while they last. Table 1.4 presents some of the common middle ear problems identified by the structures involved.

1.8.4 Hearing Loss Due to Problems in the Cochlea

Unlike problems of the outer and middle ear, which lead to conductive hearing loss, problems involving cochlear structures cause sensorineural hearing loss. Disorders of the cochlea can involve problems with the sensory cells (*i.e.* hair cells and/or cilia), fluids of the inner ear, or problems with other structures.

The most common causes of sensorineural hearing loss are related to hair cell and cilia abnormalities. Such problems may be congenital in nature, due to abnormalities in the development of these sensory cells during the embryonic and foetal stages, or due to hereditary/genetic factors leading to abnormal development of these structures. Although less common, disorders may occur

Table 1.4 Problems of the middle ear that cause conductive hearing loss.

Problem	Structure involved	Causes and treatments
Perforated tympanic membrane (hole)	Tympanic membrane	Medicine to heal; time needed for hole to close; in some cases, surgery is required to close the hole
Infection/inflammation of tympanic membrane	Tympanic membrane	Antibiotics and anti-inflammatory medicines to reduce swelling
Otitis media	Middle-ear cavity	Antibiotics if infection is present; decongestants; allergy medications if related to allergens; surgery to drain fluid
Otosclerosis	Stapes mostly footplate	Bony growth around oval window causes footplate to be immobilized; surgery to remove stapes and bony growth and replace with artificial device
Ossicular fixation	Any middle-ear ossicle	Two or more ossicles are fused or "stuck" together and cannot move; sometimes congenital; surgery to "unstick" the ossicles; sometimes surgery removes one ossicle and replaces it with artificial device
Ossicular discontinuity	Any middle-ear ossicle	Joints between ossicles break; can sometimes be congenital; surgery or device to connect ossicles

during the gestation period and lead to problems with the developing hair cells. For example, viruses that invade the mother, such as the rubella virus, can lead to hair cell abnormalities and dysfunction. Even rhesus blood incompatibility between the mother and developing foetus can cause destruction of hair cells in the newborn.

The most common causes of hair cell damage are noise and ageing. Exposure to loud sounds over long periods of time can lead to hair cell damage, especially involving destruction of cilia. This is often noted in people who work around loud noises and who do not use hearing protectors. The hearing loss associated with noise is known as *noise-induced hearing loss* (NIHL).

Presbycusis, due to the natural changes resulting from ageing, is one of the most common types of sensorineural hearing loss. It can involve a number of different structural changes in the cochlea, including hair cell deterioration, problems with blood supply leading to hair cell damage, and changes in other structures of the organ of Corti leading to transmission problems in the cochlea. Table 1.5 presents some of the most common causes of sensorineural hearing loss.

1.8.5 Problems in the Auditory (Eighth) Nerve and Central Auditory Pathways

Some problems affect only the auditory nerve, whereas others affect nerves within the central auditory pathways. In rare cases, both the auditory nerve and nerves within the central auditory system are involved. When a disorder affects the auditory nerve it is called a *retrocochlear disorder*. Such disorders

Table 1.5 Some of the most common pathologies causing sensorineural hearing loss.

Problem	Structure involved	Causes and treatments
Congenital	Hair cells, cilia, entire cochlea	Birth defects; problems picked up by the mother transmitted to the foetus; hereditary factors; rhesus factor; trauma
Neonatal	Hair cells; cilia	Infections picked up by the newborn; birth trauma
NIHL	Hair cells; cilia	Permanent hearing loss due to noise exposure
Temporary threshold shift	Hair cells; cilia	Temporary hearing loss due to noise exposure
Presbycusis	Hair cells; cilia; blood supply to cochlea	Normal changes in cochlea due to ageing
Ototoxicity	Hair cells; cilia; other cochlear structures	Drugs that are toxic to the cochlea, such as some mycin antibiotics and drugs used in cancer treatment, cause permanent hearing loss
Temporary ototoxicity	Hair cells; cilia	Drugs that are toxic to the cochlea only when high doses of the drug are in the person's system; most common is aspirin
Viruses and bacteria	Hair cells; cilia	Some viruses and bacteria can invade the cochlea and do permanent or temporary damage; one common bacterium is a form of streptococcus that leads to permanent hair cell damage and can also lead to encephalitis
Viruses and bacteria	Cochlear fluids	Some viruses and bacteria invade the intracochlear fluids, leading to dizziness and hearing loss, often temporary, only while disease is present in inner ear; sometimes referred to as labyrinthitis
Perilymphatic	Perilymph fluid	Hole (called a fistula) in the ligament holding footplate in the oval window or a hole in the membrane of the round window; loss of perilymph through the hole causes temporary hearing loss and dizziness; once hole is closed (spontaneous or by surgery), fluid returns to normal, as does balance and hearing
Ménière's syndrome or disease	Endolymph fluid	Improper absorption of endolymph leads to pressure build up in membranous channels of the inner ear, leading to dizziness and hearing loss that fluctuates with pressure changes
Advanced Ménière's	Perilymph and endolymph fluids, Reisner's membrane and hair cells	Advanced stages of Ménière's can lead to rupturing of Reisner's membrane, allowing perilymph and endolymph fluids to mix and cause ionic imbalance in cochlea that can cause permanent hair cell destruction
Cochlear otosclerosis	Perilymph, basilar membrane, hair cells	In some cases of otosclerosis the bony growth moves into the cochlea, invading the perilymph fluid and basilar membrane; can lead to damage to hair cells

cause sensorineural hearing loss (neural type). In contrast, problems in the auditory pathways of the CANS affect the ability to process and understand auditory information rather than hearing itself, *i.e.* the person can *hear* sounds but cannot *understand* them or interpret them as speech. If the problem is due to a lesion, such as a tumour pressing on one of the nerve pathways in the CANS, the disorder is called a central hearing loss. However, if the problem is merely related to interpreting auditory information in the absence of a lesion, the problem is called an *auditory processing disorder*.

The most common pathologies involving nerves relate to tumours or growths on, or that pinch, nerves, problems with blood flow to the nerves and other CANS structures, diseases (viruses or bacteria) that invade the nerves or CANS structures, or age-related degeneration of the nerve structures. These will all cause problems with the normal transmission of neurochemical substances or with nerve impulse transmission.

Trauma and accidents can lead to the destruction of nerves or CANS structures. Diseases that can cause deterioration of nerves are often referred to as *neurodegenerative diseases*. One of the most common of these neurodegenerative problems is referred to as *neural presbycusis* and is due to the natural changes and degeneration of the auditory nerves and CANS structures due to ageing.

One last site of neural problems involving central hearing loss is damage, disease, deterioration or related pathologies of the *auditory cortex* in the brain. This is the area of the brain (located above the ears) that is dedicated to the auditory sense. Hearing problems involving this area of the brain are often called *central deafness*. Table 1.6 presents some of the most common pathologies of the eighth nerve and CANS that include the brain.

Table 1.6 Pathologies of the auditory nerve and CANS pathways leading to hearing or auditory problems.

Pathology	Structure involved	Causes and treatments
Eighth nerve tumours	Auditory nerve	Abnormal cell growth of structures surrounding the auditory nerve; leads to sensorineural hearing loss; usual treatment is surgical removal, but radiation may be used to shrink them
Auditory neuropathy	Auditory nerve	Abnormal development or lack of development of the eighth nerve; wait to see if nerve pathway develops or permanent problems mostly with auditory processing
Congenital	Auditory nerve and CANS structures	Rare, but child could be born without an eighth nerve or other CANS structure including cortical; wait to see if nerve pathway develops or permanent problems, mostly with auditory processing; eighth nerve causes sensorineural hearing loss as well
Trauma/accidents	Auditory nerve, CANS structures, brain (auditory cortex)	Blows to the head; traumatic brain injury; depends on amount of injury, could be temporary, but is often permanent; auditory processing problems
Tumours of the CANS structures	Any structures in the CANS including the cortex, but excluding the auditory nerve itself	As with eighth nerve tumours, only these grow on the nerves of the CANS or in the brain (auditory cortex); surgical removal of tumour or growth; radiation or chemotherapy to shrink; leads to auditory processing problems
Cerebral vascular accidents (or stroke)	Burst blood vessel in CANS structural area or in brain (auditory cortex)	Leads to pressure in area, damage of cells in area; must wait to assess extent of damage; surgery may be tried to reduce swelling; leads to auditory processing problems

1.9 Medical and Non-medical Treatments

1.9.1 Medical and Surgical Treatment of Problems in the Auditory System

There are a number of different possible types of medical intervention. In many cases, as noted in the tables above, medical intervention involves prescribing medications and drugs to treat the diseases that affect the system. When medicines are prescribed, the hearing loss usually subsides as the symptoms are treated. In other cases, medication is unlikely to be successful because of the nature of the disorder (*e.g.* NIHL or trauma).

In addition to medicines, surgical interventions are prescribed in some cases, as noted in the tables. Usually, the surgery removes or corrects a problem, such as a tumour, but the hearing loss may still remain after the surgery. For example, if a tumour of the auditory nerve has led to a 60 dB hearing loss, removal of the tumour will leave the hearing loss at the same level. Additionally, surgery to treat or reduce serious, possibly life-threatening, problems, such as tumours, may, itself, cause greater hearing loss. For instance, removal of a tumour on the eighth nerve may require or result in partial removal or destruction of the nerve during surgery. This will have a serious effect on hearing.

When pathologies invade the nerves and CANS pathways, including the brain, radiation and chemotherapy may be tried. Again, the success of these interventions is the amount of reduction in swelling or growth, and, hopefully, total remission of the problem.

The professional who provides medical and surgical intervention is the ear, nose, and throat (ENT) physician, otologist, otolaryngologist, or otorhinolaryngologist. Some ENT physicians provide medical intervention only, but most of them can also perform surgery. Neurotologists (ear physicians specialising in disorders and surgeries of the auditory pathways) carry out surgical interventions involving the auditory nerve and CANS pathways.

1.9.2 Non-medical or Non-surgical Interventions

Audiologists are professionals who help to diagnose and provide non-medical/non-surgical treatment of disorders of the auditory system. The audiologist is trained to provide diagnostic, interpretive, and rehabilitative treatment using technological intervention, counselling, and what is called communication strategies, including the use of lip- and speech-reading.

Audiologists often evaluate, fit and even dispense or sell hearing aids. In some cases, people with hearing loss go to professionals who only fit and dispense or sell hearing aids but who are not trained in the diagnosis and rehabilitative treatment of hearing problems. These hearing health-care professionals may be called hearing-aid dispensers, dealers, fitters or audioprosthodotists. In many places, audiologists and hearing-aid dispensers are either certified or licensed (or both) to practise their professions, just as medical doctors are board certified and licensed. In some countries, individuals are able to obtain hearing aids as part of the state health system, whereas in others they have to purchase them privately or obtain them through medical insurance.

In many cases, medical or surgical treatments are not indicated or it is decided not to apply a medical or surgical treatment. For example, a person with otosclerosis for whom the surgery could be life threatening for a variety of reasons, or the degree of *otosclerotic growth* does not yet warrant surgery, could be fitted with a hearing aid. Assistive technology and various rehabilitative strategies could be used to improve communication and (auditory) access to sound.

For most people for whom medical or surgical treatment is not indicated, a hearing aid is the first step towards helping the person gain auditory access to sound. Although some people with hearing loss choose not to use hearing aids, these electroacoustic devices are still the most widely prescribe non-medical, non-surgical treatment for hearing loss.

When the hearing loss is too great to benefit from a hearing aid, but the person chooses to obtain auditory access to sound, a cochlear implant may be appropriate. These surgically implanted devices provide electrical rather than acoustic stimulation to the auditory nerve.

When a hearing aid or cochlear implant is not sufficient or for the deaf community (who prefer to remain deaf), assistive devices may be offered as well. The following chapters in this book provide a description of the devices available, including the technical principles on which they are based, and their application for persons who are deaf and hard-of-hearing.

1.10 Learning Highlights of the Chapter

The chapter began with an overview of the facility of hearing. This was explored using two themes: one scientific, in which the acoustics of sound was investigated, and the other medical, in which the functioning of the auditory system was described. This second theme led, in turn, to medical conditions giving rise to hearing impairment and deafness.

Specific learning objectives were:

- gaining a basic understanding of the acoustics of sound, including how sound is propagated;
- understanding the anatomy of the auditory system, and learning how each part of the ear functions;
- understanding how hearing loss is measured and various degrees and types of hearing loss;
- learning about the main causes of the different types of hearing loss and the possible medical and non-medical treatments.

This chapter established a context for the measurement of hearing loss and provides the motivation to use technology assist those people who suffer a hearing loss or who are deaf. In the Chapter 2, the measurement of hearing and the science of audiology is studied. In Chapter 3, the engineering and scientific aspects of electronic hearing-aid prostheses are described.

Projects and Investigations

Understanding Amplitude, Frequency, and Phase (Sections 1.2.1, 1.2.2, and 1.2.3)

1. Draw two sine waves that differ in (a) amplitude and (b) frequency. Describe how the diagrams differ in amplitude and frequency, and what changes in sound and movement of the eardrum (tympanic membrane) and middle ear bones (ossicles) due to the changes in amplitude or frequency will occur.
2. Draw two sine waves of the same frequency and amplitude, one that begins at 0° phase and the other beginning at +90° phase. On adding these two sine waves together, what will be the resultant wave and amplitude?
3. Draw two sine waves of the same frequency and amplitude, one that begins at 0° phase and the other beginning at 180° phase. On adding these two sine waves together, what will be the resultant wave and amplitude?
4. What deductions can be made about adding sine waves of the same frequency and amplitude added together that start at different phases? How can shifting phase 180° and adding the two waves together be used in a sound system?

Understanding Sound Intensity and dB (Section 1.2.4)

5. Calculate the sound pressure for sounds having the following P_m values: (a) 40 µPa; (b) 200 µPa; (c) 200,000 µPa.

Understanding Line Spectrum and Wave Envelope (Section 1.2.6)

6. (a) Draw the line spectrum and wave envelope for the two sounds with the outputs at the given frequencies in the table below.

Sound 1		Sound 2	
100 Hz	10 dB	250 Hz	100 dB
200 Hz	20 dB	500 Hz	80 dB
300 Hz	30 dB	1000 Hz	60 dB
400 Hz	40 dB	2000 Hz	40 dB
500 Hz	50 dB	4000 Hz	20 dB
		8000 Hz	0 dB

(b) What type of complex sound is present in Sound 1 and in Sound 2?

Understanding Filtering (Section 1.2.7)

7. (a) In Question 6 above, one of the two curves represents filtering. Which curve represents filtering, and what is the amount of filtering expressed in dB per octave for that curve?

   (b) For the filter curve, does effective filtering occurs at: (i) 250 Hz, (ii) 500 Hz, (iii) a frequency between 250 and 500 Hz, (iv) 4000 Hz, (v) 8000 Hz, or (vi) a frequency between 4000 and 8000 Hz.

   (c) For the filter curve, what frequencies of sound will be heard after the filtering has occurred?

Understanding Anatomical Relationships (Section 1.3)

8. Look at the various diagrams in the anatomical sections of the chapter. Identify the components that are lateral, medial, anterior, posterior, superior, and inferior.

Understanding Physiology and Pathology Connections (Sections 1.8+)

9. In each of the physiological sections on the pathologies of the auditory system, mark the specific part or parts of the ear that are affected by each pathology. Identify the parts of the ear that are affected or "go wrong" when each pathology occurs.

References and Further Reading

 Further Reading

Books

Ballou, G.M., 2001. *Handbook for Sound Engineers*. Butterworth-Heinemann.
Clark, J.G., Martin, F.N., 2002. *Introduction to Audiology*, 8th edition. Allyn & Bacon.
Denes, P.B., Pinson, E.N., 1993. *The Speech Chain: The Physics and Biology of Spoken Language*. W.H. Freeman & Co.
Katz, J., Burkard, R., Medwetsky L. (Eds), 2001. *Handbook of Clinical Audiology*, 5th edition. Lippincott, Williams & Wilkins Publishers.
Speaks, C.E., 1999. *Introduction to Sound: Acoustics for the Hearing and Speech Sciences*. Singular Publishing Group.
Zemlin, W.R., 1991. *Speech and Hearing Science: Anatomy and Physiology*, 4th edition. Allyn & Bacon.

2 Audiology: The Measurement of Hearing

2.1 Introduction: The Measurement of Hearing

Hearing is measured to determine the extent and type of any hearing loss. These measurements can be used to inform decisions on rehabilitative and other support measures. Hearing assessment can also contribute to the identification of medical conditions, tumours or other diseases of the auditory system. The measurement of hearing is important in occupational health, particularly for workers in noisy environments. It can be used to determine the effectiveness of occupational hearing conservation programmes, including whether additional measures will be required to protect hearing. The term *audiology* is used to denote the science of hearing measurement. There are a number of different tests, including pure tone audiometry, speech audiometry, immittance audiometry and electric response audiometry (ERA). However, before considering the specifics of audiology in detail, a brief introduction to measurement systems and a discussion of some of the errors associated with hearing measurement will be presented.

2.1.1 Learning Objectives

This chapter describes the various techniques used in measuring hearing, the technologies used and the principles of human-centred testing. Specific learning objectives are:

- to understand some essential terms from instrumentation and measurement science;
- to learn about the basic assessment methods and how they are used diagnostically;
- to gain knowledge of the basic equipment used to measure hearing;
- to gain an appreciation of audiology equipment design and calibration;
- to review and understand the appropriate equipment standards and related safety issues.

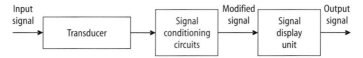

Figure 2.1 Basic components of a measurement system.

2.2 Measurement Systems

Most measurement systems can be represented by the block diagram in Figure 2.1. There are three main components:

- transducer
- signal conditioner
- display.

The *transducer* converts a variable or property that cannot be measured directly, or is hard to measure, into one that is easier to measure. A pure transducer carries out the conversion with no loss or storage of energy. The only property required of a transducer is a fixed relationship between output change and input change over the range of interest. This relationship does not have to be linear. In some cases the transducer may be referred to as the sensor.

The *signal conditioner* converts the signal output from the transducer into a form that can easily be recorded. Signal conditioners include amplifiers and filters.

The *display* presents the signal in a form from which a reading can be taken. Information can be displayed in digital, analogue or graphical form. For instance, a digital watch displays the time in numerical form, whereas an analogue watch displays it by the displacements of two (or three) pointers, called "hands". In another example, a voltmeter would display a numerical value of an analogue voltage signal, whilst an oscilloscope displays an analogue graphical representation.

2.2.1 Definitions

The science of instrumentation and measurement is a well-established branch of electrical engineering. Consequently, many of the ideas in this field have been studied and formalised as distinct concepts. Below is a small set of the most fundamental definitions that are useful in audiology studies:

- *Accuracy* is a measure of closeness to the true value of a measurement, estimate or result generated by an algorithm.
- *Absolute error* is the modulus of the difference between the true value and the measured, estimated or calculated value:

$$\text{Absolute error} = |\text{true value} - \text{measured value}|$$

- *Relative error* is the modulus of absolute error over true value times 100%:

$$\text{Relative error} = \frac{|\text{true value} - \text{measured value}|}{|\text{true value}|} \times 100\%$$

- *Resolution* of a measurement system is the smallest change it can measure.
- *Full-scale deflection* is the highest value on the scale of a scale and pointer display.
- *Zero error* is the measured value when the input is zero.
- *Tolerance* is the permitted variation in a measured value.
- *Reproducibility* or *repeatability* of a measurement is determined by the variation in displayed value when the same quantity is measured repeatedly under the same conditions within a short time.
- *Range* of a measurement system is the difference between the highest and lowest measurable values.
- *Capacity* of a measurement system is the highest measurable value.
- *Drift* is a gradual change in output for no change in input.
- *Dead zone* is a range of input values for which there is no change in the output.

2.2.2 Frequency-response Curves

Gain is a measure of the change in a system output caused by a change in the input to the system. It is measured as the simple ratio

$$\text{Gain} = \frac{\text{change in output value}}{\text{change in input value}}$$

For many simple mechanical devices, such as springs and gear trains, gain is a constant number whatever the change in the input. However, for many electronic components, such as electronic amplifiers, gain varies with the frequency of the input signal. In this case a frequency-response curve of gain against input frequency is required.

2.2.3 Gain in Decibels

In general, gain is measured in decibels (dB) rather than as a simple ratio. For a variable with gain x, the gain in decibels is defined as

$$\text{Gain (dB)} = 20 \log_{10} x$$

Using a logarithmic decibel scale has the following advantages:

- Gains of amplifiers or other components in series can be added, rather than multiplied. This can be done either numerically or graphically, by shifting the graphs.
- As frequency is plotted on a logarithmic scale, using decibels gives a log–log graph, which converts many frequency-response curves to straight lines or curves that can be simply approximated by straight lines.

2.2.4 Amplifiers

Amplifiers are devices designed to amplify a signal magnitude without changing its inherent nature. Mechanical amplifiers are passive devices that are used to amplify displacement or rotation. Mechanical amplifiers are of little interest in audiology; instead, interest focuses on electronic amplifiers. There are two main types of electronic amplifier:

- voltage amplifier
- power amplifier.

Voltage amplifiers increase the amplitude of a voltage signal, but supply negligible current. *Power amplifiers* give little or no voltage amplification, but have large output currents. Therefore, the output of a voltage amplifier should be fed into the input of a power amplifier if the output is required to do physical work, such as operating the speech coil of a loudspeaker to vibrate the air.

Passive elements do not produce energy and can only deliver energy that has previously been stored to the system. They include masses, dampers and springs in mechanical systems and inductors, resistors and capacitances in electrical systems.

Active elements can deliver external energy to a system. They include external forces and torques in mechanical systems and current and voltage sources in electrical systems.

2.3 Measurement of Biological Variables and Sources of Error

Errors are unfortunately an integral part of any measurement system. Regular calibration and checking of all the functions of the equipment, as well as the use of appropriate standards, can reduce errors. How often a calibration should be carried out depends on the type of equipment, how often it is used and whether it is stationary or mobile, but should generally not be less than once a year.

2.3.1 Types of Error

In the diagnostic context, two particular types of error are important:

- *false positive*, e.g. diagnosing that someone has a hearing loss when they do not have one;
- *false negative*, e.g. diagnosing that someone has "normal" hearing when they have a hearing loss.

These errors are analogous to type I and type II errors in hypothesis testing and statistics.

In audiology diagnosis, the terms sensitivity and specificity are used:

- *Sensitivity* is a measure of the ability of a test to detect correctly those people with hearing loss (or another condition). More formally, it is the number of true positives divided by the number of subjects with the condition (×100%).

- *Specificity* is a measure of the ability of a test not to make false diagnoses. More formally, it is the number of true negatives divided by the number of subjects without the condition (×100%).

Both sensitivity and specificity are frequently measured as percentages. A good test should have both high sensitivity and high specificity. However, in practice, increasing one tends to reduce the other. Therefore, high sensitivity will be required when (early) detection is important, for instance in the case of cerebellopontine angle tumours. This is a very serious illness that can be treated. High specificity will be required when it is important not to have false alarms, which could worry people unnecessarily, for instance in the case of otosalpingitis. This is less serious and there is no generally accepted method of treatment.

2.3.2 Physiological and Environmental Sources of Error

In assessing hearing it is often useful to determine whether there are changes over time, for instance whether hearing loss is increasing or staying the same. However, the presence of measurement errors can make it difficult to determine whether hearing has changed or not. In this case statistical tests may be required. It has been shown that there is a 95% probability (significance level of 0.05) that a change has occurred if the difference in thresholds between two tests is at least 2.8 times the standard deviation. Statistical tests generally concentrate on not falsely diagnosing a change that has not occurred rather than on missing a real change in thresholds. However, in assessing hearing it is preferable that the initial tests highlight all possible changes and then more accurate tests can be used (if necessary) to determine whether or not these changes have really occurred.

Psychoacoustic tests, such as pure-tone audiometry, require the active participation of the listener. Therefore, misunderstanding or misinterpretation of the instructions can lead to errors. Close to a threshold, people may be unsure whether they have heard a tone or just imagined it. Particularly close to the threshold, the test tones may be masked by noise in the body, *e.g.* due to the circulatory system. In addition, tinnitus can interfere with hearing test tones, particularly at higher frequencies. Using an audiometer with a pulse tone or frequency-modulated (warble) tone allows the characteristics of the test tone to be changed to make it easier to distinguish the test tones from tinnitus or environmental noise. At higher sound levels, adaptation, habituation and fatigue all make the auditory system less sensitive. This could lead to falsely elevated thresholds being recorded.

The physical and mental state of the person being tested can also affect the result. For instance, some test methods, such as brain-stem audiometry, are very sensitive to how relaxed the person is, and movement or muscular activity can disturb the results in *impedance audiometry*. Recent exposure to loud noises can temporarily raise thresholds, so, as far as possible, noise exposure should be avoided for a period of 14 hours before testing. This could require temporary transfer to another part of the workplace for workers in noisy environments.

Some people lack motivation, for instance due to being pressurised to come by family rather than having decided for themselves to have a hearing assessment. They may be worried about the results of the test, be tired or be on a course of medicinal drugs, and could find it difficult to concentrate for a number of reasons. As far as possible, distractions and noise should be eliminated from the test environment, both to avoid inattention and to avoid the test signal being masked by noise in the surroundings.

The positioning of the earphone or bone vibrator on the ear or skull or the placement of the listener relative to a loudspeaker may affect the results obtained. This is likely to vary slightly each time a test is carried out and it could lead to differences in recorded threshold values. It is important that over-the-ear earphones fit tightly, otherwise sound leakage could increase thresholds by up to 15 dB for low frequencies. Large variations in test sound levels can occur if the test-room surfaces are not anechoic so that they do not fully absorb the sound. This problem can be reduced by using frequency-modulated tones or narrow-band noise.

2.4 The Test Decision Process

In evaluating hearing loss, it is necessary to determine both the extent and type of hearing loss. In Chapter 1 there was a full discussion of the levels of hearing loss and the related medical conditions that might be causing the loss. The diagnostic process involves a sequence of steps leading to a number of diagnostic decisions. These are as follows.

Step 1. First determine whether there is:

- conductive hearing loss
- sensorineural hearing loss.

Step 2. If there is conductive hearing loss, then determine whether there is a:

- whole eardrum
- perforated eardrum with dry ear
- perforated eardrum with middle ear effusion.

Step 3. If there is sensorineural hearing loss, then determine whether it is:

- cochlear
- retrocochlear
- central.

Pure-tone audiometry, sometimes in combination with speech audiometry, can generally be used to determine whether there is a conductive or sensorineural hearing loss. Acoustic reflex tests may also be required, if there is sensorineural hearing loss with an air–bone gap, *e.g.* as with Ménière's disease. In the case of conductive hearing losses, immittance audiometry and otomicroscopic examination of the ear can be used to give further information.

In determining the type of sensorineural hearing loss, tests in the following three main categories are used:

- psychoacoustic tests, such as loudness balance, threshold tone decay tests and sound localisation tests
- immittance audiometry
- eletrophysiological tests, such as ERA.

The degree of hearing loss affects the tests that can be used. Increasing hearing loss will make it more difficult to differentiate between cochlear and retrocochlear lesions. For severe hearing losses, acoustic reflexes can generally be recorded far more easily than brain-stem audiometry, but there are also limitations on its use. In some cases, what equipment is available and whether there are personnel available who are experienced in its use will affect the choice of tests. For instance, equipment for brain-stem audiometry may not be available. The psychoacoustic methods require cooperation from the subject and generally have relatively low sensitivity in diagnosing retrocochlear lesions. The problem of low sensitivity can be solved by using several tests, but this increases the time the tests take. The trend is now to use brain-stem audiometry and acoustic reflex tests, which have higher sensitivity, possibly in combination with electronystagmography. When brain-stem audiometry cannot be used because equipment is not available or thresholds are too high, a combination of acoustic reflex tests, electronystagmography and psychoacoustic tests can be used. In the case of central and retrocochlear lesions, computer tomography (CT) scans and other radiological examinations should also be applied to check for the presence of tumours.

2.5 Pure-tone Audiometry

Pure-tone audiometry is one of the most commonly used methods of hearing assessment. It is generally the initial test. It is based on determining the thresholds of hearing, *i.e.* the minimum loudness required for audibility, at a number of different frequencies across the speech spectrum. It gives hearing sensitivity as a function of frequency. It can predict the level of speech necessary for audibility, but not whether speech at a particular level can actually be heard and understood. The term *pure tone* is used as the hearing is tested using pure tones or sounds at a single frequency.

Both air conduction and bone conduction thresholds can be obtained. Air conduction tests the performance of the whole auditory system, whereas bone conduction tests the performance of the inner ear and auditory nerve. Therefore, bone conduction thresholds are generally not significantly higher than air conduction thresholds and are not tested if air conduction thresholds are close to 0 dB, *i.e.* "normal".

2.5.1 Audiograms

The results of pure-tone tests are generally recorded on a graph called an audiogram, though a table is sometimes used in industry. This graph has the test frequency in hertz on the abscissa or horizontal axis and the hearing level in decibels on the ordinate or vertical axis. The scales should be chosen so that

Table 2.1 Audiogram symbols.

	Threshold	Masked threshold
Right ear, air conduction	O (in red)	Δ (in red)
Left ear, air conduction	X (in blue)	□ (in blue)
Right ear, bone conduction	<	[
Left ear, bone conduction	>	]

the distance between one octave on the frequency scale is equal to the distance of 20 dB on the hearing-level scale. The 250, 500, 1000, 2000, 4000 and 8000 Hz frequencies are generally marked on the frequency axis of the audiogram and the 3000 and 6000 Hz frequencies indicated. The air conduction and bone conduction thresholds at the different frequencies for the right and left ears are marked on the graph and joined by straight lines. Both masked and unmasked thresholds can be shown. Masking is explained in Section 2.5.4. The symbols used on an audiogram are shown in Table 2.1.

Sensorineural, conductive and mixed sensorineural and conductive hearing loss have different types of audiogram. A pure conductive loss is indicated by "normal" bone conduction thresholds (close to 0 dB) and raised air conduction thresholds. A pure sensorineural loss is indicated by equally raised bone and air conduction thresholds, *i.e.* both thresholds are greater than 0 dB and about the same. A mixed loss is indicated by raised thresholds, with an *air bone gap*, *i.e.* both thresholds are clearly non-zero and the air conduction threshold is higher than the bone conduction threshold. The graph of a conductive hearing loss is also generally much flatter than that of sensorineural hearing loss, where hearing loss increases sharply towards the higher frequencies and thresholds may be approximately "normal" for low frequencies. The air and bone conduction thresholds for sensorineural, conductive and mixed hearing losses are shown in Figure 2.2(a)–(c) respectively.

2.5.2 Noise

Background noise will generally interfere with the tests and increase thresholds, so it is important that the test area is as quiet as possible. Tables have been drawn up giving the maximum permissible ambient noise levels for thresholds not to be increased by more than 2 dB due to ambient noise when the lowest tone level used is 0 dB HL. The maximum permissible noise levels are generally considerably lower for bone conduction than air conduction and are also frequency dependent. There are a number of commercially available sound rooms with double-wall examination rooms to give additional attenuation of outside noise.

2.5.3 The Test

In the test the person being tested listens to a series of pure tones. A clinical audiometer, as shown in Figure 2.3, generates these tones. The test frequencies are presented in the following order: 1000, 2000, 4000, 8000, 1000, 500 and 250 Hz. The 1000 Hz test is repeated to give a measure of the reliability of the

Audiology: The Measurement of Hearing

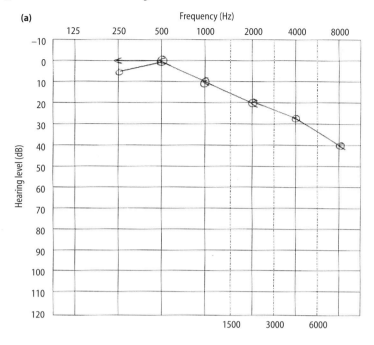

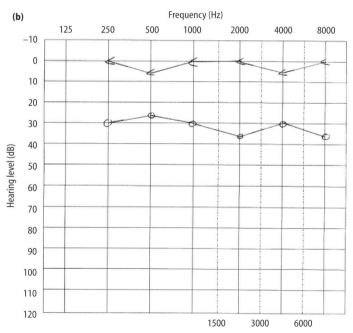

Figure 2.2 (a) Sensorineural hearing loss (right ear); (b) conductive hearing loss (right ear); (c) mixed hearing loss (right ear).

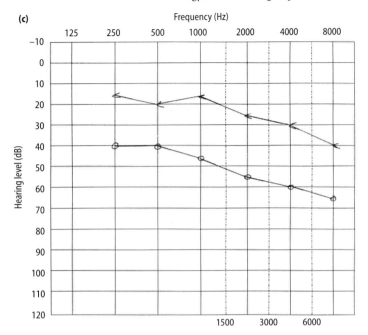

Figure 2.2 (*continued*)

results. If the threshold values obtained in the two tests at 1000 Hz differ by more than 10 dB, then the other tests are repeated. Hearing is sometimes also tested at 125 Hz. The intermediate frequencies of 750, 1500, 3000 and 6000 Hz should be tested if a difference in sensitivity of at least 20 dB is obtained between adjacent test points. This will give additional information about where the change in sensitivity is occurring. The 3000 and 6000 Hz frequencies should be tested if there is a possibility of a compensation claim.

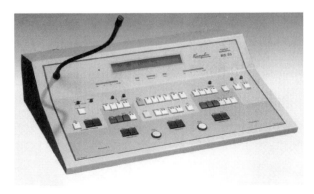

Figure 2.3 A clinical audiometer.

In the air conduction test the test sounds are presented through high-quality earphones with appropriate attenuation properties. The better ear is tested first, if this can be established, for instance by asking the person being tested or from previous tests. For each frequency, hearing thresholds are obtained by either an ascending or descending procedure. In the ascending procedure the test tones are increased in intensity until an audible signal is found, whereas in the descending procedure the test tones are decreased in intensity until the signal is no longer audible. The threshold is the first level at which three responses are obtained. The intervals between signals should be varied to avoid people guessing when the tone is due rather than actually hearing it.

Pure-tone bone conduction testing is generally carried out after pure-tone air conduction testing. The procedure is very similar. The sound is now presented through a bone vibrator, which is placed either on the mastoid process of the outer ear or occasionally on the forehead. The ear with the poorer air conduction threshold is generally tested first.

2.5.4 Masking

Masking may be used to stop the non-test ear affecting the hearing evaluation. The idea is to prevent crossover hearing, in which the test signal is heard in the non-test ear. Crossover hearing generally occurs by bone conduction even when air conduction is being tested, as the vibration of the earphone against the skull stimulates the cochlea of the non-test ear by bone conduction. The skull attenuates air-conducted tones by 40 to 80 dB and bone-conducted tones by an insignificant extent, assumed to be 0 dB. Therefore, in bone conduction tests the pure tones will generally be heard in both ears and masking will be required unless the threshold in the non-test ear is less than in the test ear. In air conduction tests the sound is attenuated by the skull. Therefore, masking will only be required if the bone conduction threshold in the non-test ear is more than 40 dB greater than the air conduction threshold in the test ear. The lower limit of skull attenuation is used, as the amount of attenuation is generally not known exactly. Masking may be required at some frequencies and not at others, and different amounts of masking noise may be required at different frequencies.

Masking is generally achieved using narrow-band noise input through earphones to the non-test ear. Narrow-band noise is obtained by filtering white noise (which has equal energy at all bandwidths) to obtain bands centred round each test frequency. It is given the symbol Z. This indicates the level to which the threshold of the masked ear is shifted. Therefore, the effect of masking noise is to raise the level of the threshold of the non-test ear so it is too high for crossover hearing.

Care has to be taken to give sufficient masking while avoiding over-masking, in which the masking noise affects the threshold of the test ear as well as the non-test ear. In some cases, particularly when there is severe hearing loss in only one ear, the required masking noise could be uncomfortably loud. The presence of masking can sometimes distract the person being tested or lead to confusion between the test signal and the noise. Therefore, it is not always possible to use masking noise.

Example

Thresholds at 1000 Hz:

- air conduction threshold in the right ear, 70 dB HL
- air conduction threshold in the left ear, 40 dB HL
- bone conduction threshold in the right ear, 60 dB HL
- bone conduction threshold in the left ear, 25 dB HL.

Masking will not be required when the left ear is tested, as the bone conduction threshold in the right ear is higher than both thresholds in the left ear.

Masking will be required when air conduction in the right ear is tested, as the air conduction threshold in the right ear (70 dB) is greater than the bone conduction threshold in the left ear (25 dB) by more than 40 dB (specifically by 45 dB). Masking will also be required when bone conduction in the right ear is tested.

Masking noise is required to raise the bone conduction threshold in the left ear:

- to at least 70–40 dB, say 35 dB, *i.e.* by at least 10 dB when carrying out air conduction tests on the right ear;
- to at least 60 dB, say 65 dB, *i.e.* by $60 - 25 = 35$ dB when carrying out bone conduction tests on the right ear.

2.5.5 Instrumentation

Commercially available pure-tone audiometers range from simple portable models for school testing to more elaborate instruments that can be used in research or to administer a wide range of tests in addition to pure-tone audiometry. Figure 2.3 shows a typical clinical audiometer. Most pure-tone audiometers will provide for air and bone conduction testing and masking. The pure-tone audiometers currently in use generally provide discrete frequency tones at octave and mid-octave intervals. There are also sweep-frequency instruments; these provide a tone that varies continuously over frequency. The hearing-level dial is generally graduated in 5 dB steps, though many audiometers have intensity controls in 1 or 2 dB steps. However, in practice, this fine tuning is rarely used.

The main controls are as follows:

- power switch
- frequency selector
- attenuator or hearing level control
- output selector (air or bone conduction, right or left ear)
- interrupter switch
- switch and attenuator for masking noise.

If speech and pure-tone audiometry are combined on one instrument, then the audiometer should provide at the least the following facilities:

- inputs
  - microphone
  - turntable
  - stereo tape deck with delayed auditory feedback
  - pure tone generator (preferably two)
  - masking noise generators – narrow band for pure tones and white noise or speech noise for speech
- two input channels
- selector switches for choosing inputs for each channel
- volume control for each input
- volume indicator meters – preferably separate meters for each channel, otherwise one meter that can be used with both channels
- amplifiers
- attenuators
- outputs
  - air conduction earphones
  - bone conduction vibrator
  - preferably two loudspeakers
- output selector switches for selecting either or both input channels for any of the outputs
- monitoring and patient talk-back system, including microphone for the patient amplifier, attenuator and earphone and/or loudspeaker for the examiner
- patient signalling device – switch and light.

As the maximum output available generally varies across the spectrum, the maximum output in dB HL is indicated for each frequency. The interrupter switch can generally be used to turn the tone either on or off when depressed. It is either spring loaded or non-mechanical, so that it returns to the other position when released.

2.5.6 Technical Description of an Audiometer

The general functional structure of an audiometer is shown in the simplified diagram of Figure 2.4. The translation of this structure into a working instrument is

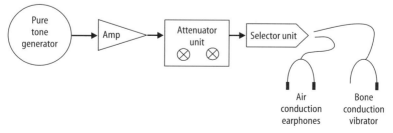

Figure 2.4 Basic structure of the audiometer.

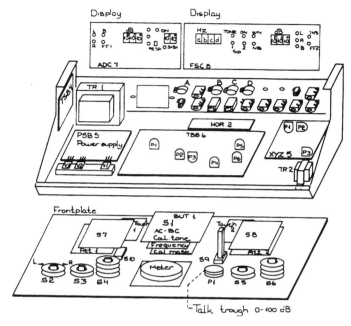

Figure 2.5 Cutaway view of an audiometer (analogue technology).

the task of the engineer. Currently, both analogue and digital instruments are available, with the more recent entries to the market being based on digital technology and computer systems.

Older audiometers, still in use, are based on a mixture of analogue and digital components. Figure 2.5 illustrates a cutaway of the case and part of the analogue circuit for an older design of audiometer. It should be noted that the pure tones are generated by oscillators, rather than by the digital signal processor found in more recent models.

More modern instruments are based on digital electronics, digital signal processing and computer systems technology. Typically, the main components include:

- a central processing unit (CPU)
- keyboard
- printer
- RS232 interface
- display
- digital signal-processing unit
- talk forward
- two channels of output.

The keyboard, printer, RS232 interface and liquid-crystal display are all connected directly to the CPU, whereas the other components are connected indirectly to it through dual-port random access memory.

Audiology: The Measurement of Hearing

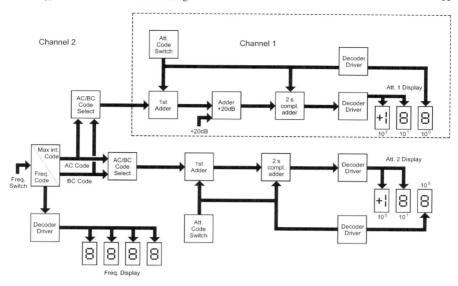

Figure 2.6 A typical implementation for a digital audiometer.

All operations are controlled from the CPU, which can receive input from the keyboard. Pure tones are generated in a digital signal processor. Variable and fixed attenuators are used to give the desired output intensity. A table of the maximum output intensity at each frequency is given in Section 2.5.7. A low-pass filter with a cut-off frequency of 20 kHz is used to remove high-frequency noise and the higher harmonics.

One digital signal processor generates the pure tones for both channels, but the two channels have separate attenuators and low-pass filters. Both channels can be connected to either the left or right earphone or the bone vibrator and can also include a masking noise. The digital signal processor also generates the signal for the talk forward for communicating with people being tested.

The RS232 interface is designed to transmit data from the audiometer to a computer and control the audiometer from a computer. Typically the computer and audiometer both have 25- and 9-pin plugs. There are pins for received and transmitted data, clear to send, data set ready, signal ground and data terminal ready. The logic levels used are data "1" and "0" at −12 V and +12 V respectively. Control off and on is also given by −12 V and +12 V respectively. Data, consisting of one start bit, eight data bits, one parity bit and two stop bits with even parity, are transmitted asynchronously to the audiometer. The baud rate can be selected internally as 9600, 19,200 or 28,400 baud. A schematic of a typical digital implementation is given in Figure 2.6.

2.5.7 Technical Specifications

A typical modern audiometer must satisfy international and US standards, IEC645-1-1991 and ANSI 3.6, 1996 respectively, and the international safety standard IEC 601-1. Calibration is carried out according to ISO R389 third

Table 2.2 Values of the maximum intensity for frequency versus headphone options.

Frequency (Hz)	Air conduction (dB HL)		Bone conduction (dB HL)	
	Supra-aural	Insert	B71	A20
125	90	90	–	–
250	110	105	45	40
500	120	110	65	60
750	120	115	70	70
1000	120	120	70	70
1500	120	120	70	70
2000	120	120	75	70
3000	120	120	80	70
4000	120	120	80	60
5000	120	115	80	60
6000	120	100	55	50
8000	110	95	50	40

edition for air conduction and ISO 7566 or ANSI 3.26-1981 for bone conduction. Most audiometers have an external power supply and can be used with either a 110–120 V or 230–240 V, 50–60 Hz mains supply, but will require different fuses, for instance T 250 mA in the first case and T 125 mA in the second. Audiometers are generally designed to be used at temperatures of 15–35 °C and relative humidities of 30–90%. This covers a wide range of climate conditions. A special design may be required in some cases to allow the audiometer to be used in more extreme climactic conditions. Warm-up time is typically 3 min.

Values of the maximum intensity for different frequencies are given in Table 2.2 for air conduction with super-aural (over-the-ear) and insert headphones and two bone conduction options.

Tone presentation options include manual, reverse, and multiple and single pulses of 250–5000 ms duration. Typically, the attenuator is able to produce −10 to 120 dB HL in 1 and 5 dB steps. Communication with the person being tested is through 0–110 dB SPL talk forward, which is continuously adjustable on the operations panel.

2.6 Immittance Audiometry

2.6.1 Definitions

In *immittance audiometry* the acoustic impedance or admittance of the middle ear is recorded. Impedance is a general term for resistance against motion. In the auditory system the motion of interest is the vibration of air molecules caused by sound pressure. This vibration is measured in terms of the velocity of a given volume of air, *i.e.* volume velocity. Therefore, the acoustic impedance of an ear is a measure of the sound pressure that is required to make the air molecules in the auditory system vibrate with a certain volume velocity. It is defined as the ratio of sound pressure to volume velocity in pascal seconds per metre cubed (Pa s m^{-3}). Admittance is a measure of mobility and, therefore, *acoustic admittance* Y_a is the reciprocal of acoustic impedance Z_a. It is defined as the ratio of volume velocity to sound pressure. The "a" in the symbol indicates acoustic and is often omitted; it is also sometimes written on the line rather than as a subscript.

At each frequency the acoustic impedance can be expressed as a complex number with real and imaginary components. It is a combination of the friction component, *acoustic resistance* R_a and the mass and spring components *acoustic reactance* X_a. Therefore

$$Z_a = R_a + jX_a$$

This is analogous to an electrical system with resistance R, inductance L and total impedance Z given by

$$Z = R + j\omega L$$

Similarly, acoustic admittance has the real and imaginary components *acoustic conductance* G_a and *susceptance* B_a:

$$Y_a = G_a + jB_a$$

There is a resonant frequency at which reactance is zero, making impedance purely real and so impedance has a minimum value and admittance a maximum. The term *immittance* is sometimes used to refer to both impedance and admittance. Each instantaneous change in ear-canal pressure has an associated valued of acoustic admittance.

2.6.2 Measurement

It is generally admittance rather than impedance that is measured. This has a number of advantages. In particular, admittance has a linear relationship with pressure, and so two admittances in series can be added, whereas there is a non-linear relationship between the corresponding impedances and they cannot be combined by simple addition. This is analogous to combining resistors in series and in parallel.

Three main techniques for measuring acoustic immittance are used clinically:

- static acoustic immittance of the middle ear
- tympanometry
- acoustic reflex testing.

When acoustic impedance is measured, an acoustic impedance bridge is used to compare the sound pressure level in the ear canal in volts to a pre-set standard (Figure 2.7). The sound pressure level due to the acoustic admittance of the ear canal is initially balanced with the standard. Changes due to changes in ear-canal pressure or contraction of middle-ear muscles can then be measured by rebalancing with the standard. The sound pressure required to rebalance the bridge is directly proportional to the change in acoustic impedance. In tympanometry (see Section 2.6.4), when the ear-canal pressure is swept across the measurement range, balancing is generally omitted, giving the result in arbitrary units.

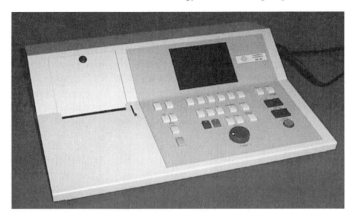

Figure 2.7 A clinical impedance audiometer.

2.6.3 Static Acoustic Immittance

It is generally the admittance of the middle ear that is required to be measured, but in practice this has to be obtained from the admittance of the total and outer ears. The admittance of the middle ear can be obtained by subtracting outer-ear admittance from total-ear admittance, so that

$$Y_2 = Y_T - Y_1$$

where Y_1, Y_2 and Y_T are the admittances of the outer-, middle- and total-ear.

Static acoustic admittance measures the ease of flow of acoustic energy through the middle ear and is generally expressed in terms of equivalent volume in cubic centimetres. The static acoustic immittance of the outer ear is measured with an ear-canal pressure of +2 or −4 kPa, as the tympanic membrane is very stiff at +2 and −4 kPa and essentially excludes the middle ear from acoustic immittance measurements. The admittance of the outer ear is then subtracted from that of the combined middle and outer ears. The error in calculating the static acoustic admittance of the middle ear by subtracting the static acoustic admittance of the outer ear from that of the whole ear is small, being about 2%.

For low-frequency probe tones, such as 226 Hz, the phase angle of the admittance vector is close to 90° and so its magnitude is close to that of the imaginary component, the susceptance vector and therefore measurements are often performed at this frequency.

2.6.4 Tympanometry

A *tympanogram* is a recording of the mobility of the middle ear as a function of air pressure when air pressure is varied from +2 to −4 kPa. It indicates the stiffness of the middle-ear mechanism relative to "normal". It gives a measure of the Eustachian tube function by measuring the air pressure in the middle-ear space. A probe, generally with probe tone of 226 Hz, is placed in the ear canal. The air tightness of the fit is then checked automatically or by increasing the pressure to about 2 kPa and checking that the pressure is not reduced by air leakage. Introducing this positive pressure makes the middle-ear mechanism very stiff.

The pressure in the ear canal is then reduced using a moderate sweep rate of $0.2\,\text{kPa s}^{-1}$ to -2 kPa. If a compliance maximum has not been observed, then the pressure is reduced further until a maximum is reached, but not lower than -6 kPa. The pressure is then slowly returned to zero. The tympanogram is usually recorded automatically by a built-in or external recorder or is displayed on an electronic display. The air-pressure value for maximum compliance and the middle-ear compliance, *i.e.* the difference between the compliance at peak and $+2$ kPa, should be recorded.

2.6.5 Acoustic Reflex Threshold

The *acoustic reflex threshold* is defined as the lowest sound intensity required to make the middle-ear (stapedius) muscle contract. Intense sound (in either ear) leads to contraction of the middle-ear muscles. It also causes a temporary increase in the impedance of both middle ears. The acoustic reflex is generally measured in the ear canal opposite to the ear being stimulated. A headphone is placed on one ear and the immittance meter probe assembly inserted into the other ear. When the signal from the earphone is sufficiently intense, middle-ear stiffness increases in both ears, leading to increased reflection of sound from the eardrum. This increase in sound pressure can be measured on the immittance meter. The reflex threshold obtained is generally considered to be that of the ear being stimulated, not the ear in which the reflex is measured. It is therefore called a contralateral (other or opposite) reflex threshold.

2.7 Electric Response Audiometry (ERA)

Sound waves stimulating the ear give rise to electrical activity in the neurons in the auditory pathways. This electrical activity can be measured using variations in the electrical potential difference between two appropriately placed electrodes. Test methods based on recording this potential difference are called ERA. The electrodes are placed on the skull, in the ear canal or in the middle ear according to which part of the auditory system is being investigated. ERA equipment is generally more complex and expensive than other audiometric equipment. It consists of three main components: a signal generator; an amplifier and filter; and a central processing and computing unit. The recording unit consists of electrodes, an amplifier, filters and an analogue-to-digital (A/D) converter.

The signal generator generates a signal of the desired type, for instance, click, tone pip or tone burst. A broadband click, which is generated by feeding an electrical pulse lasting 0.1–0.2 ms to the earphone, is often used.

The electrical signal from the signal generator is transmitted to the person being tested by the earphone or loudspeaker. Conventional audiometer earphones are generally used. Electromagnetic radiation can be reduced by the use of µ-metal shielding or electrostatic or piezoelectric earphones with a negligible magnetic field. A loudspeaker can be used for people who have problems with earphones, but its calibration is less reliable and the additional travelling time from the loudspeaker can influence the results obtained.

The amplifier requires a gain in the range of 10^5–10^6 to amplify the electrode signals of less than a microvolt to the order of a few volts at the input to the A/D converter. A differential amplifier with two stages is generally used to give low sensitivity to external interference. It has three input connections: non-inverting or positive; inverting or negative; and common, which acts as a reference. The differential amplifier has the advantage of amplifying only the difference in potential between the positive and negative inputs. Therefore, it suppresses unwanted biological signals and external interference.

The amplification of about 10^5 is obtained from the second stage of the amplifier. The output of the second stage is passed through a band-pass filter to increase the signal-to-noise ratio before signal averaging. The filter range is chosen to reject background activity unrelated to the potential. Digital filters are increasingly replacing analogue ones in ERA, as phase distortion occurs with analogue filters, particularly close to the cut-off frequency.

Good quality disposable electrodes are frequently used, as reusable electrodes must be carefully cleaned and sometimes re-chlorided to maintain their electrical characteristics. All the electrodes should have low (less than 5 kW) and approximately equal impedances to avoid excessive noise generation and increased sensitivity to external interference. The non-inverting electrode is often placed on the vertex (top of the skull) or upper forehead, with the latter placement generally more comfortable. The inverting electrode is placed on the mastoid or earlobe on the same side as the stimulation. The common electrode is placed on the mastoid, earlobe or neck on the other side from the ear being stimulated. The earphone and its cable should be kept as far as possible from the electrode cables (which should be kept close together) in order to minimise inductive interference from the earphone.

The third component, the common control unit or signal averager, carries out all processing and analysis, including signal averaging. Averaging is required to increase the signal-to-noise ratio sufficiently for the response to be identified.

The system may be housed in a portable self-contained unit, which has a limited number of controls and includes a small recorder for printouts. Alternatively, the unit may be closer in design to a small computer, with the stimulus generator and amplifier added as extension units and the printouts provided by a separate plotter. Data are entered through the keyboard and there is greater flexibility. In plotting the response, the non-inverting and inverting leads, generally from the vertex (or the forehead) and ipsalateral (same side) ear lobe or mastoid, are usually connected to the positive and negative inputs respectively. This gives an upward deflection on the oscilloscope. This is referred to as "vertex positive and up". Two channel recordings simultaneously from both ears can facilitate identification of the different peaks of the response. Contralateral (opposite side) masking should be used.

2.7.1 Electrocochleography

Electrocochleography is used to assess the function of the inner ear. Its main applications are the estimation of hearing thresholds and the evaluation of the peripheral auditory function in children. It gives useful clinical information for people with mixed hearing loss, including when there are masking problems, as it tests each ear separately and does not require masking.

Two different types of recording technique are used. In one approach, a transtympanic needle electrode is used with its tip on the promontory of the middle ear, with a highest signal amplitude of up to 10–20 µV. The other approach uses ear-canal electrodes on the eardrum or inner part of the ear canal, where response amplitudes can reach a few microvolts. There are a number of ear-canal electrodes that do not penetrate the eardrum. These have the advantages of avoiding infection and mechanical damage (though the risk is small), but the disadvantage of recording electrical activity further away from the cochlea and so giving a lower response amplitude. The filter generally has a range of 20–300 Hz to 1000–3000 Hz. Broadband unfiltered clicks, filtered clicks or brief tone bursts are generally used as the stimuli.

2.7.2 Brain-stem Response Audiometry

Brain-stem audiometry is used for the clinical evaluation of sensorineural hearing disorders and can be used to estimate thresholds for children and people with multiple disabilities who are difficult to test. It is also used to diagnose suspected brain-stem lesions, with or without auditory symptoms. The auditory brain-stem response is of very low amplitude, of the order of a few hundred nanovolts at high stimulus levels. Therefore, care is required to minimise noise and other interfering electrical activity. Disposable silver/silver chloride surface electrodes are generally used. One recording electrode is placed on the vertex or high on the forehead and the other close to the test ear.

The filter range is normally 20–300 Hz to 1000–30,000 Hz. A broadband click generated by either a rectangular or half sinusoid electrical pulse lasting 0.1–0.2 ms is generally used to give the auditory brain-stem response. The use of magnetic shielding on the earphones reduces the risk of stimulus artefacts. Short tone bursts can be used and give greater frequency specificity, but lower response amplitude. A stimulus repetition time, not related to the mains frequency, in the range 10–20 s is recommended. Click calibration should be specified in dB SPL; dB HL can be used, but threshold estimation is less reliable at higher sound levels. There is a possibility of phase distortion, especially when close to the cut-off frequencies. Therefore, test results should always be compared with a set of "normal" results obtained on the same equipment and with the same filter settings.

2.8 Standards

The performance specifications of audiometers and the equipment used to calibrate and test them are stated in a number of national and international standards. International standards are maintained by the International Electrotechnical Commission (http://www.iec.ch) and the International

Organisation for Standardisation (http://www.iso.ch) and given IEC and ISO numbers respectively. New standards are sometimes added and standards are updated and sometimes given new numbers.

The IEC 60645 series specifies the minimum performance requirements for audiometers. Part 1 of the series has just been revised. OIML Recommendation R 104 is based on it and specifies requirements for the pattern evaluation and verification of pre-tone audiometers and lists a set of recommended routine checks for audiometers.

All the standards in the series have been adopted as dual-numbered BS EN standards. However, the OIML recommendation illustrates the good calibration practices already adopted in other countries. Minimum performance requirements for acoustic impedance meters are specified in IEC (BS EN) 61027. This standard is being revised and will become IEC 60645-2.

The current international (IEC) and UK (BS EN) standards are as follows:

- IEC 60645-1:2001 and BS EN 60645-1:1995. Audiometers – Part 1: Pure-tone audiometers.
- IEC 60645-2:1993 and BS EN 60645-2:1997. Audiometers – Part 2: Equipment for speech audiometry.
- IEC 60645-3:1994 and BS EN 60645-3:1995. Audiometers – Part 3: Auditory test signals of short duration for audiometric and neuro-otological purposes.
- IEC 60645-4:1994 and BS EN 60645-4:1995. Audiometers – Part 4: Equipment for extended high-frequency audiometry.
- IEC 61027:1991 and BS EN 61027:1993. Instruments for the measurement of aural acoustic impedance/admittance.
- OIML International Recommendation R 104:1993. Pure-tone audiometers.

A pure-tone audiometer is used to measure hearing threshold levels relative to a reference threshold sound pressure level or vibratory force level. These reference levels are defined internationally in terms of the sound pressure at an audiometric earphone or the force levels set up by a bone vibrator coupled to an artificial ear or mastoid. All the equipment involved in these definitions must meet appropriate international standards.

The ISO 389 series of standards specifies the zero reference level for the calibration of audiometric equipment. Part 1 (ISO 389-1:1998) and part 2 (ISO 389-2:1994) specify the reference equivalent threshold sound pressure levels for pure tones with supra-aural (over the ears) and insert earphones respectively. Part 3 (ISO 389-3:1994) specifies the reference equivalent threshold sound force levels for pure tones and bone vibrators and part 4 (ISO 389-4:1994) specifies the reference levels for narrow-band masking noise.

2.9 Audiometric Equipment Design and Calibration

The importance of regular calibration is discussed in Section 2.3. The basic equipment for checking output levels should include:

- a measuring amplifier with input for a condenser microphone or a sound-level meter that meets IEC 651 type 1;
- a sound-level meter, a spectrum analyser, or microphone preamplifier and measuring amplifier;
- 6cc and 2cc acoustic couplers (artificial ears) that meet IEC 60318-1:1998 (IEC 308 and IEC 126);
- a 2.54 cm (1 in) pressure field condenser microphone for the couplers, which meets IEC 1094-1;
- a 500 g weight;
- a mechanical coupler for bone-vibrator measurements (artificial mastoid) that meets IEC 373;
- a general-purpose frequency counter;
- a general-purpose digital multimeter.

Other useful equipment includes a storage-type oscilloscope to trace and monitor the signals, a graphic level recorder, a frequency analyser and/or a distortion meter. All this equipment must be reliable and stable.

Both hardware and software should be calibrated. Hardware calibration includes calibration of the attenuators on both channels. This requires an AC voltmeter with a 1000 Hz band-pass filter. The angle of the liquid-crystal display should be adjusted to give clear readings. Software calibration requires:

- adjustment of the sound-level meter and modification register;
- calibration of the left and right earphones;
- calibration of the left and right bone conduction and masking outputs;
- calibration of the tone, narrow-band and white-noise inputs.

The ambient noise levels in the test room should be checked using a sound-level meter that is sufficiently sensitive to allow testing to 8 dB SPL. Ambient noise levels should be checked every 6 months and, additionally, if changes occur in the external environment or noises are heard in the test booth.

2.9.1 Earphone Calibration

Earphones can be calibrated using a sample of young adults with "normal" hearing, but the use of an artificial coupler is much easier. The 6cc coupler was originally used, but its impedance characteristics are the same as those of a human ear over only part of the frequency range. The IEC 318 coupler was developed to resolve this problem. Although an improvement on the 6cc coupler, its impedance characteristics are also different from those of a real ear.

A 500 g mass is placed on top of the earphone, which is placed on the coupler. The output in volts is read and then transformed to decibels. It can sometimes be read directly in decibels. The earphone is placed on the coupler and then a low-frequency tone (125 or 250 Hz) is introduced. The earphone is readjusted on the coupler until the highest output intensity is reached. The output can then be compared with the expected values, which are given in ISO 389-1:1998 and ISO 189-2:1998 for supra-aural and insert earphones respectively.

2.9.2 Calibration of Pure-tone Audiometers

In pure-tone and speech audiometry the three parameters of frequency, intensity and time (both phase and signal duration) should be checked regularly. Frequency should be checked initially and then at yearly intervals. The permitted tolerance is ±3% of the measured value. Harmonic distortion should be less than 3% at specified frequencies for earphones and 5% or less for the probe tube transducer or insert receiver. Gross attenuation and distortion problems should be detectable by listening to the audiometer, which should be done daily. In digital audiometers much of the calibration can be done in software.

Tone intensity in pure-tone audiometers is usually calibrated by varying the resistance in the output circuits of the oscillators that generate the pure tones, so that the desired output at the earphone is obtained on an artificial ear. The earphone is placed on one side of the coupler and the sound-level meter microphone on the other. The audiometer is set at the prescribed hearing level for a particular frequency. The oscillator for that frequency is adjusted until the output measured by the sound meter agrees with the specified value for that frequency and hearing-level dial setting.

An audiometer can also be calibrated using a second audiometer that is known to be in calibration. The calibrated audiometer is set at a given frequency and hearing level. Then the hearing-level control on the other audiometer at the same frequency setting is adjusted until the tone loudness of both audiometers is approximately equal.

Pure-tone audiometers are calibrated at 125, 250, 500, 750 1000, 1500, 2000, 3000, 4000, 6000 and 8000 Hz. The calibration is generally accurate to 0.2 dB. If possible, the audiometer potentiometers or programming adjustments should be used to recalibrate the audiometer. When this is not possible, or when different earphones will be used with the same audiometer, a calibration correction card can be used if the corrections are less than 15 dB. If the error is more than 15 dB at any frequency or is 10 dB at three or more frequencies, then the audiometer should be recalibrated by the manufacturer.

2.9.3 Calibration of Couplers and Sound-level Meters

A mechanical coupler system consisting of a coupler and a sound-level meter or measuring amplifier should be calibrated at the following frequencies: 250, 500, 750 1000, 1500, 2000, 3000 and 4000 Hz. Calibration is based on the meter reading when a static force of 5.4 N and a known vibratory force are applied together to the dome of the coupler. The coupler should be maintained at a temperature of 23 ± 1 °C, as its sensitivity is highly temperature dependent. Calibration accuracy is 0.3 dB at a confidence level of 95%. Earphones can be calibrated by being connected to a reference coupler or artificial ear and a known voltage applied. Measurements are made at 125, 250, 500, 750, 1000, 1500, 2000, 3000, 4000, 6000 and 8000 Hz and the meter readings recorded. These measurements can be repeated at later times to check that the same results are still obtained.

Before being used, the sound-level meter should itself be calibrated. Values for the parameters to be measured are given in the relevant IEC standard.

Observation of harmonic distortion requires a sound-level meter and an octave band-filter set. The earphone is put over the coupler and the intensity is set to the level specified for the frequency by the standard. The difference in levels between the primary signal and the second harmonic is compared with the standard specification. The second harmonic is produced by setting the filter one octave higher than the audiometer signal, so that the fundamental is rejected by the filter and the second harmonic passed, *i.e.* a signal of 2000 Hz is passed for a 1000 Hz signal. The difference between the levels of the primary signal and the second harmonic can then be compared with the standard specification. In checking attenuator linearity the earphone is set over the coupler and the attenuator settings are reduced in 10 dB steps. The values on the sound-level meter are noted at each stage to determine whether the reduction in sound pressure level is linear.

2.9.4 Calibration of Bone Vibrators

The preferred procedure for calibrating bone vibrators uses a mechanical coupler or artificial mastoid, which should meet IEC 60373:1990 (to become 60318-6). The standard is based on unoccluded ears with masking on the opposite ear. When calibrating both earphones and bone vibrators, the distortion and overall intensity through the transducer should be checked. Distortion can be measured directly with a distortion meter connected to the output of the artificial mastoid or with a frequency analyser. The distortion meter approach is more accurate. Distortion values for bone vibrators are not quite as stringent as they are for earphones.

2.9.5 Calibration of Acoustic Immittance Devices

A frequency counter can be used to check the frequency of the probe signal(s) to acoustic immittance devices, which should be within ±3% of the nominal value. The harmonic distortion measured in an HA-1 2cc coupler (see Section 2.9.2) should not be more than 5% of the fundamental and the probe signal measured in the coupler should not be greater than 90 dB. The accuracy of acoustic immittance measurements can be checked by connecting the probe to the test cavities and checking the output accuracy at specified temperatures and air pressures. It should be within ±5% of the indicated value or ±10^{-9} cm^3 Pa^{-1}, whichever is greater. Air pressure can be measured by connecting the probe to a manometer and measuring water displacement for changes in the immittance-device air pressure. Air pressure should not differ by more than ±1 kPa or ±15% from the stated value, whichever is greater. The reflex activating system should also be checked.

2.10 Artificial Ears

Artificial ears are man-made ear simulators used in audiometric calibration. The existing standards for seven different types of ear and mastoid simulators used in the calibration of audiometers are being revised. These standards are being brought together in the IEC 60318 series of standards on electro-acoustics – simulators of human head and ear. Parts 1, 2 and 3, all dated 1998, give the respective specifications for acoustic couplers to be used in the calibration of supra-aural earphones, for audiometric earphones in the extended high-frequency range and for supra-aural earphones to be used in audiometry.

IEC 60711:1981 (which will become 60318-4) is for an occluded ear simulator for the measurement of insert earphones; IEC 60126:1973 (which will become 60318-5) is for a reference coupler for the measurement of hearing aids using insert earphones; IEC 60373:1990 (which will become 60318-6) is for a mechanical coupler for measurements on bone vibrators and IEC 60959 TR (which will become 60318-7) is for a provisional ear and torso simulator for acoustic measurements on air conduction hearing aids.

Ear simulators are used to determine earphone response, measure hearing-aid gain and performance and for other quantities that require simulation of the sound transmission characteristics of an external ear. They are intended to provide sound pressure data that are equivalent to sound pressures at the eardrum of a real human ear. The ear simulator should provide acoustic impedance and sound-pressure distributions that approximate those in a median adult human ear between an earmould and eardrum. The ear simulator should be constructed from rigid, non-porous, non-magnetic and stable material. Ear simulators designed according to the US ANSI standards have a specific acoustic characteristic impedance of 9.2 MPa s m^{-3} at an ambient temperature of 23 °C and pressure of 10 Pa.

2.10.1 The 2cc Coupler

The 2cc hard-walled coupler was originally designed to provide:

- a means of quality control for different units of the same hearing-aid model;
- a consistent electroacoustic measurement standard for the exchange of data between laboratories.

The 2cc coupler was never intended to be used in the selection of hearing aids for a particular hearing loss for the following reasons:

- its internal volume is greater than that of a human ear;
- its impedance does not approximate the acoustic impedance of a human ear.

However, non-speech-based approaches to hearing-aid selection have used a 2cc coupler rather than real ear gain and output measurements.

The tympanic membrane is simulated by a calibrated pressure microphone on one face of the coupler, which is about 2.5 cm across. Sound from the hearing-aid receiver enters the 2cc cavity at the centre of the opposite face. The HA-1 earphone coupler is the most generalised form. It has a relatively large opening, which allows it to be used with most aids. The aid is mounted on the coupler with a formable seal. The end of the tubing, earmould tip or hearing aid should be centred and flush with the upper face of the cavity.

The original form of the 2cc coupler, the HA-2 earphone coupler, was designed to test button-type receivers on body aids. Results from this coupler can differ from those with the HA-1 coupler, due to differences in the length and diameter of the tube from the receiver nub. The HA-2 tube has a standardised length of 18 mm and diameter of 3 mm. The HA-3 is a particular form of the HA-1 coupler with a rigid or flexible sealing construction. It can be used to test the module portion of modular in-the-ear hearing aids and/or non-battery (insert)-type receivers. The tube length from the module or receiver is generally 10 mm and the diameter 1.93 mm.

Its high volume and lack of acoustic resistance makes the 2cc coupler unsuitable for testing hearing aids with vented earmolds, unless the vents are closed. The microphone response declines rapidly above about 8000 Hz. Therefore, the coupler should not be used for tests above 7000 Hz without correcting for the microphone response. The response curves obtained with the 2cc coupler are absolutely reproducible, making the coupler very useful for inspection control, and the design is simple and robust. The coupler has performed well for its original purpose, *i.e.* the comparison of hearing aids.

2.10.2 Zwislocki Coupler

The Zwislock coupler was developed owing to problems in the use of the 2cc coupler for clinical hearing-aid measurement and to predict sound levels at the tympanic membrane when a hearing aid is used. It has a volume of 1.2 cm^3, which is close to the remaining volume of an average adult human ear when the auditory meatus (ear canal) is blocked with an earmould. Its impedances are similar to those of a typical adult ear.

The coupler consists of an approximately 1.27 cm (0.5 in) condenser microphone and four side-branch resonators. The microphone represents the tympanic membrane and the branch resonators have inertance (mass), resistance, capacitance (volume) and compliance. They have approximately the same acoustic impedance variations as occur in real ears. The mean pressure in a typical ear and in the Zwislocki coupler are considered to differ by no more than 2 dB and to be essentially identical below about 800 Hz. The tip of a hearing-aid earmould ends at the entrance to the ear simulator. There is a type M 1.27 cm (0.5 in) condenser microphone at the other end.

The Zwislocki coupler can be used with either vented or open canal earmoulds. It has adapters that simulate HA-1, HA-2 and HA-3 type connections. This allows it to be used in a similar way to the 2cc coupler for closed earmould measurements in a hearing-aid test box, though the results are not identical. Its main application is in the Knowles Electronics Mannikin for Acoustic Research (KEMAR). It can also be used for hearing-aid measurements in a sound box. Comparison of the responses of the Zwislocki and 2cc couplers with hearing-aid receivers has shown that the response of the 2cc coupler is lower at all frequencies. The difference is about 4 dB at the lower frequencies and increases to about 15 dB at 10 kHz.

2.10.3 KEMAR

The KEMAR consists of a head and a torso, proportioned like an adult human and designed to give lifelike test conditions for acoustic measurements. It is fitted with one or two Zwislocki couplers to represent human ears. These couplers were designed according to the international standard IEC 711 and US standard ANSI S3.25. The sound pressure at the microphones of the ear stimulators is intended to correspond approximately to the sound pressure at the human eardrum. The pinnae (ear lobes) are flexible, removable and human type and come in four different sizes. Testing hearing aids on KEMAR or a similar figure provides much better information on its gain-frequency and directional characteristics than carrying out tests in a sound box, as using KEMAR takes account of the diffraction of the body and head. This can significantly change the input sound pressure to a hearing-aid microphone.

2.11 Learning Highlights of the Chapter

In engineering and measurement systems, the technology is becoming more sophisticated and flexible. To be able to organise this information at different levels of abstraction is an important skill. Using such general tools as block diagrams, a good conceptual grasp of the structure of the instrumentation equipment and operation becomes easier to obtain. This chapter describes the various techniques used to measure human hearing and the technologies to implement these techniques. Some development of the principles of human-centred testing was also presented. At the conclusion of this chapter the student should be able to:

- understand the general structure of a measurement system and some essential terms from measurement science;
- understand the basic principles of the main hearing assessment methods and their use diagnostically;
- appreciate the different technological solutions for hearing measurement equipment, particularly pure-tone audiometers;
- understand the importance of technical standards for audiology equipment design;
- appreciate the broader issues for equipment calibration, and related safety issues.

Acknowledgements

We are grateful to Peter McKenna (University of Glasgow) for redrawing Figures 2.5 and 2.6, and to PC Werth for permission to use the audiometer figures.

Projects and Investigations

These projects could be combined with a visit to a hospital audiology department.

- Arrange a visit to a hospital audiology department and discuss the procedures in place for audiology measurements with

adult subjects. Identify parts of the procedure designed to minimise or eliminate measurement error. Use a pure-tone audiometer to measure hearing loss for a number of students and plot the results on an audiogram. Discuss the results obtained.
- Arrange a visit to a hospital audiology department and discuss the procedures in place for audiology measurements made with children. Identify parts of the procedure designed to minimise or eliminate measurement error. Consider how the design of the audiometer is dependent on the person being tested. What are the differences and where do they occur?
- Draw up design specifications for an audiometer and discuss how these specifications vary according to where it will be used, who will be using it and in what context. Compare and contrast the design specification for an audiometer that is to be used in different global locations.
- Design, build and test a computerised pure-tone (and immittance) audiometer that has facilities for storing audiometric records, printing out audiograms and self-testing.
- Discuss the advantages and disadvantages of self-testing, compared with testing by a trained audiologist.
- Design and build an ear simulator.
- What are the Technical Standards systems? Why are they useful? How would an electrical engineer use the standards system? Obtain the international standards for an audiometer and comment on them. Obtain national standards and compare them with the international ones.

References and Further Reading

Further Reading

Books

Arlinger, S. (Ed.). *Manual of Practical Audiometry*, vol. 1. Whurr Publishers Ltd, London and New Jersey.
Arlinger, S. (Ed). *Manual of Practical Audiometry*, vol. 2. Whurr Publishers Ltd, London and New Jersey.
Arnst, D., Katz, J. (Eds), 1982. *Central Auditory Assessment: The SSW Test, Development and Clinical Use*. College Hill Press.
Bess, F.H., Humes, L.E., 1990. *Audiology, the Fundamentals*. Williams and Wilkins, Baltimore.
Gelfand, S.A., 1997. *Essentials of Audiology*. Thieme, New York.
Hodgson, W.R., 1980. *Basic Audiologic Evaluation*. Williams and Wilkins, Baltimore and London.
Katz, J., Burkard, R., Medwetsy, L. (Eds.), 2001. *Handbook of Clinical Audiology*, 5th edition. Lippincott, Williams and Wilkins, Baltimore.
King, P.F., Coles, R.R.A., Lutman, M.E., Robinson, D.W., 1993. *Assessment of Hearing Disability*. Whurr Publishers, London and New Jersey.
Martin, F.N., 1997. *Introduction to Audiology*, 6th edition. Allyn and Bacon, Boston.
Martin, M. (Ed.), 1987. *Speech Audiometry*. Taylor and Francis, London, New York and Philadelphia.
McCormick, B. (Ed.), 1993. *Paediatric Audiology 0-5 Years*. Whurr Publishers Ltd, London and New Jersey.
Newby, H.A., 1979. *Audiology*, 4th edition. Prentice Hall, New Jersey.

Newby, H.A., Popelka, G.R., 1992. *Audiology*. Prentice Hall, New Jersey.
Silman, S., Silverman, C.A., 1991. *Auditory Diagnosis Principles and Applications*. Academic Press Inc.
Tucker, I., Nolan, M., 1984. *Educational Audiology*. Croom Helm, Beckenham.

Technical Papers

Goemans, B.C., 1992. Audiometry environment remote control system. *Medical and Biological Engineering and Computing* 645–650.
Haughton, P., 1998. Present day methods in clinical audiometry. *Acoustics Bulletin* (July–August), 7–14
Job, A., Buland, F., Maumet, L., Picard J., 1996. Visaaudio: a Windows software application for Bekesy audiogram analysis and hearing research. *Computer Methods and Programs in Biomedicine* 49, 95–103.
Kujov, H., Madsen, P., Sukolov Y., Sukolova, O., 1997. Comprehensive audiological assessment system. *Canadian Acoustics* 25 (4), 37.
McBride, D., Calvert, I., 1994. Audiometry in industry. *Annals of Occupational Hygiene* 38, 219–230.

Web Sites

htttp/academics.uwww.edu/bradleys/ohc/puretone.html.
http://www.microaud.com
http://www.pcwerth.co.uk/kamplex
http://physicianequipment.com

3 Hearing-aid Principles and Technology

3.1 Learning Objectives

The general features of a hearing aid, and brief résumés of some technical terms, features of human hearing, sensorineural impairment, and hearing-aid prescription are first presented in an introductory section. Standard hearing-aid classifications and a brief history of the development of electronic hearing aids follow. Next, the ear as an environment for which hearing aids are to be designed considers some effects of both aid-on-body and body-on-aid. Signal-processing strategies for hearing aids form a major section, featuring discussion of single channel and multiple channel schemes, including: equalisation, control of acoustic feedback, non-linear compression, speech detection, spectral subtraction, sinusoidal modelling, spectral enhancement, frequency mapping, directional microphones, microphone arrays, and adaptive noise cancellation (ANC). The technology of modern electronic aids is then discussed, focusing on digital devices. A concluding discussion follows, with projects and further reading to close the chapter. Thus, the learning objectives of the chapter may be given as

- to establish a classification for current hearings aids and understand their main functional differences;
- to review the historical trends in electronic hearing-aid development;
- to understand the major ergonomic and engineering issues associated with hearing aids;
- to appreciate the main features of various signal-processing schemes used in, or proposed for, hearing aids;
- to examine the technology and signal-processing schemes used in modern commercially available hearing aids.

3.2 Introduction

The modern hearing aid is an electronic device, the main parts of which are the microphone, the signal processor, the receiver, the battery and the controls, as shown in general in Figure 3.1 and as in a conventional behind-the-ear (BTE) aid in Figure 3.2.

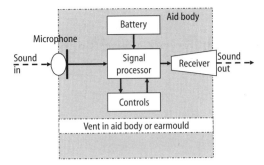

Figure 3.1 A general hearing-aid schematic.

The microphone converts incident sound into the sympathetic variation of an electrical signal. The signal processor modifies the electrical signal in some way to attempt to compensate for the wearer's hearing deficiency, *e.g.* by amplifying the sound frequencies at which the wearer has low sensitivity. The receiver converts the processed signal back to sound (loudspeaker action), or in some cases to synthetic nerve signals or mechanical vibration. The battery provides power to all of these units. The controls allow the dispenser and/or the user to adjust the aid either at time of fitting or in daily use. The vent provides a narrow passage for air to avoid complete blockage of the ear. In addition to its ventilation function it reduces the audible effect (occlusion effect) noticeable on the wearers own voice, and modifies the low-frequency response of the aid.

A useful hearing aid must reduce the perceptual deficit caused by the individual's hearing loss, and an aid's performance with speech signals is of particular interest because of their importance for communication. The aim of hearing-aid research into the development and incorporation of new technology and new signal-processing schemes (algorithms) is to maximise the aid's supportive interaction and minimise its interference with the individual's residual hearing.

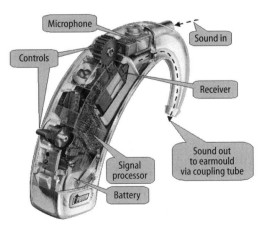

Figure 3.2 BTE hearing-aid schematic (image courtesy of Phonak).

3.2.1 Review of Technical Terms

The amplification or "gain" of a signal processor is the ratio of the change in output signal magnitude to the respective change in the input signal magnitude. Gain may be different at:

- different frequencies, *e.g.* boosting signals at certain frequencies (filter action);
- different signal amplitudes, *e.g.* amplifying large-amplitude signals less than small-amplitude ones (compressor action).

The phase relationship between two signals is a way of representing their relative time relationship as a function of frequency. The transfer function describes the variation with frequency of both gain and phase, imposed by a system on signals passing through it.

The ratio of "desired signal" power to "undesired signal" power is referred to as the signal-to-noise ratio (SNR). Although systems with low SNRs are likely to damage intelligibility, SNR should be used solely as an *engineering* measure of the "goodness" of a hearing-aid system, since it has no intrinsic relationship to the intelligibility of the signal. Gain, transfer function modulus, and SNR are commonly expressed using the logarithmic units of decibels (dB).

The amplitude of signal received at the microphone will vary from moment to moment. Often, parts of a signal-processing system are required to respond, not to instantaneous signal values, but to the trend in amplitude changes, and some form of averaging scheme is employed. A commonly used measure is the square root of the average of the squared signal, known as the root-mean-square (RMS) value.

3.2.2 Human Hearing Viewed from an Engineering Perspective

Human hearing covers a range of frequencies from about 20 Hz to 20 kHz and can respond to an enormous range of sound levels, within which lies those generated by conversational speech; Figure 3.3 shows a rough guide to the separation in frequency and level between vowel sounds and consonants.

The lowest sound pressure level (SPL) that humans can hear varies with frequency and is called the hearing threshold, with the greatest sensitivity normally in the range 1 to 4 kHz (Figure 3.3). An SPL of 0 dB is defined as the minimum audible sound level of a 1 kHz tone and has been standardised at a value of 20 µPa. The highest sound level that humans can tolerate with discomfort is around 120 dB SPL, *i.e.* 10^{12} times the minimum detectable. Hearing level (HL) in decibels is measured relative to the standardised "normal" hearing threshold at each of the measurement frequencies (Ballantyne, 1990). Of course, the hearing threshold of any individual or group is likely to deviate from this standard; *e.g.* the average of 18 "normal" ears is shown in Figure 3.4, but things are still classed as "normal" if the deviation is within a range of about −10 dB to +20 dB about 0 dB HL.

An example of a raised threshold due to sensorineural impairment is shown in Figure 3.5, relative to the "normal" threshold and the average SPL range of conversational speech.

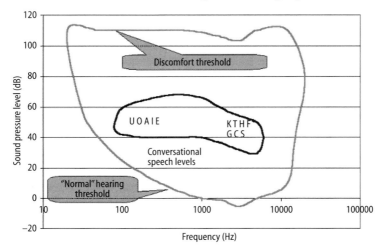

Figure 3.3 Human hearing and speech data.

The ratio of uncomfortable loudness level (UCL) to the hearing threshold is known as the dynamic range, which varies with frequency and is normally expressed in decibels. This defines the maximum range in which auditory cues can safely be delivered to a listener. It can be seen that the dynamic range is being severely compromised, particularly at high frequencies, and that much of the high-frequency content of speech, which is a particularly important contributor to intelligibility, will be below threshold even under ideal listening conditions. When background noise is present, *e.g.* the automobile cabin noise level shown in Figure 3.6, the frequency range that is above threshold contains signals that are at low or negative SNRs that damage intelligibility.

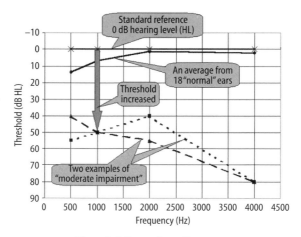

Figure 3.4 Example audiograms.

Hearing-aid Principles and Technology

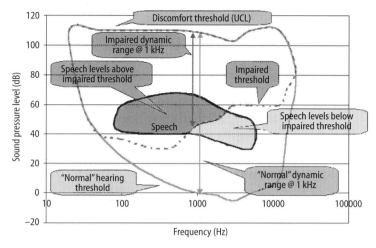

Figure 3.5 Effect of impaired threshold.

The processing functions from the outer ear to the auditory nerve leaving the cochlea (Figure 3.7) are accepted (in engineering terms) as being transduction, filtering, amplification, non-linear compression, impedance matching and spectral analysis (Figure 3.8).

Sound pressure waves are transformed into electrochemical nerve signals in each cochlea and these are then processed by the auditory brain stem and the higher functions in the auditory cortex of the brain.

The external ear (pinna) and the ear canal act as a guide, directing sound waves that vibrate the eardrum. The acoustic transfer functions formed by the shape, size and position of the head and pinna also provide information on the relative direction of the sound source. The roughly horn-shaped pinna and ear canal create an acoustic transfer function that is directionally sensitive and

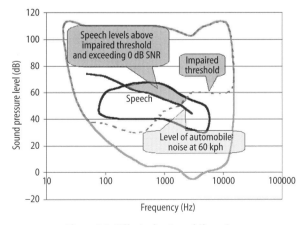

Figure 3.6 Effect of automobile noise.

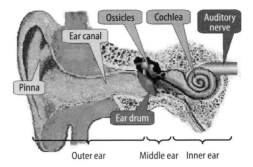

Figure 3.7 Sectional view of the ear.

also amplifies sound at certain frequencies, *e.g.* 10 to 20 dB gain around 2.5 kHz.

The vibration of the eardrum is transferred through the chain of small bones (ossicles) in the middle ear. These, in turn, vibrate the oval window of the cochlea. This impedance-matching chain of transmission acts to reduce power loss as the airborne vibrations are transferred to the fluid medium in the cochlea. Excessive movement of the ossicles is constrained by a neuromuscular feedback mechanism that acts to prevent damage due to loud sounds. Vibration of the oval window produces pressure waves in the cochlear fluid; these stimulate the cochlear structures that perform a spectral analysis. Sensor "hair" cells within the cochlea cause neurons connected to the auditory nerve to "fire" and transmit timing, amplitude and frequency information to the auditory brain stem, where a hierarchy of neural processing commences. Within this hierarchy, current interpretations of experimental evidence identify the separation of: left from right ear signals, low- from high-frequency signals, timing from intensity information; and their reintegration at various processing centres and levels.

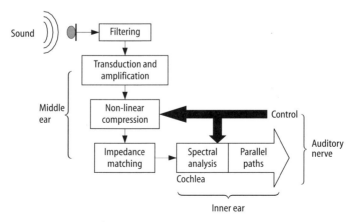

Figure 3.8 The auditory periphery.

Hearing-aid Principles and Technology

This chain of communication may be disrupted at various places and interfere with hearing to a greater or lesser degree. Two main hearing deficits were previously considered appropriate for treatment by a hearing aid: conductive loss due to problems in the outer or middle ear, and sensorineural impairment resulting from damage to the cochlea. Owing to advances in surgical instruments and techniques for tackling conductive loss, sensorineural impairment is now the more important for consideration here.

Sensorineural hearing loss appears to exhibit two main features that hearing-aid designers attempt to address:

1. Loudness recruitment, *i.e.* the reduction of dynamic range between the raised threshold of hearing and the often normal UCL. This results both in a loss of sensitivity to soft sounds and the apparent rapid growth of loudness with increase of stimulus intensity.
2. Reduced frequency and temporal resolution due to spectral gaps or widened auditory filters producing a "smearing" of audio information into adjacent frequency bands.

These factors can affect amplitude, time and frequency resolution, resulting in a reduced ability to hear clearly. Even when sufficient amplitude is available to be *detected*, the sound may not be *intelligible* due to the degraded resolution. This is particularly disturbing when listening to speech in the presence of background noise, especially competing speech (cocktail party problem), and in noticeably reverberant environments. During periods of low SNR, a person with normal binaural hearing can compensate to a much greater degree than those with sensorineural hearing loss, who appear to experience a "blurred" acoustic signal making conversations in noisy environments difficult.

3.2.3 Hearing-aid Prescription (in Brief)

The audiometric data traditionally used to prescribe an aid are hearing threshold (HT), most comfortable loudness level (MCL) and UCL. The latter places a limit on the maximum output SPL of the aid; however, in practice, the upper limit of hearing-aid output is usually selected between the UCL and the MCL. The former is used to set an appropriate level of gain and compression taking account of the available dynamic range in each frequency band in which adjustment is available. This direct approach is a classical equalisation method, where the aid is viewed simplistically as a device for compensating dips in the user's auditory transfer function. An unsophisticated example of compensation by a wide-band gain of +30 dB is shown in Figures 3.9 and 3.10 applied to the illustrations of Figures 3.5 and 3.6.

The amplified speech is now above the illustrated threshold; but, because the gain was applied across the whole frequency range of speech, the louder speech sounds may be pushed above the MCL. As shown in Figure 3.10, the background automobile noise of is now amplified to levels that would be, at least, extremely fatiguing, and the SNR has not been improved. The application of different gains in two bands (see Figure 3.11: +10 dB below 1 kHz, and +30 dB above 1 kHz) avoids pushing the higher amplitude low-frequency speech sounds above the MCL.

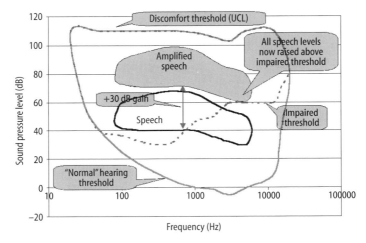

Figure 3.9 Effect of wide-band +30 dB gain.

In altering the relative level of the high- and low-frequency speech sounds the variation of speech amplitude with time (temporal modulation) will be changed, which may adversely affect intelligibility. In fitting an aid, the audiologist is seeking to balance these and other factors, *e.g.* the so-called "upward spread of masking" (Moore, 1995).

An alternative approach is to allow the user to compare several aids under controlled test conditions. This is both time consuming (in setting up and evaluating each aid) and it may not be appropriate for candidates who have difficulty in reporting consistently, *e.g.* young children.

Prescriptive methods apply the audiometric data within a formula, of which there are several, to estimate the required gain at various frequencies. The aim is to supply a gain profile that will deliver conversational speech at the MCL.

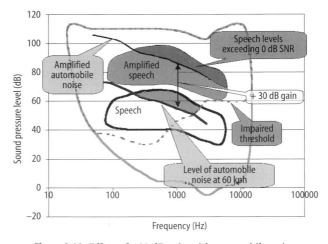

Figure 3.10 Effect of +30 dB gain with automobile noise.

Hearing-aid Principles and Technology

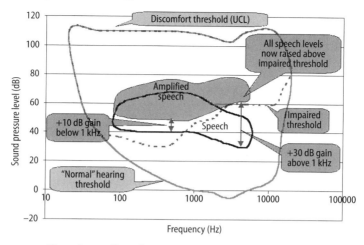

Figure 3.11 Effect of gain applied in two frequency bands.

For example the NAL(R) scheme (Byrne and Dillon, 1986) calculates a compensating gain at a set of frequencies f, based on the formula

$$G(f) = 0.31\text{HT}(f) + 0.05[\text{HT}(500) + \text{HT}(1000) + \text{HT}(2000)] + C(f)$$

where HT(f) is the measured hearing threshold at frequency f, and $C(f)$ (dB) is tabulated against f (Hz) in Table 3.1.

However, there are many other important considerations to be addressed, and the reader is directed to other texts for these (*e.g.* Ballantyne, 1990; Martin, 1997; Sandlin, 2000).

A major factor in the success of delivering benefit to a hearing-aid user is the relevance of the performance data of the aid, the audiometric data from the user, and the fitting procedure. In particular:

1. The laboratory tests used to characterise the performance of an aid may not accurately reflect the aid's performance when in daily use.
2. Audiometric measurements made on the ear without the aid in place are not guaranteed to be relevant once the aid is inserted.
3. The human auditory system has been shown to adapt to the presence of an aid over a period of several weeks.

In addition to these concerns, modern digital aids offer many possible fitting adjustments to take advantage of their multiple frequency bands and choice of compression scheme within each band group. Such aids are not necessarily best adjusted using the prescriptive methods that have regularised the fitting process for conventional aids (Kuk and Ludvigsen, 1999). The manufacturer Widex has developed an aid *in situ* fitting procedure that combines the hearing test and the aid fitting. This addresses parts of items 1 and 2 above: not

Table 3.1 NAL prescription offsets.

f (Hz)	250	500	750	1000	1500	2000	3000	4000	6000
$C(f)$ (dB)	−17	−8	−3	1	1	−1	−2	−2	−2

only are the obvious adjustments of gains and compression features made, but also the adjustment of the response of the automatic feedback cancellation scheme. Ideally, an aid would include a self-calibration feature that could be initiated by the user; however, as yet this is not possible.

3.3 Categories of Electronic Aids

Hearing aids have historically been categorised by their fitting position on or in the wearer's body, and commonly used terms are: body worn (BW), behind the ear (BTE), in the ear (ITE), in the canal (ITC), completely in the canal (CIC), spectacles, middle-ear implant and cochlear implant. Since there is intimate contact at some point between the wearer's ear and the aid, all these devices require some part to be specifically tailored to fit an individual. This implies either a custom earmould connected to the processor, or a custom moulded casing for in-ear devices.

A categorisation that has recently arisen is the distinction between conventional analogue and digital signal processing (DSP) hearing aids. The majority of commercial hearing aids in use today are still analogue electronic devices. In these, the continuous time signals from the microphone are processed as a continuum (Figure 3.12) with no discretisation in time or quantisation of amplitude, much as signals are in a public address system.

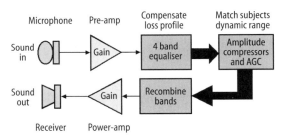

Figure 3.12 A typical analogue hearing-aid system.

In a fully digital hearing aid (Figure 3.13) the continuous time signals from the microphone are filtered to reject frequencies outside of the required range,

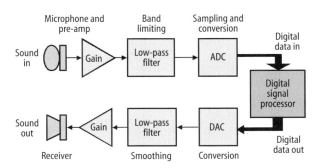

Figure 3.13 A typical DSP hearing-aid system.

Table 3.2 Summary of aid features (typical).

Aid type	Frequency range	Maximum gain (dB)	Maximum output (dB)	Battery life (h)	Telecoil
CIC	4 to 5 octaves starting in the region 100 to 500 Hz	45 ± 10	100	100	No
ITE		45 ± 10	100	100	Few
BTE		65 ± 10	130	200–500	Most
BW		85 ± 10	140	1800	Most

sampled (*i.e.* discretised in time) and converted (*i.e.* quantised in amplitude), then processed as a stream of digital (binary) numbers.

This digitally processed data is returned to a continuous time signal by the combination of a digital-to-analogue converter and a smoothing filter. Table 3.2 summarises the typical features of the most common aid types, and these apply to both analogue and digital instruments.

3.3.1 Body-worn Aid

BW aids place the receiver (loudspeaker) in an earmould, and in some cases the microphone, at the users ear. These are connected, usually by fine wires, to the other components contained in a small box worn on the body. Until substantial miniaturisation of the electronic components and batteries was achieved, this was the standard type of aid supplied. Nowadays, it tends to be supplied only to people having trouble using the more commonly prescribed aids, or for cases where a very high gain (*e.g.* 60 to 95 dB) is required and physical separation of the microphone and the receiver is beneficial to avoid acoustic feedback. It has practical advantages, in that the controls for gain and mode of operation can be conveniently sized and located, and that a larger battery can be accommodated, giving a long operating life of around 1800 h.

3.3.2 Behind-the-ear Aid

Since the early 1970s this has been the most commonly prescribed aid. The microphone, receiver, electronics and battery are contained in a plastic casing (Figures 3.14 to 3.17) that is designed to sit, partially hidden, above and behind the ear, hanging on the pinna by a detachable flexible plastic tube that channels sound from the receiver to the earmould fitted into the external part of the ear canal.

This location allows the user to alter the gain and switch modes (MTO switch) to select either microphone operation (M), telecoil operation (T) for use with a telephone or induction loop broadcast system (some aids provide an MT combination setting), or off (O) to save battery energy. A removable panel usually provides access to the pre-set controls (trimmers) for fitting adjustment, or in newer aids a small hatch allows a cable connection to a computer for the same purpose. Since the earmould is the only tailor-made item, the aid body can be manufactured as a standard part and be easily replaced if damaged. Typically, the gain provided is <70 dB with a battery life <500 h.

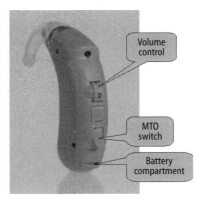

Figure 3.14 BTE aid showing user controls (image courtesy of Siemens).

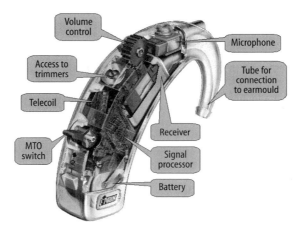

Figure 3.15 A BTE hearing aid (image courtesy of Phonak).

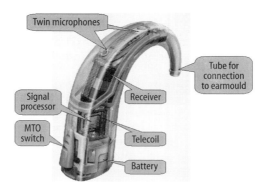

Figure 3.16 A digital directional BTE hearing aid (image courtesy of Phonak).

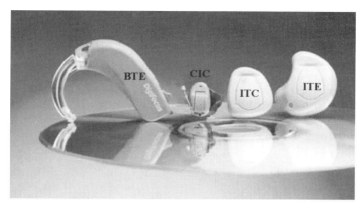

Figure 3.17 Comparative size of aids (image courtesy of Oticon).

3.3.3 Spectacles Aid

This is essentially a variant of the BTE aid in which the device is built into one leg of a pair of spectacles linked to an earmould by a plastic tube. The freedom to increase separation of the microphone from the earmould allows greater amplification before feedback becomes a problem, *e.g.* gains of >60 dB.

In addition, for subjects with a severe unilateral hearing loss, contralateral routing of signals (CROS) operation can be conveniently supported by a spectacles-aid system. The one-sided nature of their hearing loss is exacerbated by the acoustic shadow cast by their head towards the "good" ear. This shadow is frequency dependent and particularly affects the higher speech frequencies that are important contributors to intelligibility. This effect can be ameliorated by a CROS system in which a microphone is positioned on the spectacle frame at the severely affected ear with its signal connected, by fine wires hidden in the frame, to an aid supplying the contralateral ear. Pollack (1975) features an extended discussion of CROS.

3.3.4 In-the-ear Aid

This configuration incorporates all the aid components into a custom-made casing that is located ITE, partially ITC, or CIC (Chasin, 1997). Each of these styles is necessarily smaller than the foregoing one (Figure 3.17), and thus proides cosmetic benefit at the cost of smaller components and controls. The dif - ficulty of adjusting small controls (Figure 3.18) can be overcome by employing wireless remote control systems or automatic volume control (AVC; Figure 3.19). The very close proximity of the microphone and receiver also requires careful system design to avoid feedback.

Whereas ITE aids may provide telecoil operation, ITC and CIC aids normally do not, since their location in the ear canal allows near-normal use of a telephone handset. Locating the CIC aid well within the shelter of the ear canal provides some protection from wind noise, and benefit is claimed in terms of a

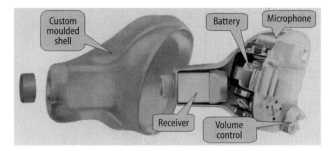

Figure 3.18 ITE aid construction (image courtesy of Siemens).

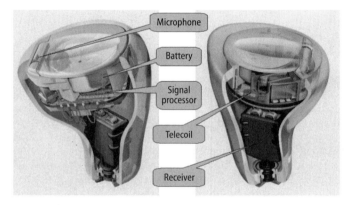

Figure 3.19 An AVC ITE aid (image courtesy of Phonak).

more natural sound quality and directional judgement. The custom-made casing requires a deep canal impression mould. The small size causes difficulties with battery replacement, and being located inside the ear canal these devices require a tether (and a steady hand) to remove and insert the aid. Compared with the BTE aid, the CIC aid's smaller battery size (and thus smaller stored energy) restricts the achievable amplification (since high gain implies higher battery drain and thus shorter usage time). However, CIC and ITC aids benefit from their deeper location in the ear canal, since the smaller enclosed air volume allows a lower gain aid to generate higher SPLs. Typically, the gain provided is <50 dB with a battery life <100 h.

3.3.5 Bone-conduction Aid

The bone-conduction aid has been especially useful for subjects with conductive hearing loss or gross occlusion of the ear canal where surgical intervention is judged inappropriate. In essence, the aid is different only at the receiver that delivers vibration to the skull, effectively bypassing the middle ear to affect the cochlea directly. The other components may be placed in a BW, spectacles or a BTE package.

3.3.6 Middle-ear Implant Aid

This type of prosthesis can be considered a recent variant of the bone-conduction aid. Instead of clamping or screwing a vibration transducer to the skull, a surgical operation locates the transducer such that it can act directly on an ossicle. Both magnetic and piezoelectric transducers are being investigated. Hüttenbrink (1999) provides a useful review.

The system developed by Symphonix requires the attachment of a small magnetic vibrator, consisting of an electromagnet coil and a permanent magnet, to an ossicle using a titanium clip or an adhesive. The electromagnet is connected by fine wires to a radio receiver implanted under the subject's skin, usually just above the external ear and powered by a rechargeable battery. An external processor, magnetically secured over the implant site, contains the microphone and electronics to transmit a radio signal to the receiver.

A slightly less invasive version places a driving coil, microphone and amplification electronics in the ear canal as with a CIC aid. However, the larger separation of the coil and the magnet limit the efficiency of this approach.

An even less invasive approach, the ear lens (Goode, 1989), involves placing a thin magnetic disk on a film of oil sprayed on the eardrum. The disk, held by surface tension to the eardrum, is set into motion using an amplifier/coil inserted in the ear canal. Obviously, this requires a functional eardrum and ossicles.

A piezoelectric system developed by Implex (Leysieffer *et al.*, 1997) uses a piezoceramic transducer that changes its dimensions in response to an applied electric field, in the same manner as the vibrating crystals used in "quartz" watches. This transducer is implanted in the mastoid cavity and connected to an ossicle by a titanium driving-rod. A microphone implanted under the skin of the ear canal is connected to the implanted receiver. A particular advantage of this approach is the low power consumption compared with magnetic systems.

3.3.7 Cochlear Implant Aid

The cochlear implant (Loizou 1998) requires a tiny flexible linear electrode array to be surgically implanted inside the spiral chamber of the cochlea (Figure 3.20).

The array of (at present) less than 30 electrodes is connected to an implanted receiver as for the middle-ear implant devices discussed above. The distribution of the electrode array is an application of the "place theory", which describes the operation of the cochlea as a spectrum analyser that converts detected frequency into position along the basilar membrane. In addition to inserting the device, the surgeon manipulates its position within the cochlea to ensure that the electrodes are brought suitably close to the auditory neurons it is intended to stimulate, and checks that sufficient functioning neurons are stimulated.

In use, a BTE or BW processing unit picks up and processes the acoustic signal; this is then transformed by one of several possible algorithms into a pattern of pulses suitable for directly stimulating the auditory neurons. The

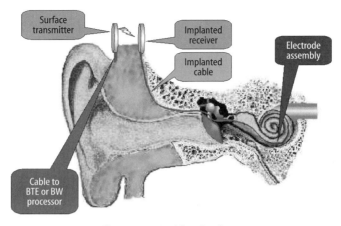

Figure 3.20 Cochlear implant.

signal is transmitted to the implanted receiver, which relays it to the cochlear array, where the temporally and spatially distributed pattern of electrical pulses directly stimulates auditory neurons. For example, the SPEAK algorithm (Seligman and McDermott, 1995) selects the six to ten loudest frequency components and routes the pulse train representing the highest frequency component to the electrode stimulating the high-frequency area of the cochlea, and so on down to the lowest frequency component.

In practice, significantly fewer stimulation channels than the number of electrodes are usually achieved. And since the number of electrodes is orders of magnitude less than the number of neurons, the wearer can only experience a much less rich auditory experience than "normal" listeners. However, the devices have been successful in providing profoundly deaf individuals with useful acoustic information.

3.3.8 Auditory Brain-stem Implant Aid

Development work is under way to provide a solution for persons without a functional cochlea or with a damaged auditory nerve (http://www.cochlear.com/). This is a surgically invasive hearing-aid system that completely bypasses the cochlea and directly stimulates the neurons of the cochlear nucleus located in the auditory brain stem. Mapping of the response to sound of the nerve fibres in this region has established that they appear to be physically organised by frequency. Thus, the signal-processing approaches used in cochlear implants are candidates for this device. Preliminary trials indicate that implanted subjects are able to detect sound and can demonstrate some improved lip-reading skill. This work is equivalent to, and is at roughly the same stage as, that on the eye, which is attempting to replace a damaged retina by an electronic photosensitive device with direct connection to the optic nerve (Peachey and Chow, 1999).

3.4 Historical Background

Hearing aids using electrical microphone/receiver devices appeared towards the end of the 19th century following the invention of the telephone in 1876 by Alexander Graham Bell. Based on carbon granule microphones, these aids were either static or portable but cumbersome. These devices amplified only a narrow band of frequencies, typically peaking at gains of around 40 dB at 1 kHz, and suffered from distortion and noise due to physical movement.

Electronic amplification became possible with the invention of the triode vacuum tube in 1907, and a hearing-aid design using this was patented in 1921. Developments in vacuum-tube technology allowed portable BW aids to be developed; however, although the level of undistorted amplification was satisfactory in many cases of conductive hearing loss, the cosmetic considerations, physical size and power consumption limited the attractiveness and usefulness of these devices. By the 1930s, an electrical bone-conduction device had been devised, and this approach was able to benefit from subsequent developments in electronics.

The trend to miniaturisation and reduction of power consumption was given a huge boost by the invention of the transistor at Bell Labs in 1947. BTE and spectacle-frame hearing aids using transistors appeared commercially in the early 1950s, and by the end of that decade ITE and ITC instruments were available due to improvements in battery, microphone and receiver technology. In 1964, the first BTE hearing aid using an integrated circuit became commercially available. Driven mainly by cosmetic considerations, the miniaturisation trend has continued since the 1960s to the present day, with current technology providing CIC instruments.

Over most of the period described, the signal-processing operation had been confined principally to providing amplification. Later, a degree of shaping of the frequency response was introduced in an attempt to equalise the subject's audiogram. In 1969, the first hearing aid incorporating a directional microphone became commercially available. Non-linear compression appeared in an integrated-circuit hearing aid of 1972, and in the 1980s further developments of analogue integrated-circuit electronics extended and diversified this feature.

Digital electronic hearing aids were developed in the late 1980s, but these were initially available only in the form of digitally controlled analogue processing instruments, as distinct from digital-processing instruments. These hybrids allowed features such as the amount of amplification in each frequency band to be programmed, either during the fitting procedure or, in some cases, by the wearer using a wireless remote control to select a pre-set programme "in the field".

True DSP BTE hearing aids became commercially available during the 1990s. This approach allowed the use of algorithms that would either be difficult or impossible to implement using analogue-based designs. Features such as adaptive sound cancellation (Davanox Genius, 1990), speech detection (Siemens PRISMA) and automatic gain control (AGC) (Oticon Multifocus, 1991) have been implemented, and a CIC DSP device (Widex, 1997) has been achieved.

Experiments with direct electrical stimulation of the auditory nerve in the late 1950s led to the development of systems in the mid-1970s in which an electrode array is inserted into the cochlea. This "cochlear implant" device is presently only prescribed for relatively small numbers of profoundly deaf subjects because of the invasive and expensive operation required. Apart from materials developments, the main technological contributors to improvement of this aid's performance have been developments in the DSP algorithms and the increase in the number of elements in the electrode array from less than ten to currently around the mid-20s.

A middle-ear implant is currently under development following work reported in the late 1980s. The main technological developments associated with this approach are in the magnetic or piezoelectric transducer, which imparts mechanical motion directly either to the eardrum or to one of the ossicles.

3.5 The Ear as an Environment

The ear has the potential to be harmed by contact with foreign bodies and the body has evolved mechanisms for neutralising or rejecting them. Sometimes this may involve direct reaction with part of a hearing aid, *e.g.* as an allergic reaction to a material used in the aid's construction. Sometimes the aid is just the unfortunate recipient of accumulations of materials produced in the natural self-cleaning process of the ear. Inserting the aid, or part of it, into the ear also disturbs the acoustic properties of the ear and the aid to some extent. So aid-on-body and body-on-aid effects are important to hearing-aid design.

3.5.1 Aid-on-body Considerations

In fitting a device on to or into the body a risk is assumed, and this must be minimised. It is obvious that any such aid should be designed to fail safe, so that further damage to the body is prevented. For a hearing aid, this requires a system design that will inherently limit the sound intensity that the aid can deliver and a structure and materials that are compatible with their location on or in the body and that are capable of being kept clean.

Insertion of an aid into the ear restricts the natural ventilation processes, and this, in conjunction with the heat generated by power dissipation in the device, can raise the local temperature to the point where sweating becomes a source of discomfort and irritation.

A particular case of importance to aid design is the disturbance caused by the inserted aid to the acoustical properties of the ear canal, which normally provides a significant gain at around 2.5 kHz.

Common battery compounds employ the toxic metals zinc and mercury; thus, leakage is an obvious concern. However, modern hearing-aid battery construction offers a very high degree of integrity. Part of the hearing aid may be in non-invasive surface contact with the skin, as with an earmould, whereas some forms of aid involve the implantation into, or the cementing or clipping of objects to, the cochlea, the eardrum, the ossicles, and the skull. In all cases, the materials and the fit are critical to avoiding discomfort and to reducing the likelihood of abrasion, allergic reaction, chemical reaction, toxicity and infection. Various plastics, both hard and pliable, are well characterised from this point of view, *e.g.* Lucite, a hard acrylic used for earmoulds. Metals offer a much more limited choice, with titanium and gold being medically graded. Certain implant devices utilise relatively inert piezoceramic-type materials. In addition, the materials used in implants must be considered from the point of view of their possible effect on the body due to stimulation by external energy sources. An earmould material that deforms in hot weather or that reacts with the salt in sea spray is avoidable, but an implanted electrical device in which no part reacts significantly with the intense magnetic field of a magnetic resonance imaging body scanner is a tall order; and less extreme but more common radiating sources are magnetic security systems and mobile phones.

The signal path from microphone to receiver to eardrum to ossicles to cochlea is not the only path by which acoustic energy can reach the cochlea. Subjects with a functional cochlea can hear by bone conduction, and blocking your ears with your fingers while speaking demonstrates this and the change in voice quality due to the occlusion effect. On removing your fingers as you continue to speak the character of your voice returns to normal, as the air-borne sound is allowed to reinforce the bone-conducted sound. So, aid wearers will hear their own voice both through the aid and by bone conduction.

In order to reduce the occlusion effect and to prevent discomfort caused by pressure difference build up, due to an aid blocking the ear canal, it is common to incorporate a narrow passage (vent) for air, around 1 mm diameter, which connects the inner part of the ear canal to the outside air. In addition to its ventilation function it also provides a degree of acoustic filtering, and modifies the low-frequency response of the aid. Thus, the signal paths through a well-fitted aid are the electronic one and the acoustic one through the vent (Figure 3.1).

Visual information can also be of great value to the hearing impaired. It is not necessary to reach the level of skill required for true lip reading in order to appreciate our sensitivity to, and use of, lip synchronisation information. Most people unconsciously increase their visual concentration on the desired speaker's lips as the background noise level increases, especially background speech (the "cocktail party" problem).

Last, but not least, there are duplicate signal paths through the other ear, and the combined (inter-aural) signals are important both for locating sound sources and improving detection and intelligibility under noisy conditions.

Since the electronic path performs a filtering action it must inherently introduce a frequency-dependent phase shift to the signals. Thus, the hearing aid will introduce a time delay between the electronic path and all the other paths discussed above. The effect of a time delay on our audio communications may vary from unnoticeable to devastating, *e.g.* having your own voice fed back to your ears with a time delay of a few hundred milliseconds can induce major stuttering and hesitation in your speech. If an equal time delay could be inserted in all the other signal paths, and its value was not such as to be obvious during a conversation, then time delay in the electronic path would not be such an important restriction. For example, the minimum detectable inter-aural time delay (ITD) is in the range of 10 to 40 µs. To require a monaurally fitted electronic aid to have a delay of less than 10 µs would be incompatible with the processing operations required, but binaural fitting of aids could compensate for the modified ITD otherwise introduced. This, however, is not practical for the visual path or the bone-conduction path. Thus, any time delay introduced must be kept below a value that would cause significant problems in the more sensitive of these two paths. Summerfield (1992) reported that a delay of audio relative to visual of 80 ms and above would reduce the intelligibility of speech. Stone and Moore (1999) found that "the auditory effect of delays between bone-conducted sound and aid-conducted sound are likely to become disturbing for delays exceeding 20 ms. Somewhat longer delays may be tolerable for moderate to severe hearing losses".

Thus, a hearing aid should ideally introduce a time delay of less than 20 ms; so, in implementing signal-processing schemes, low-delay structures are important, and binaural fitting should be considered to avoid upsetting ITD judgements.

3.5.2 Body-on-aid Considerations

At a superficial level, the placement of the microphone may expose it to wind noise or clothing-generated noise and so some form of physical shielding may be required. At a deeper level, the body is an aggressive environment for electronic devices. The conductive components, in particular, are prone to corrosion and must be protected by the design of the aid casing. The skin of the ear canal sweats, secretes wax, and sheds its dead cells, all of which should be transported out of the ear by normal processes. In order to function well, most conventional hearing aids require a close fit to the ear canal. However, when an aid is fitted, a major part of which obscures the ear canal, the vent and the receiver outlet may become blocked by the accumulation of debris that can then interfere with the aid's functioning. It has been reported by Oticon that "[o]ne third of all hearing instrument breakdowns are caused by problems with earwax".

Another effect on the aid of it being located on or in the ear is the restriction on achievable gain due to acoustical feedback. A conventional hearing aid can be thought of as a miniature public address system. It is a common experience that, when the gain is high, such systems can go into oscillation and "howl". This is due to a coupling path allowing acoustic energy from the speaker system to be fed back to the microphone with an amplitude and phase that sustains the oscillation at some characteristic frequency. The design of the aid has to take this into account, since the separation between the microphone and the receiver in an ear-worn aid can be very small (less than 15 mm), and the gain may be high (greater than 40 dB). In the case of a hearing aid, we can broadly classify the possible feedback paths (Hellgren *et al.*, 1999) as internal paths and external paths (Figure 3.21).

The internal paths could include electrical feedback within the processing electronics and acoustic feedback. The latter may occur either through the aid body mechanically coupling receiver-generated vibration to the microphone or through airborne acoustic transmission within the aid, a special case of which is acoustic coupling through the vent. In the semi-sealed environment of an ear with a well fitted conventional aid, a balance requires to be struck between the performance requirements of venting and gain to avoid "howl around" feedback.

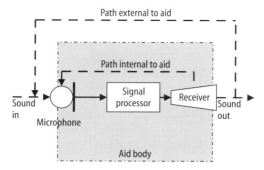

Figure 3.21 Acoustic feedback paths.

The external paths can include a leakage path around either the earmould (BTE, ITE) or the aid body (CIC) due to imperfect fitting, and in BTE instruments airborne transmission from vibration of coupling tube walls, cracks in tubing and via gaps at tubing joints. In well-designed modern aids, the care taken in materials selection and electrical design means that many of these paths only develop in instruments damaged by "wear and tear". However, not all possible feedback paths can be engineered out, or blamed on "out of specification" devices. The presence of a vent provides an unavoidable potential feedback path; and for devices being inserted and removed by the wearer on a daily basis, the fit of the earmould or aid body is likely to vary daily. In addition, items coming close to the ear, such as hat brims or a telephone handset, can create potential acoustic feedback paths.

3.6 Processing Strategies

Processing strategies are presented here as single-channel or multiple-channel methods. Some authors use channel to refer to a band of frequencies; here, though, channel will refer to a monaural signal that may, if appropriate, consist of a group of frequency sub-bands. Thus, a stereo or binaural processing system will be a two-channel system. Single-channel processing methods may, of course, be applied to the individual channels of a multiple-channel approach. Although the strategies discussed here could be implemented by analogue signal-processing techniques, the more complex ones are only practicable using DSP.

3.6.1 Single-channel Processing Schemes

Equalisation

The signal-processing function of electronic hearing aids was historically that of providing compensation for the attenuation measured by the audiologist in units of dB HL, usually by pure-tone audiometry and displayed as an audiogram; see Figure 3.4.

The logic was that if, relative to "normal", a subject exhibited, say, a 30 dB higher threshold at 1 kHz, then 30 dB of amplification at 1 kHz would enable them to detect sounds close to the "normal" threshold. In engineering terms, the audiologist performed a system identification experiment to provide transfer function information in the form of an audiogram. Engineers may view this as the magnitude part of a Bode plot of the subject's hearing threshold. The job of the hearing aid was to equalise that magnitude plot, returning it to the "normal" range.

A major shortcoming of this simplistic equalisation approach is that the identification is being performed on a human subject: a complex, non-linear, adaptive, time-varying system. The methodology adopted by the audiologist attempts to control some of these factors; however, even assuming that a simple engineering model of the system is valid, non-linearity and adaptation play important parts in its normal operation.

Most currently prescribed hearing aids allow the audiologist to set the amplification in only a few frequency bands. Even when more bands are available, simple linear amplification is not a sufficient remedy for significant sensorineural hearing loss, since loudness recruitment and decreased spectral resolution are not addressed. For example, the existence of the UCL places a ceiling on the amount of gain that can be employed. If our example subject had a UCL of 100 dB, then more than 30 dB of compensation gain would make uncomfortable a loud speech level of 70 dB, and levels above 70 dB would have to be suppressed, *i.e.* limited.

Although, in practice, fitting procedures do not usually attempt compensation solely by this crude equalisation criterion, the approach essentially views the aid as a miniaturised version of the "graphic equaliser" common in domestic music systems, in which the gains in each band have been fixed.

Amplitude Compression

The reduced dynamic range of the impaired ear may be matched to that of the "normal" ear by a non-linear compression scheme. The crudest form of this is to place an upper "hard" limit on the maximum SPL allowed, to avoid exceeding the UCL, and below this level to provide a linear gain function. However, a "hard" non-linearity can introduce significant unpleasant harmonic distortion, just as "clipping" does in an audio amplifier. By replacing the linear gain characteristic with a curvilinear or piecewise linear gain function, as shown in Figure 3.22, low sound amplitudes can be expanded and high sound amplitudes can be compressed into the impaired dynamic range.

So-called "multi-channel compression", in our terms multi-band compression, applies a separate compression function in each selected frequency band, since a subject's dynamic range often differs in different frequency bands, as seen in Figure 3.5.

Fixed compression schemes result in the aid wearer frequently adjusting the volume control in an attempt to keep the sound level in the vicinity of the MCL, so automatic schemes have been devised known as AVC, AGC and syllabic compression (SC). These dynamic schemes involve a feedback or feed-forward system that estimates the present required gain based on a measure of the

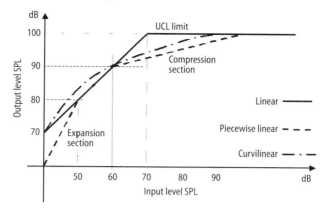

Figure 3.22 Static compression curves.

input signal magnitude. Kuk and Ludvigsen (1999) provide a useful discussion on the implications of various schemes.

The aim of AVC is to remove the necessity on the wearer to adjust the volume control manually for relatively slowly changing listening situations, such as going from a normal to a whispered conversation. This is done using a long time-scale measure of the signal magnitude. Figure 3.23 shows an oscilloscope trace of the behaviour of a compression scheme to a step change in the amplitude of an 800 Hz tone. The times associated with the gain decrease (attack time) and the gain increase (release time) do not need to be identical.

In the case of AGC and SC, a short time-scale measure of the signal magnitude is used. AGC schemes attempt to perform fast reduction of gain in response to sudden large increases in sound level, *e.g.* when someone nearby coughs, and to restore the gain quickly when the loud sound has ceased. Within a few hundred milliseconds, speech content may change from a relatively high-power low-frequency event, typically a voiced sound such as a vowel, to a wide-

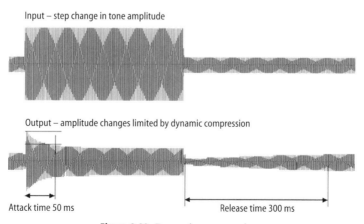

Figure 3.23 Dynamic compression.

band event that may be 10 to 20 dB lower, *e.g.* an unvoiced sound such as a consonant. SC attempts to boost the weaker speech sounds, which are very important contributors to intelligibility, but reduce the gain fast enough to prevent over amplifying the higher amplitude sounds in speech.

The difference between these gain-control schemes essentially comes down to the magnitude and the speed of gain change that is allowed. AVC typically operates in times of between 10 s and several hundred milliseconds, whereas AGC and SC typically have operation times in the range of 1 to 100 ms. Often, a short attack time is combined with a long release time to reduce the likelihood of obvious amplitude pulsations known as "pumping"; *e.g.* the Siemens PRISMA device provides for selection of all three of these compression schemes.

AGC and SC schemes have been criticised (Plomp, 1988, 1994; Drullman *et al.*, 1996) on the grounds that fast-acting wide-band compression will tend to reduce the natural temporal modulation of speech, and fast-acting multi-band compression will tend to reduce spectral contrast, both of which may be important cues for the hearing-impaired. To counter these criticisms, more complex compression schemes have been devised.

The compression functions in the most recent digital aids may be combined and distributed through the signal-processing chain, and many multi-band digital hearing aids now apply compression schemes either independently to groups of frequency bands, or dynamically link the compression functions across neighbouring bands. One example, shown in Figure 3.24, is the OTICON Digi-Focus II (Naylor, 1997). This splits its frequency range (0 to 5.5 kHz) to implement a seven-band digital equalisation of the hearing loss, then groups the three lower bands (0 to 1.5 kHz) to apply SC, using short attack and release times, to the high-energy voiced speech components. The four higher frequency bands (1.5 to 5.5 kHz) are grouped to apply AGC, using short attack and long release times, to the low-energy unvoiced components.

Another example, the Siemens SIGNIA, splits its frequency range to support an eight-band equalisation, then implements two successive AGC operations. The first groups the eight bands in pairs into four bands, each of which is

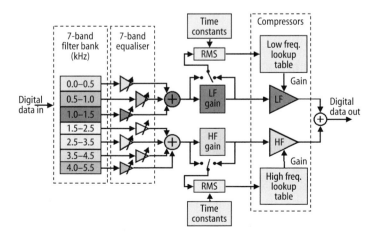

Figure 3.24 The "Digifocus" signal processor (after Naylor (1997)).

subjected to its own AGC; a subsequent four band AGC system with different characteristics from the first is then applied. An insight can be gained into the care required when comparing and assessing a variety of such systems in Stone *et al.* (1999).

The enhancement operation performed by compression schemes can be visualised as a "graphic equaliser" in which the gains in each band are time varying and derived from non-linear functions of some measure of the in-band signal magnitude (*e.g.* signal RMS) formed over a time neighbourhood.

Spectral Contrast Enhancement

Subjects with sensorineural hearing loss exhibit reduced frequency selectivity, often described in terms of broadened auditory filters, resulting in a smoothing of the peaks and valleys of the spectral envelope. In addition, background noise sets a noise floor and can be visualised as tending to raise the valley floors and thus reduce the prominence of the spectral peaks. Spectral contrast enhancement (Moore, 1995) is an equalisation scheme performed in the frequency domain by applying a time-varying local pre-emphasis to the spectral shape. Typically, a spectrum (Figure 3.25) is obtained at a point in time, either by a filter-bank or a transform method, such as the fast Fourier transform (FFT) (Denbigh, 1998).

The magnitude spectrum is then examined and modified using a function that exaggerates the difference between the peaks and valleys of the speech spectrum. The gain in each band is thus time varying and depends on the difference in spectral amplitude compared with neighbouring bands. The wideband spectrum is then reconstituted from the modified frequency bands and the corresponding contrast-enhanced time-domain signal is recovered. As with other spectral magnitude modification schemes, the basic enhancement operator may need to be limited to prevent negative, zero or overlarge spectral magnitudes being produced.

The enhancement function is an approximation to a differential operator, *e.g.* Moore obtained the magnitude spectrum using a 128-point FFT then, after some smoothing, the 128-point spectrum was convolved with a filter having a difference of Gaussians (DoG) impulse response

$$\text{DoG}(\Delta f) = G_1(\Delta f) - G_2(\Delta f)$$

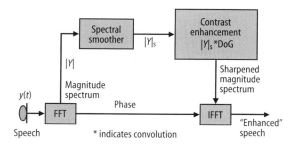

Figure 3.25 Spectral contrast enhancement.

where each Gaussian function has the form

$$G_m(\Delta f) = \frac{1}{\sqrt{2\pi}} \frac{1}{m} \exp\left[\frac{-(\Delta f/mb)^2}{2}\right]$$

and parameter b sets the bandwidth of the DoG function and Δf is the frequency shift required for the convolution operation.

This particular operator is often used in digital image enhancement because the Gaussian shape is preserved under a Fourier transform operation and the smooth shape yields filter functions with low levels of "ringing", which could appear as artefacts in the processed signal. It has also been claimed to exhibit similar characteristics to the early neural processing of human vision (Jones, 1982).

The enhancement operation can be visualised as a "graphic equaliser" in which the gains in each band are time-varying functions of some measure of the in-band signal magnitude formed over a frequency neighbourhood.

Reduction of Unwanted Signals

Whilst the single channel schemes discussed so far can raise the sound level above the threshold for detection, they act identically on desired and undesired signals. In addition, since the background noise contributes to the total signal being processed by the aid, the noise will influence any automatic amplitude compression system. Thus, the dynamic range ideally required by the desired signal may be eroded by the presence of noise, or schemes such as SC may be confused by the time variation of the noise component. The sound may be made audible, and intelligibility improvements achieved for one-to-one conversation in quiet low reverberation environments, but the SNR is not improved in everyday environments. This is a common source of complaint, and word recognition studies have shown that hearing-aid users require between 5 and 20 dB improvement in SNR, dependent on noise character, to match the scores of "normal" hearing subjects. Various attempts have been made to improve the SNR available to the impaired ear, including directional microphones, spectral subtraction and voice activity detection (VAD) schemes.

Sub-band processing is required for flexibility in the equalisation and compression processes, where each frequency band can be given the desired gain and compression; but it is also increasingly being used in conjunction with speech-detection schemes. The logic is that if a sub-band is being dominated by non-speech-like signals, then there is no point amplifying it during that period; rather, it should be de-emphasised and the overall SNR thus improved. The Siemens PRISMA instrument is one aid in which this approach is used. The inherent parallelism of the sub-band approach also allows for implementation by parallel processors.

It should be kept in mind that what is annoying noise in one situation may be the desired signal in another situation, *e.g.* when switching attention between speakers in a multi-speaker scenario, or the importance of traffic noise when sitting at a roadside café compared with crossing the road. Schemes that reject certain types of signal should ideally be under the control of the user and provide automatic reversion to a "safe-mode".

Directional Microphones

The majority of commercial hearing aids are monaural devices using an omnidirectional electret microphone. Such microphones have a suitably wide and relatively flat frequency response with a directional sensitivity that does not vary strongly with angle of incidence of sound. However, the placement of the microphone will influence the directional sensitivity of the aid, *e.g.* due to the head shadow effect.

If the desired signal comes from a single sound source then the SNR at the aid can be improved by, on average, around 3 dB (Wouters *et al.*, 1999), by employing a directional microphone to reject interfering sources lying off the axis between the desired source and the listener.

Simple directional microphones consist of an omnidirectional microphone having two ports, one leading to each side of the microphone's pressure-sensing diaphragm. The diaphragm thus responds to the pressure difference communicated through the two ports (Figure 3.26).

The port positions and path lengths to the diaphragm are arranged such that sound from the undesired directions, *e.g.* incident sound wave A in Figure 3.26, arrives at either side of the diaphragm in-phase and tends to cancel out. By varying the path properties the directivity can be modified and the effective frequency range controlled to some extent. This approach yields, among others, the so-called cardoid-type directivity pattern, and this was exploited in a Willco electronic hearing aid in 1969. The disadvantage of this approach is that the directivity pattern and frequency range are fixed during manufacture, and a less directional response may be required at some times for safety reasons.

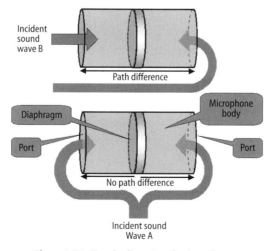

Figure 3.26 Simple directional microphone.

A more flexible way to achieve directionality uses two microphones whose outputs are combined via an electronic time-delay network. Both microphones may be omnidirectional, or one may be directional. The user can then be allowed to select the directivity pattern that best suits their acoustic environment, *e.g.* selecting an omnidirectional pattern when crossing the road, a partly directional pattern when in a group discussion, or a strongly directional pattern when conversing one-to-one in a noisy environment. Devices from Phonak and Siemens utilise such a dual-microphone system. These approaches are mainly provided in BTE configurations, since the directivity pattern would be greatly modified by an ITE fitting.

Spectral Subtraction and Sinusoidal Modelling

In spectral subtraction the magnitude spectrum of the noise is estimated during a non-speech period, the noise spectrum is then subtracted from the spectrum of the succeeding noisy speech (Vary, 1985; Virag, 1999). The estimate of the noise spectrum may be periodically updated during pauses in speech to allow some adaptation to changing background noise characteristics. The method is related to an adaptive form of Wiener filtering, and the assumptions made in this approach are:

1. the existence of an effective strategy for VAD to allow reliable estimates of the noise spectrum;
2. the estimate of the noise spectrum made during any period will be valid over the subsequent processing period, *i.e.* the noise is assumed to be quasi-stationary;
3. the noise signal is independent of the speech signal;
4. the corruption process is additive.

Under these conditions, one form of spectral subtraction based on the power spectra results in a processing system like that shown in Figure 3.27.

The success of the process is dependent on the validity of the assumptions, and especially on having reliable VAD. Spectral subtraction can be very successful if the interfering noise is principally deterministic and periodic, which

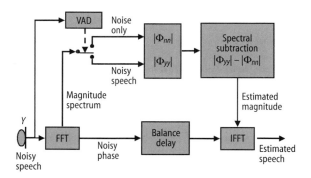

Figure 3.27 Spectral subtraction.

implies a constant spectrum; a good example is a rotary fan. However, if the noise is stochastic or statistically non-stationary, then the noise spectrum estimated during the non-speech period differs from that during the noisy speech period and the subtraction leaves a distracting residual noise that is perceived as a characteristic "burbling" sound called "musical noise". So the method can result in the replacement of one type of noise disturbance by another, and although various schemes have tried to suppress this musical noise, spectral subtraction has not yet been shown in practice to improve *intelligibility* for hearing-aid wearers. There is some evidence that it may improve *quality* for some listeners, but only at relatively high SNRs, say greater than 15 dB.

Sinusoidal modelling can be considered as a variant of spectral subtraction, in which the subtraction is continuously performed and leaves only a selected number of the highest energy tones. Typically, this is achieved by using an FFT or filter bank to analyse the signal spectrum, then sorting the frequency components by magnitude, selecting say 16 with the largest supra-threshold magnitude and passing these to any further processing units. This assumes that the major tonal components will come from the desired speech signal and that the subset will be sufficient to allow intelligible speech to be discerned. Surprisingly intelligible speech can be achieved with around 16 tones, in spite of the fact that the method must inherently degrade particularly the unvoiced components of speech, which are generally accepted as having a major impact on intelligibility. However, the presence of either competing speech or background noise with a strong periodic component will seriously compromise simple implementations of sinusoidal modelling. The SPEAK algorithm (Seligman and McDermott, 1995) used in some cochlear implant processors is an example application of this approach.

The psychoacoustics model used in MPEG audio coders is essentially a more sophisticated approach to selecting the perceptible components of an audio signal. A useful review article is that by Noll (1997).

Although, as yet, spectral subtraction methods have not been able unequivocally to justify inclusion in hearing aids, the property of changing the noise character may yet be of use. Human hearing exhibits a feature known as masking, which means, for example, that a narrow band of noise centred on a fixed frequency will tend to reduce the perceptibility of a neighbouring signal tone. The larger the frequency separation is, the less is the masking effect, which has a greater influence towards the high-frequency side of the masker, the so-called "upward spread of masking" (Moore, 1995). Thus, any processing method that modifies the characteristics of the noise is also likely to modify its masking effect, and it may be possible to exploit this.

The spectral subtraction enhancement operation can be visualised as a "graphic equaliser" in which the gains in each band are time varying and derived from some measure of the in-band noise signal magnitude formed over a time neighbourhood.

Voice Activity Detection

In general, both speech and environmental noise are intermittent signals. When noise is not present, or we have a high SNR, then amplification and compression may be sufficient for many hearing-aid wearers. When speech is not present, or there is a very low SNR, then it may be possible to obtain a "picture" of the noise signal that can be used during subsequent processing when the speech returns, as in spectral subtraction. There is some evidence that "normal" human hearing makes use of "listening in the gaps" to improve intelligibility scores.

Various approaches to detecting the presence or absence of speech in a signal have been attempted based on rather gross features of speech. The existence of harmonically related energy in the normal range of speech formant frequencies suggests a "harmonic sieve" approach to confirming the presence of voiced speech. That is, one would check for the presence of significant signal amplitude at frequencies in the range 50 to 500 Hz, note them and then search for peaks close to second and third harmonics. If a fundamental and first and second harmonics are present, and the frequencies and relative amplitudes match pre-stored voiced phonemes, then speech presence is assumed. The presence of low-amplitude high zero-crossing rate activity has also been used to signal the presence of unvoiced speech. Obviously, both of these relatively simple approaches are likely to be fooled by some types of background noise and give false detections.

Another approach is based on the characteristic amplitude modulation present in a speech signal. The modulation spectrum can be obtained by spectral analysis of the envelope of the speech signal from the output of a standard envelope detector scheme. Typical speech modulation frequencies lie in the range 1 to 8 Hz, related to the rate at which syllables are uttered, with an average across speakers peaking at about 4 Hz (Plomp, 1988). Thus, a speech activity detector can be constructed by analysing the modulation frequency profile of the current sound signal and taking the absence of a strong peak around 4 Hz as an indication that speech is not present. The Siemens PRISMA DSP hearing aid applies this approach by splitting the digitised speech signal into four frequency bands, detecting the envelope of each band, analysing it for frequency content around 4 Hz and, if below a threshold, attenuating the signal in that band.

The presence of speech-like modulation frequencies can also be used in conjunction with other methods, such as the two mentioned above, with a majority voting scheme, fuzzy logic or "expert system" making the decision on whether or not speech is assumed to be absent. The scheme, as described, would still fail with competing speech; however, a multi-channel approach could be used to confirm voice activity from a defined location by monitoring inter-channel correlation/coherence (Agaiby and Moir, 1997). Figure 3.28 illustrates the performance of such a multi-channel VAD scheme.

The top waveform is the original "clean" speech signal shown for comparison purposes. The centre waveform shows the speech signal contaminated by a spatially separated noise signal, the long-term spectrum of which has been shaped to mimic that of the speech. Although some of the speech activity is still visible, much has become submerged in the noise and is now at a low or negative SNR. The bottom waveform shows the decisions made by the VAD when presented only with the noisy speech signal. It can be seen that the VAD decisions (zero equates to speech absent) compare well with the presence or absence of speech in the top waveform.

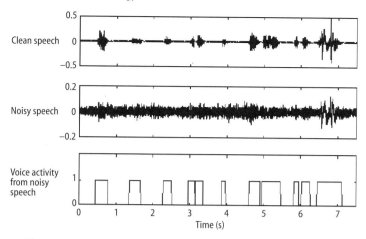

Figure 3.28 Voice activity detection (after Agaiby and Moir (1997)).

Control of Acoustic Feedback

Any amplification system may become an oscillator if a suitable feedback path (loop) exists between output and input. This occurs frequently in simple hearing aids, usually at frequencies in the range 1 to 4 kHz, and is both annoying and wasteful of battery energy. The conditions for oscillation to become established are expressed in the well-known Nyquist stability criterion (Oppenheim and Willsky, 1983). The oscillation can be suppressed by the wearer turning down the volume control to reduce the loop gain; however, this is inconvenient, it defeats the purpose of the aid, and it is uncertain, in that the presence of the hand near the aid microphone can modify the feedback path. A more embarrassing social situation is that the aid wearer may not be aware that the aid has entered an oscillation operating region and cannot actually hear the "howl".

In the case of a hearing aid, we previously classified the possible feedback paths as internal paths and external paths, as shown in Figure 3.21. The aid could be designed to ensure that the gain was low in the problematic frequency range, but this would compromise the usefulness of the aid for many users. Incorporating a fixed notch filter to reduce gain, at or around the likely oscillation frequency, is a slightly more focused version of this approach, but its success depends on the stability of the frequency of oscillation. An adaptive notch filter that tracks the oscillation frequency is a more advanced and flexible approach, and a related scheme patented in 1990 (Goodings *et al.*, 1990) was incorporated in the "Genius" aid from GN Danavox. Owing to the complexity of this on-line identification scheme, present technology requires a digital implementation. The structure of such a system is shown in Figure 3.29.

The aid processing is that necessary to compensate for the subjects hearing loss, but to the output of this processor is added a pseudo-random "probe" signal at a level ideally inaudible to the user. This known signal is injected

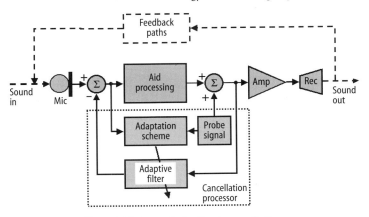

Figure 3.29 Acoustic feedback cancellation.

to allow characterisation of the feedback path transfer function from receiver to microphone. Assuming an additive process, the microphone signal thus consists of the incident external sound plus the undesired feedback with its probe component modified by the feedback path transfer function. Using the known input probe signal, a correlation operation extracts the effect of the feedback path on the probe component in the microphone signal and modifies the adaptive filter using the least-mean-square ANC scheme (Widrow and Stearns, 1985; Haykin, 1996). Use of this scheme by Danavox allowed aids to provide a gain up to 10 dB above that of previous aids and to increase the aid bandwidth, without the continual feedback "whistle" that would previously have been inevitable. The scheme did require a finite time to perform the calculations that characterised the feedback path; thus, users had to accept a few seconds of feedback "whistle" from time to time.

Frequency Transposition

The discussions so far have made an implicit assumption that the subject's cochlear function has retained useful sensitivity over all frequency ranges of interest. In some cases, the degree of damage may be so severe in some regions that amplification cannot compensate; the subject effectively has gaps in their frequency range or, in engineering terms, deep notches in their frequency response. Knowing the location of the functioning regions, information can be transposed from frequencies in the gaps, down or up the frequency range and into a region of sensitivity. This is the technique used in electronic "voice changers" and obviously results in what may be, initially at least, a strangely different sounding world. However, some degree of adaptation will take place and the benefits may outweigh this drawback for some persons.

In practice, the transposition is most flexibly accomplished by digital techniques using an FFT to provide the signal spectrum. Signal amplitudes in a "notch" region are then mapped into a sensitive region, and some form of mixing has to be performed with any coexisting spectral content.

3.6.2 Multiple-channel Processing Schemes

Multiple-microphone schemes provide multiple signal channels to the processing system, the most obvious arrangement being to mimic the two ears of human binaural hearing. Binaural hearing is most obviously connected with the ability to locate an acoustic source and has been shown superior to monaural hearing at maintaining the intelligibility of speech in the presence of reverberation and noise. Binaural hearing does not simply perform coherent addition of the signals received at the two ears. The "binaural unmasking" or binaural masking release effect (Moore, 1995) acts to lower the hearing threshold and appears to utilise the correlation properties of the signals at the two ears to de-emphasise an undesired signal.

Engineering possibilities for utilising multi-channel processing to enhance a desired signal include the following:

- Source separation through lateralisation, *e.g.* by correlation (Bodden and Blauert, 1992), and characterisation, supporting construction of a map of the auditory scene. Although this appears a possible engineering operation to perform, there is evidence that human hearing utilises this approach for map formation as distinct from signal enhancement (Culling and Summerfield, 1995).
- Coherent addition using a microphone array (Hoffman *et al.*, 1994).
- ANC (Widrow and Stearns, 1985).

At present these schemes are the subject of research activity and are not available in commercial hearing aids.

Microphone Array Systems

The formation of a directional instrument using two microphones, as previously discussed, is a special case of a microphone array. Linear arrays of microphones with their outputs combined via a progressive delay network can provide a more directional response than simple cardoid microphones. Experiments with microphone arrays mounted on spectacle frames, either along the leg "end-fire" arrays or above the lens "broadside" arrays (Soede *et al.*, 1993a), have reported improvements in speech reception threshold (SRT) of 7 dB average, relative to a single omnidirectional microphone (Soede *et al.*, 1993b). In binaural listening experiments, the classic equally spaced transducer fixed linear arrays have achieved 2 to 4 dB improvements in SRT over cardoid microphones (Desloge *et al.*, 1997). One disadvantage of such arrays is their size, which requires that they be mounted on a structure such as a spectacle frame; this may be cosmetically unacceptable for many people. Another disadvantage is that the directivity pattern varies with frequency and requires more complex processing than a delay-sum beamformer approach if side-lobe interference is to be minimised.

A further refinement and increase in complexity comes with adaptive array systems. In these an adaptation scheme is incorporated to detect automatically an interfering (jammer) signal and attempt to modify the directivity pattern to reduce its influence relative to the desired (target) signal. This presupposes that the target or jammer directions are known *a priori* or can be determined, *e.g.* by the VAD scheme discussed previously. Schemes that have been investigated for hearing-aid application mainly use two microphones and generally assume that the target will be at 0° azimuth.

Kollmeier *et al.* (1993) reported a binaural frequency-domain processing technique related to spectral subtraction and beamforming approaches. Frequency bands are selected with phase and amplitude corresponding to a desired target direction, and can be modified to suppress reverberation. However, the subjective assessment by hearing-impaired listeners did not demonstrate an unequivocal improvement in speech intelligibility in reverberant surroundings. As with related spectral subtraction methods, audible artefacts of the processing can become distracting.

Adaptive Noise Cancellation

ANC (Haykin, 1996) is capable of estimating a channel transfer function or separating signals on the basis of their correlation. In Figure 3.30, the signals S1 and S2 are assumed to have some correlated components, *e.g.* both contain the same speech signal but statistically independent additive noise contamination.

The adaptive scheme in the ANC structure automatically adjusts the filter coefficients in such a way as to reduce the RMS error between S2 and the filtered version of S1. This it can only do if the filter is driven to extract from S1 the components that are correlated to components of S2. In the case described here, this will extract (enhance) the speech signal, assuming that the filter has enough coefficients to model the relationship between the correlated components. The ANC scheme has structural similarities to the equalisation and cancellation model (Durlach, 1972; Durlach *et al.*, 1986) proposed to explain binaural unmasking.

An engineering implementation of ANC offers the possibility of performing "binaural unmasking" outside the body, providing signals of improved SNR to a hearing-aid system. One such approach combines multi-microphone methods with intermittent adaptive processing and diversity of processing within sub-bands (Toner and Campbell, 1993). It allows noise features within sub-bands during a detected "noise only" period to influence the subsequent

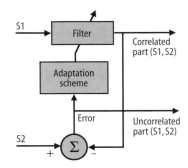

Figure 3.30 ANC as correlation separator.

Hearing-aid Principles and Technology

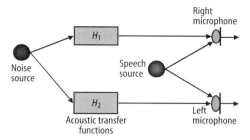

Figure 3.31 Two-sensor acoustic model.

processing during the "noisy speech" period. A signal model is shown in Figure 3.31, and assumes the desired speaker is close to the listener for simplicity.

Two microphones at average human ear separation are used in a sub-band ANC scheme (Figure 3.32) involving the identification of a differential acoustic path transfer function, involving H_1 and H_2, during a "noise only" period in intermittent speech.

A noise power and correlation/coherence estimate can be made by a sub-band processor (SBP) during the "noise only" period allowing subsequent processing decisions based on the relationship in a sub-band between noise power and a chosen noise power threshold, or inter-channel noise correlation/coherence and a chosen threshold. Three suggested tests and decisions are:

- If the noise power or noise-to-signal ratio is less than a predetermined threshold in a sub-band, then set that sub-band transfer function to unity until the noise exceeds some threshold.
- Else, if the inter-channel noise correlation is less than a noise correlation threshold, then perform the adaptive cancellation approach of Ferrara and Widrow (1981).

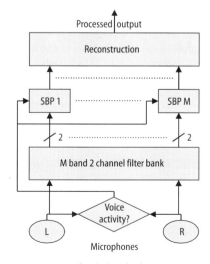

Figure 3.32 Binaural sub-band adaptive processing.

- Else, perform standard ANC in sub-bands during the "noise only" period, freeze the adaptation when speech is detected, and process the noisy speech with the frozen filter.

Assuming reliable operation of the speech/noise detector and an appropriate choice of threshold, then the first option, which is similar to that used in the Siemens PRISMA instrument, will obviously improve the overall SNR; so, research effort has concentrated on examining the latter two options (Shields and Campbell, 1998).

Close spacing of the microphones reduces the required order (complexity) of the adaptive filter (and thus the sub-band computational load) both for adaptive and intermittent fixed processing. Sub-band operation has other advantages, including faster adaptation through the freedom to use different adaptive step-sizes, and make separate decision on the appropriate form of processing in each band (Mahalanobis *et al.*, 1993). The scheme is dependent on a reliable VAD, otherwise it will attempt to cancel the speech rather than the noise, and requires that the acoustic transfer functions H_1 and H_2 are not identical.

3.7 Modern Hearing-aid Technology

3.7.1 Analogue Hearing Aids

The technology is essentially that contained in the signal-processing units of a personal cassette recorder, namely a microphone, preamplifier, automatic recording-level control or AVC, amplitude compression to accommodate the limited dynamic range (of the audio tape), tone controls or "graphic equaliser", power amplification and earphones. Using the available manufacturing technology to miniaturise these functions, mainly to satisfy the cosmetic pressure for low visibility hearing aids, necessarily limits the complexity of the instruments. The balancing act required to provide all these basic necessary functions means that compensation can only be provided over a few (typically, one to four) relatively wide frequency bands, and the number of selectable processing schemes, or "comfort programmes" is very limited.

In addition, issues of internal self-generated electrical noise levels, current consumption, the size of battery and user controls all placed severe limitations on any further development. Given that present-day analogue technology is not capable of addressing user dissatisfaction with the performance of hearing aids, a technology shift was required. Thus, signal processing by digital electronics was introduced, and this is now generally accepted as the likely way forward. For this reason, analogue electronic hearing aids are not considered further; the analogue electronics of the personal cassette recorder are giving way to the digital electronics of the personal "Mini-disc" recorder.

3.7.2 Digital Hearing Aids

Modern digital hearing aids are technically advanced instruments that have to perform their function of compensating for a hearing loss under extraordinarily restrictive conditions, while attempting to satisfy contradictory requirements. They must:

- be lightweight and portable, small enough to be situated in or on the ear, but allow the user to control selected features;
- have very low power consumption, giving reasonable battery life, but provide high gain;
- perform sophisticated real-time signal-processing algorithms, but keep processing delay to low levels.

In theory, the precision of DSP systems is limited only by the analogue-to-digital conversion (ADC) process at input and the digital-to-analogue conversion (DAC) at the output. In practice, sampling rate and digital word length restrictions (number of bits) modify this. However, the increasing operating speed and word length of modern digital logic is allowing many more areas of application. Digital systems are inherently less susceptible than analogue systems to electrical noise (pick-up) or component tolerance variations. Adjustments for electrical drift and component ageing are essentially removed, which is important for complex or difficult to access systems. Practicably inappropriate components, like physically large capacitors or inductors, can be avoided. Modern digital aids can provide filter banks with five times as many frequency bands as analogue devices (if desired), provide steep filter transition bands, and incorporate linear phase-shift characteristics that support simple sub-band to wide-band signal reconstruction. Programmability allows upgrading and expansion of the processing operations, without necessarily incurring large-scale hardware changes, and practical systems with desirable time-varying and/or adaptive characteristics can be constructed.

Technology has reached the stage where small hearing aids incorporating custom DSP devices are able to sample sound at high frequencies, process the data digitally at high throughput rates, provide gain values equal to or better than conventional analogue aids, and aim to achieve high fidelity. A typical modern DSP hearing aid digitises the acoustic signal to a resolution of 16 bits or greater at a sampling frequency of 16 kHz or greater, employs a core processor performing over 150 million instructions per second (MIPS), incorporates a speech detection scheme or twin microphones to reduce the amount of background noise received, AVC, an amplitude compression and equalisation scheme, and automatic anti-whistle feedback suppression. Such devices often initially digitise the input signal using a high sampling rate single-bit ADC for implementation efficiency and noise shaping. A high data rate, single-bit output stage (Class D) reduces the complexity and power consumption associated with the DAC process when combined with appropriate design of the receiver unit to attenuate the unwelcome harmonics of the bit stream.

Products using such technology are available from all the major hearing-aid manufacturers in a variety of fitting types, and the reader is encouraged to access their Web sites for the most up-to-date technical specifications. Some of these products are almost completely automatic, whereas others have selectable settings dependent on the acoustic environment and offer remote controls for adjustment. A summary of the features of such aids is available on the RNID Web site, and Engebretson (1994) provides a useful review of the likely benefits of digital hearing aids. At present, the cost of digital hearing aids is the main deterrent to their greater market penetration. The pitfalls for the potential wearer in using the technical specifications of devices as a guide to likely benefit are well summarised by Andersen et al. (1999).

The major drive in the development of DSP microprocessors has been to increase processing power. Comparing two BW speech-processing units developed a decade apart highlights the improvements. Engebretson et al. (1986) used the Fujitsu MB8764 DSP processor, operating at a clock frequency of 5 MHz. A unit reported by Raas and Steeger (1996) used a Motorola DSP56002 processor running at 40 MHz. Taking into account the increase in architecture efficiency through utilisation of on-chip memory, wider data word length, extended Harvard architecture, cache, hardware multipliers and pipelining, the number of MIPS also increased and the true performance increment was around 100:1. In confirmation that the trend continues, the recently announced TMS320C64x DSP processor core uses a 1.1 GHz clock delivering 8800 MIPS.

Raw speed is not the only requirement for a hearing aid DSP device, and although integration and fabrication technology have reduced both the size and number of components, a major factor dictating overall unit size is the battery, e.g. see Figure 3.19.

Modern battery chemistries have increased their energy densities significantly; but this does not necessarily mean that the battery size will be reduced, since longer battery life is also an important area for improvement. DSP cores can now operate at 2.5 V, and incorporate power-saving features such as "sleep modes" for selected units, but the potential reduction in power consumption has been offset to an extent by the trend of increasing processor clock frequency to provide more computational power. However, the development pressure surrounding portable computing and communication devices is resulting in processors operating from even lower voltage supplies. For example, TI has announced an 800 MIPS DSP core requiring a 1 V power supply and consuming 0.05 mW/MIPS.

3.7.3 Portable Speech Processors

Present-day commercial digital hearing aids allow a greater degree of flexibility than analogue systems; however, this flexibility is provided within an essentially fixed processing strategy. They are not in any substantial sense reprogrammable, so they cannot benefit from progressive improvements that may be made in signal-processing algorithms. Reprogrammability is a feature that is particularly useful when the effectiveness of a processing scheme is being experimentally assessed.

In an attempt to provide an ear-worn device with some reprogrammability, Oticon developed the JUMP-1 device (Naylor and Elberling, 1997) and offered it to approved academic researchers. This completely digital BTE instrument featured the technology used in the DigiFocus aid, and support software was provided to allow reprogramming. The device was a laudable attempt to allow realistic assessment of different signal-processing schemes over an extended wear period in normal daily use. However, while allowing variations on a theme, the device architecture placed significant limitations on more speculative approaches.

At present, BW processors are the main vehicles combining advanced signal-processing potential with the advantage that they can be completely reprogrammed when a new signal-processing algorithm becomes available. Extracorporeal binaural processing requires two binaurally fitted aids to communicate and share signal information. At present, the development and assessment of such approaches is only practicable through a cable connection to a BW central processor, but recent computer communications advances may soon provide wireless systems.

3.8 Conclusion and Learning Highlights of the Chapter

Improvements in component integration, transducers and batteries have resulted in small, sensitive, relatively low-power consumption hearing aids. Some of these can be inserted completely inside the ear canal, rendering them virtually invisible, providing a more natural quality of sound and interfering less with the natural directional properties of the ear. Some hearing aids employ microphone systems that allow the degree of directionality to be altered.

Although such aids have had some success, they do not satisfy the majority of people who might be expected to benefit, and present-day analogue electronic technology appears to have reached its limits.

Hearing aids using DSP are a recent development raising hopes of better performance and increased user satisfaction. The technology and processing schemes have not yet matured and much challenging development and assessment work remains to be done. There are very few truly independent studies of the performance of commercial DSP hearing aids. One is currently being carried out with support from the RNID, and information will become available from their Web site.

When compared with analogue approaches, features of DSP hearing aids that have improved wearability are:

- the lower level of internally generated electronic noise;
- stability of performance;
- better AVC;
- more successful acoustic feedback cancellation techniques to counter "howl around squeal";
- user-selectable hearing programs;
- better immunity to noise radiated into the aid from cellular telephones;
- the recent provision of a low voltage indication by "beep" tones generated within the aid to alert the user that battery replacement is necessary (emphasising the importance of considering the "less-sophisticated" but vital functions).

Among features implemented in DSP hearing aids, but not yet unequivocally proven as worthwhile from the user's perspective, are the following:

- the facility to incorporate a greater number of programmable filters than analogue systems, and thus more accurately equalise an individual's hearing loss;
- the ability to support a greater choice of amplitude compression schemes, allowing a variety of ways to address the problem of loudness recruitment;

- the incorporation of schemes for actively removing noise from the signal prior to presentation to the ear (since these require a reliable method of distinguishing between speech and undesired sounds), but such schemes are not yet mature and are of current research interest both for hearing aids and other communication devices.

Although some experimental work has shown that more accurate equalisation can deliver some benefit, the fact that there is no significant consensus among manufacturers on the optimum number of frequency bands, the form of compression to be used, or the most suitable VAD scheme indicates that significant work remains to be done in assessing the multitude of approaches being implemented. Any other processing strategy described in Section 3.6 should be considered as an area of current research.

3.8.1 Current Research

The implementation of non-linear compression schemes essentially accepts the need to provide externally a functionality that normally lies within the human hearing system. So, if hearing-impaired persons have lost, through cochlear damage, their access to the neural pathways that allow others to perform, for example, binaural unmasking, then we should not be discouraged from investigating approaches that aim to usurp and externalise such deeply embedded functions.

3.8.2 A Future Possibility?

As long as the signal processing takes place within an ear-worn aid, the limitations on size, battery life, *etc.* will impact the processing schemes used. An alternative approach would be to devise a system where the ear-worn device relays audio information by short-range radio to a BW unit, which processes the audio information and relays it back to the ear-worn device. Although personal earmoulds would still be required, standardisation of the electronic component of the ear-worn transceiver could allow mass production, with its associated cost reduction. The processing unit, its power supply and user controls would no longer be severely compromised by physical size. Standardisation of the processing-unit hardware could also take place, the commercial interests of different manufacturers becoming mainly vested in their software. Arbitration and coding schemes could allow several such aids to operate in the same location without interference, and could even support a form of local networking between hearing-aid wearers, or direct broadcasting to replace induction-loop technology.

3.8.3 Learning Highlights of the Chapter

This chapter began with a review of technical terms that led to understanding hearing as an engineering process. This engineering context was fundamental to the remainder of the chapter, in which we learnt:

- to classify electronic hearing aids based on their physical location on the wearer, and by the use of analogue or digital technology;
- to appreciate that hearing aids have a long history, but that the most significant developments have depended on the electronic technology of the last 50 years;
- to understand the engineering implications of designing a prosthesis for the ear as part of the human body;
- to understand how digital hardware and the developments in DSP were used to make today's advanced digital hearing-aid technology so successful.

The chapter closed with a look at even more-advanced technologies that might be employed in future solutions for human hearing loss compensation.

Acknowledgements

Author Douglas R. Campbell wishes to express his appreciation for the contribution of materials and permission for their use to: Stephan Launer and Hans-Ueli Roeck (Phonak), Carl Ludvigsen (Widex), Graham Naylor (Oticon), Cal Pearson (Westone Laboratories, Inc.), Matthias Wesselkamp (Siemens Audiologische Technik).

Projects and Investigations

Projects

The following projects assume the availability of MATLAB Simulink and the DSP Blockset toolbox (www.matlab.com).

1. *Amplitude compression.* Dynamic range compression is available as a MATLAB Simulink demonstration in Demo\Blocksets\DSPblockset. Investigate and report on its characteristics.
2. *Speech signal robustness.* Set up a MATLAB Simulink simulation to subject a speech signal to each of the effects: outer clipping, centre clipping, and low-pass, high-pass and band-pass filtering. Define an error measure, *e.g.* RMS; then, starting at zero effect in each case, gradually increase the effect until the speech becomes unintelligible. Record the final error measure for each effect. Consider the various problems that arise in making unbiased assessments of speech quality and discuss your results.
3. *Sinusoidal modelling.* Set up a MATLAB Simulink simulation to perform sinusoidal modelling based on the frequency-domain processing block diagram of Figure 3.33. Use a successive approximation approach to decide on the smallest number of tones that will give intelligible speech of acceptable quality.
4. *Frequency transposition.* Set up a MATLAB Simulink simulation to perform frequency transposition based on the frequency domain processing block

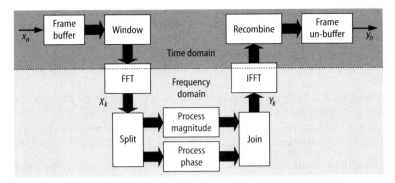

Figure 3.33 Frequency-domain processing.

diagram of Figure 3.33. Devise and investigate at least two mixing strategies.

5. *Simulated hearing aid.* Design, construct and test a MATLAB Simulink simulation of the "Digifocus" hearing aid using data from Naylor (1997).

Investigation

This investigative project is considered suitable for an MSc/MEng-level project or may be divided and/or simplified to give undergraduate projects. Hardware and/or software design elements may be included, as the supervisor thinks relevant.

Perform a feasibility study on a hearing-aid system that uses a very short-range radio system to communicate between an ear-worn device and a BW processing unit.

The ear-worn device may consist of three parts: a microphone, preamplifier, coder and radio transmitter section; a separate radio receiver, decoder, amplifier, and "loudspeaker" section; and a battery power-supply unit.

Starting from first principles, estimate the energy budget for such a device and relate this to present and projected battery technologies. Consider the possibility of trickle recharging the battery via a radio link to extend its wearing time.

The signal-processing section is to be located elsewhere on the body, *e.g.* in a pocket or handbag, and communicates with the ear-worn transceiver over the very short-range radio link. Thus, the processing unit, its power supply and user controls are no longer severely compromised by physical size. Identify components to allow construction of a bench demonstrator prototype. Specify the requirements to allow software upgrading by download from an Internet site.

A recent example of such a short-range radio link system is the "Bluetooth" scheme, which allows several computer peripherals to communicate with a personal computer system without the necessity for wire or optical links. Investigate arbitration and coding schemes to allow several such hearing aids to operate in the same location without interference. Investigate the feasibility of a form of local networking between hearing-aid wearers in the same room, or radio broadcasting as a replacement for induction-loop technology.

Although this concept is critically dependent on solving the technological problems of providing such an ear-worn device with an acceptable battery life, there are also important international standardisation issues. These arise from legislation associated with the allocation of the radio spectrum and from health and safety issues, since the radiating device is in such intimate contact with the body. Identify the appropriate national and international standards and controlling authorities. Consider the impact of the standards on the system design.

References and Further Reading

References

Agaiby, H, Moir, T.J., 1997. Knowing the wheat from the weeds in noisy speech. In: *Eurospeech 97*, Rhodes, Greece, pp. 1119–1122.
Andersen, HH, Ludvigsen, C, Troelsen, T., 1999. Signal processing hearing instruments: description of performance. In: *Danavox Symposium*, September.
Ballantyne, D., 1990. *Handbook of Audiological Techniques*. Butterworth-Heinemann Ltd, London, UK.
Bodden, M, Blauert, J., 1992. Separation of concurrent speech signals: a cocktail party processor for speech signals. In: *ESCA ETRW on Speech Processing in Adverse Conditions*, Cannes–Mandelieu, France, pp. 147–150.
Byrne, D, Dillon H., 1986. The National Acoustics Laboratories' (NAL) new procedure for selecting the gain and frequency response of a hearing aid. *Ear and Hearing* 7, 257–265.
Chasin, M., 1997. *CIC Handbook*. Singular Publishing Group Inc., San Diego, CA, USA.
Culling, J, Summerfield, Q., 1995. Perceptual separation of concurrent speech sounds: absence of across-frequency grouping by common interaural delay. *Journal of the Acoustical Society of America* 98 (2), 785–797.
Denbigh, P., 1998. *System Analysis and Signal Processing*. Addison-Wesley, Longman Ltd., Harlow, UK.
Desloge, J.G., Rabinowitz, W.M., Zurek, P.M., 1997. Microphone-array hearing aids with binaural output – part I: fixed processing systems. *IEEE Transactions on Speech and Audio Processing* 5 (6), 529–542.
Drullman, R., Festen, J.M., Houtgast, T., 1996. Effect of temporal modulation on spectral contrasts in speech. *Journal of the Acoustical Society of America* 99 (4, Pt 1), 2358–2364.
Durlach, N.I., 1972. Binaural signal detection: equalization and cancellation theory. In: Tobias, J.V. (Ed.), *Foundations of Modern Auditory Theory*, vol. II. Academic Press, London.
Durlach, N.I., Gabriel, K.J., Colburn, H.S., Trahiotis, C., 1986. Interaural correlation discrimination: II. Relation to binaural unmasking. *Journal of the Acoustical Society of America* 79 (5), 1548–1557.
Engebretson, A.M., 1986. A wearable pocket sized processor for digital hearing aid and other hearing prosthesis applications. In: *ICASSP'86*, Tokyo, vol. 1, pp. 625–628.
Engebretson, A.M., 1994. Benefits of digital hearing aids. *IEEE Engineering in Medicine and Biology* (April/May), 238–248.
Ferrara, E.R., Widrow, B., 1981. Multichannel adaptive filtering for signal enhancement. *IEEE Transactions on Acoustics, Speech and Signal Processing* 29 (3), 766–770.
Goode, R.L., 1989. Current status of electromagnetic implantable hearing aids. *Otolaryngologic Clinics of North America* 22, 201–209.
Goodings, R.L.A., Sensieb, G.A., Wilson, P.H., Hansen, R.S., 1990. Hearing aid having compensation for acoustic feedback. *European Patent Publication No. 0 415 677 A2*.
Haykin, S., 1996. *Adaptive Filter Theory*, 3rd edition. Prentice-Hall, NJ, USA.
Hellgren, J., Lunner, T., Arlinger, S., 1999. System identification of feedback in hearing aids. *Journal of the Acoustical Society of America* 105 (6), 3481–3495.

Hoffman, M.W., Trine, T.D., Buckley, K.M., Van Tasell, D.J., 1994. Robust adaptive microphone array processing for hearing aids: realistic speech enhancement. *Journal of the Acoustical Society of America* 96 (2, Pt 1), 759-770.

Hüttenbrink, K.-B., 1999. Current status and critical reflections on implantable hearing aids. *American Journal of Otology* 20, 409-415.

Jones, N.B. (Ed.), 1982. *Digital Signal Processing*. Peter Peregrinus Ltd., UK.

Kollmeier, B., Peissig, J., Hohmann, V., 1993. Binaural noise-reduction hearing aid scheme with real-time processing in the frequency domain. *Scandinavian Audiology* 38 (Suppl.), 28-38.

Kuk, F.K., Ludvigsen, C., 1999. Variables affecting the use of prescriptive formulae to fit modern nonlinear hearing aids. *Journal of the American Academy of Audiology* 10, 458-465.

Leysieffer, H., Baumann, J.W., Muller, G., Zenner, H.P., 1997. An implantable piezoelectric hearing aid transducer for sensorineural hearing loss. Part II: clinical implant. *HNO* 45 (10), 801-815.

Loizou, P.C., 1998. Mimicking human ear. *IEEE Signal Processing Magazine* (Sept.), 101-130.

Mahalanobis, A., Song, S., Mitra, S.K., Petraglia, M.R., 1993. Adaptive FIR filters based on structural subband decomposition for system identification problems. *IEEE Transactions on Circuits and Systems II - Analog and Digital Signal Processing* 40 (6), 375-381.

Martin, M., 1997. *Speech Audiometry*. Whurr Publishers Ltd., London, UK.

Moore, B.C.J. (Ed.), 1995. *Hearing*. Academic Press Ltd, London, UK.

Moore, B.C.J., 1995. *Perceptual Consequences of Cochlear Damage*. Oxford University Press, Oxford, UK.

Naylor, G., 1997. Technical and audiological factors in the implementation and use of digital signal processing hearing aids. *Scandinavian Audiology* 26, 223-229.

Naylor, G., Elberling, C., 1997. The JUMP-1 scheme: an example of industry providing academia with something other than money. In: *European Acoustics Association Symposium, Psychoacoustics in Industry and the Universities*, Eindhoven, January.

Noll, P., 1997. MPEG digital audio coding. *IEEE Signal Processing Magazine* (Sept.), 59-81.

Oppenheim, A.V., Willsky, A.S., 1983. *Signals and Systems*. Prentice-Hall International (UK) Ltd, London.

Peachey, N.S., Chow, A.Y., 1999. Subretinal implantation of semiconductor-based photodiodes: progress and challenges. *Journal of Rehabilitation Research and Development* 36 (4), 371-376.

Plomp, R., 1988. The negative effect of amplitude compression in multichannel hearing aids in the light of the modulation transfer function. *Journal of the Acoustical Society of America* 83 (6), 2322-2327.

Plomp, R., 1994. Noise, amplification, and compression: considerations of three main issues in hearing aid design. *Ear and Hearing* 15, 2-12.

Pollack, M.C. (Ed.), 1975. *Amplification for the Hearing Impaired*. Grune and Stratton, New York, USA.

Rass, U., Steeger, G.H., 1996. Evaluation of digital hearing aid algorithms on wearable signal processor systems. In: *Proceedings of EUSIPCO-96*, vol. 1, pp. 475-478.

Sandlin, R.E. (Ed.), 2000. *Textbook of Hearing Aid Amplification*. Singular Publishing Group Inc., San Diego, CA, USA.

Seligman, P., McDermott, H., 1995. Architecture of the Spectra 22 speech processor. *Annals of Otology, Rhinology and Laryngology* 166 (Suppl.), 139-141.

Shields, P.W., Campbell, D.R., 1998. Intelligibility improvements obtained by an enhancement method applied to speech corrupted by noise and reverberation. *Speech Communication* 25, 165-175.

Soede, W., Berkhout, A.J., Bilsen, F.A., 1993a. Development of a directional hearing instrument based on array technology. *Journal of the Acoustical Society of America* 94 (1), 785-798.

Soede, W., Bilsen, F.A., Berkhout, A.J., 1993b. Assessment of a directional microphone array for hearing impaired listeners. *Journal of the Acoustical Society of America* 94 (1), 799-808.

Stone, M.A., Moore, B.C.J., 1999. Tolerable hearing aid delays. I. Estimation of limits imposed by the auditory path alone using simulated hearing losses. *Ear and Hearing* 20 (3), 182-192.

Stone, M.A., Moore, B.C.J., Alcantara, J.I., Glasberg, B.R., 1999. Comparison of different forms of compression using wearable digital hearing aids. *Journal of the Acoustical Society of America* 106 (6), 3603-3619.

Summerfield, Q., 1992. Lip-reading and audio-visual speech perception. *Philosophical Transactions of the Royal Society of London, Series B* 335, 71-78.

Toner, E., Campbell, D.R., 1993. Speech enhancement using sub-band intermittent adaptation. *Speech Communication* 12, 253-259.

Vary, P., 1985. Noise suppression by spectral magnitude estimation - mechanism and theoretical limits. *Signal Processing* 8, 387-400.

Virag, N., 1999. Single channel speech enhancement based on masking properties of the human auditory system. *IEEE Transactions on Speech and Audio Processing* 7 (2), 126–137.

Widrow, B., Stearns, S.D., 1985. *Adaptive Signal Processing*. Prentice-Hall, Englewood Cliffs, NJ.

Wouters, J., Litiere, L., van Wieringen, A., 1999. Speech intelligibility in noisy environments with one- and two-microphone hearing aids. *Audiology* 38, 91–98.

Further Reading

Books

Vonlanthen, A., 2000. *Hearing Instrument Technology for the Hearing Healthcare Professional*, 2nd edition. Singular Publishing Group Inc., San Diego, CA, USA.

Web Sites

General
http://www.deafworldweb.org/
http://www.hei.org/
http://www.ilo.ucl.ac.uk/ddeaf/
http://www.rnid.org.uk/

History
http://www.oticon.com/HeAiHi/HeAiHiPG.html
http://www.entnet.org/hearing.html

Aid Manufacturers
http://www.advancedhearing.com/hearaids.htm
http://www.cochlear.com/
http://www.gnresound.com/
http://www.implex.de
http://www.nl.hearing.philips.com/
http://www.oticon.com/
http://www.phonak.com/
http://www.siemens.de/med/d/gg/sat/index.html
http://www.symphonix.com
http://www.viennatone.com/
http://www.widex.com/websmain.nsf/pages/1Widex

DSP Processor Manufacturers
http://www.motorola-dsp.com/
http://www.ti.com/

4 Induction-loop Systems

4.1 Learning Objectives

Audio-frequency induction-loop systems were introduced in 1950 as a pickup system for telephone use. They have been widely accepted as the most common wireless system for hearing-aid use since then. The main advantages are simplicity, no current consumption for the receiver and early standardisation. The disadvantages are interference from other electronic appliances due to lack of modulation. However, though they are simple, induction-loop systems do need to be installed properly and installation without measurement or calibration will generally give poor performance.

The hearing aid can be considered to be a prosthesis; it attempts to compensate for physical hearing loss. In this chapter, the first assistive technology *per se* is described, namely induction-loop technology. The learning objectives for this chapter are:

- to understand the basic electrical engineering principles of loop systems;
- to learn about the individual components and physical effects present in a loop system;
- to appreciate the factors that need to be considered in the installation of an induction-loop system;
- to review the application areas and the need for international induction-loop system standards.

4.2 Audio-frequency Induction-loop Systems

One of the most important aspects of speech recognition is the acoustic environment. It is easy to discriminate and interpret speech in a good acoustic environment. Understanding speech is much more difficult in a poor acoustic environment with interference from noise, reverberation and echo-effects. People with hearing impairments are generally more dependent on a good acoustic environment for understanding speech than are other people. People with "normal" hearing generally require a signal-to-noise ratio (SNR) of –6 dB or greater, whereas hearing-aid users require an SNR of 0 to 15 dB to understand speech. This means that people with normal hearing can understand speech in a

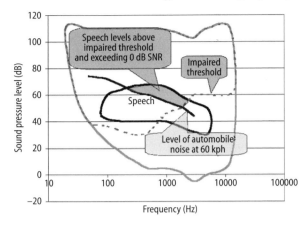

Figure 4.1 Thresholds for understanding speech in a noisy environment.

noisy environment, where the noise is louder than the speech, whereas people with hearing impairments require the speech to be louder and sometimes considerably louder. This phenomenon was first met in Chapter 3, where an understanding of speech and the hearing process was important for hearing-aid design. In that chapter, Figure 4.1 was introduced to illustrate the effects of noisy surroundings on understanding speech. The sound intensity of only a small part of the conversational speech frequencies is

- above threshold
- greater than the noise sound intensity, so that the SNR is positive.

Therefore, noise will severely reduce the ability of someone with a hearing impairment to understand speech.

The role of the induction loop is to present the speech signal directly to a person with a hearing impairment (through a hearing aid). This bypasses (most of) the noise and reverberation and, therefore, gives a good SNR and improves intelligibility. This is illustrated in Figure 4.2, which shows amplitude versus time measurements from an acoustic coupler, or artificial ear, connected to a hearing aid. The noisy environment comprises speech and noise. There are competing conversations at 4 m distance from the voice signal that is being listened to. The signals within the noisy environment are identical in all three cases. Figure 4.2(a) shows the voice and noise in an environment with a reverberation time of 2 s; it can be seen that the voice signal is completely hidden. If the reverberation time is reduced to 0.5 s, as shown in Figure 4.2(b), then the voice signal begins to appear. However, if the loop system is used, then the hidden voice signal clearly emerges from the background noise, as can be seen in Figure 4.2(c).

4.3 The Electromagnetic Principles of a Loop System

The basic principles of the loop system are found in the physics of electromagnetic fields. When a current flows through a conductor, a magnetic field is created. The field has direction and magnitude. The magnitude increases when

Induction-loop Systems

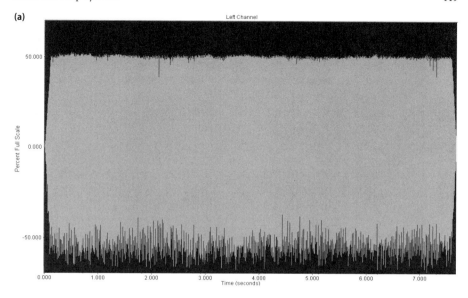

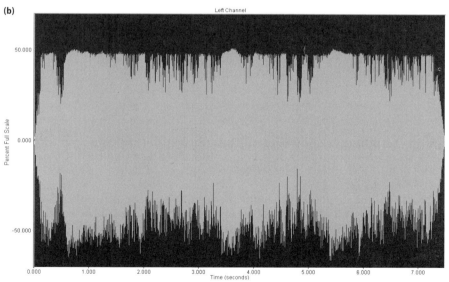

Figure 4.2 Speech signal in a noisy environment with reverberation time of (a) 2 s, (b) 0.5 s and (c) 0.5 s and a loop system in use. (*Continued overleaf*)

several wires with the same current are made into a loop. In Figure 4.3(a), the current *I* is flowing through a wire conductor. The lines on the "card" are those of the magnetic field.

Figure 4.3(b) shows that the field strength due to a current *I* in a conductor creates a magnetic field at a distance from the conductor. The magnet field *H* is resolved into the vertical and horizontal components H_v and H_h respectively.

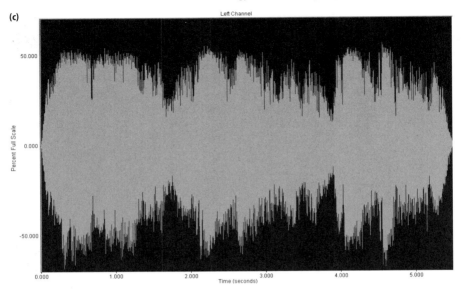

Figure 4.2 (*continued*)

The vertical field H_v is the one experienced, for example, by the telecoil in the hearing aid and induces a current in the telecoil. The magnetic field generated by the loop is measured in amperes per metre and has its strength given by

$$H_v = \frac{I}{2\pi r}\cos(\alpha) \qquad (4.1)$$

where r is the radius of the loop and α is the angle of the point P at which the field strength is measured. The magnetic field inside the loop of conductor wires is almost constant in strength; see Figure 4.4. This consistency gives this technology its utility.

To increase the strength of the magnetic field in a loop, multiple turns of the conductor wires can be used, as shown in Figure 4.5, where a double loop is shown.

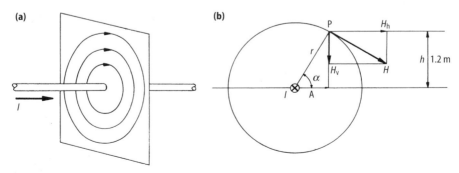

Figure 4.3 (a) Conductor and electromagnetic field lines. (b) Geometry of the electromagnetic field.

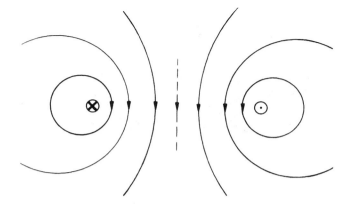

Figure 4.4 The constant magnetic field inside a loop.

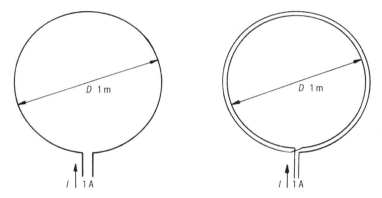

Figure 4.5 A loop system with multiple turns of the conductor wire.

4.4 Induction-loop Systems

The principle of generation of a magnetic field by an electric current in a loop of wire is used in induction systems as a transmission method. A coil of wire is placed around the listening area. Since the coil is horizontal it creates an approximately vertical magnetic field. The term *loop plane* is used to denote the height above the floor of the horizontal plane containing the loop. The loop amplifier converts the voltage from the signal source to constant current in the defined frequency range, 100 to 5000 Hz.

4.4.1 Hearing-aid Receiver or Telecoil

The hearing aid contains a telecoil, which consists of a coil with multiple turns and an iron core. Multiple turns and the iron core increase the sensitivity, with the iron core acting like a magnetic amplifier. The receiver picks up the

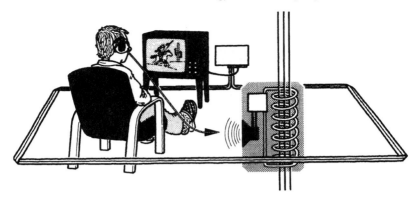

Figure 4.6 Listening to the TV with an induction-loop system.

magnetic field and transforms it back to electric current. This current is then converted to voltage. This conversion has a flat frequency response. The signals are subjected to analogue or digital processing in the hearing aid and transformed to an analogue audio signal. The combination of telecoil and induction loop is still used in modern hearing aids owing to its simplicity and zero power consumption at the aid. However, there is ongoing research to improve performance; for instance, by:

- using modulation
- reducing sensitivity to the angle of the hearing aid
- making the performance of the loop system more uniform within the listening area
- increasing the number of channels.

The term *listening plane* is used to denote the level of the receiver (telecoil) in the hearing aid. This is taken to be about 1.2 m above floor level as a compromise between sitting and standing positions, but it will depend on the height and body proportions of the hearing-aid wearer. For example, this listening height may not be a good compromise for children. Figure 4.6 illustrates the implementation of an electromagnetic transmission with an induction-loop system. The TV is connected to the loop amplifier that transmits current into the surrounding wire. This creates a magnetic field that fluctuates in sympathy with the audio signal being transmitted. The telecoil in the hearing aid responds to this fluctuating magnetic field and produces an audio signal directly in the hearing-aid earpiece.

4.4.2 The Effect of Different Materials and Loop Shapes

The magnetic field of the loop system propagates freely through electrically insulating materials, including walls made of wood, stone or brick. Electrically insulating materials do not affect the magnetic field strength. However, the magnetic field will be affected by electrically conducting materials, with the effect depending on the shape of the materials. For instance, concrete is often reinforced by small squares of metal and long rods. This creates small parasitic loops that partially absorb the magnetic field. There is a coupling effect, similar to that in a transformer, between the loop wire and the metal close to the loop. As a result, both the spatial and frequency distributions change, so that the middle of the loop has the weakest field and high frequencies are damped more than lower ones, though all frequencies are absorbed to a certain extent. Therefore, the distance between the shortest sides of a loop should preferably not be greater than 10 m. However, reinforced concrete also increases the listening area and smoothes out irregularities.

In general, it can be difficult to predict the effect of different shapes and types of metal on the field strength. It may be distorted, increased or decreased in magnitude and changed in direction. There are no simple formulae to determine what will happen.

4.4.3 Magnetic Field Strength

The term magnetic field strength indicates the magnitude of the magnetic field. The field strength at the telecoil in a hearing aid is determined by current strength and loop height. The current in the loop wire is directly proportional to the current delivered by the amplifier through the loop. It is also directly proportional to the acoustic level in the hearing aid (if it is working in a linear mode). As already indicated, the induction-loop system may have more than one turn. In the case of a single-loop system the output current is the same as the loop current, whereas in a two-loop system, with wires in phase, the output current, and hence the magnetic field, will be approximately doubled in strength.

The term *loop height* is used to denote the distance between the loop plane and the listening plane. When the loop plane is at floor level the term *listening height* is sometimes used and generally assumed to be 1.2 m; see Figure 4.7. Field strength decreases as loop height increases. The magnitude of the field strength is the same above and below the loop plane.

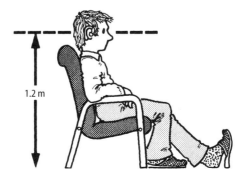

Figure 4.7 Listening height for the loop system.

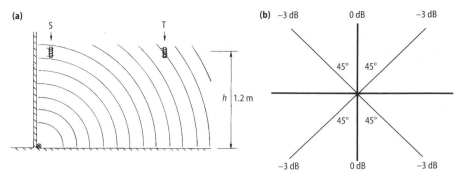

Figure 4.8 (a) Magnetic field direction in a room geometry. (b) Field strength related to angular direction of the telecoil.

4.4.4 Magnetic Field Direction

The electromagnetic field direction is shown in the Figure 4.8, where the loop is at floor level, and the listening plane is at a height 1.2 m.

The sound source is denoted by S and the telecoil denoted by T. As shown in Figure 4.8(a), the field is generally vertical at the listening region in the location of T, but it becomes more horizontal closer to the loop wire itself. Figure 4.8(b) shows the relationship between sound level and the angle of the telecoil to the magnetic field. Hearing aids are generally designed so that the telecoil is vertical when the user is upright. This gives the maximum field strength and sound level, as the telecoil is parallel to the magnetic field in this position. However, people tend to move their heads around, and this will change the angle and reduce the sound level. From Figure 4.8(b) it is possible to see that a tilt of 45° causes a 3 dB loss in field strength and a concomitant reduction in sound level.

4.4.5 Magnetic Field Distribution

The sound level in the hearing aid is directly proportional to the vertical magnetic field. Therefore, the field strength is often measured in decibels.

A typical industry standard sets the 0 dB reference level to 100 mA m^{-1} so that 12 dB corresponds to 400 mA m^{-1}. This uses the formula for Z (dB) as

$$Z(\mathrm{dB}) = 20\log\frac{X}{100} \tag{4.2}$$

where field strength is measured as X mA m^{-1} and the reference value is 100 mA m^{-1}.

In the IEC standard the reference value 0 dB is set as 1 A m^{-1}, then the field strength Z (dB) would be obtained as

$$Z(\mathrm{dB}) = 20\log X \tag{4.3}$$

where X is the field strength in amps per metre. Doubling the magnetic field strength corresponds to increasing it by 6 dB, and decreasing it to half of its value is the same as reducing it by 6 dB.

Induction-loop Systems

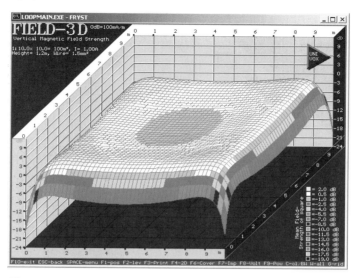

Figure 4.9 Vertical magnetic field strength distribution in a room loop.

Figure 4.9 shows the vertical magnetic field strength (Z dB) distribution in a room loop, with area 100 m² between the coordinates (0, 0) and (10, 10). As the figure shows, the field strength is approximately constant inside the loop, but becomes very low close to the loop conductor wire itself.

The field outside the loop decreases with increasing distance. Figure 4.10 shows the field strength at 6 m outside the loop is reduced to about −24 dB. Figure 4.10(a) shows the three-dimensional distribution and Figure 4.10(b) displays a cross-section.

Both the magnitude and distribution of the vertical magnetic field strength change as the loop height, *i.e.* the distance between the loop and listening plane, increases. This is shown in the Figure 4.11. The loop height increases from 0.25 to 2.0 m in steps of firstly 0.25 m and then 0.5 m. The sequence of figures shows that the electromagnetic field strength or magnitude initially increases and then decreases with increasing loop height.

Note that the distribution of the magnetic field is always symmetrical around the loop plane, so that the vertical magnetic field strength is exactly the same above and below the horizontal loop plane.

A smaller loop is more sensitive to different loop heights than a larger loop. As shown in Figure 4.12, a loop of area 25 m² has the same distribution 1.0 m above the loop plane as the loop of area 256 m² at 2 m above the loop plane. At 3 m from the loop plane the field strength has reduced approximately 10 dB in the smaller loop, but only about 5 dB in the large loop.

A common misunderstanding is that the vertical magnetic field is always zero above the loop cable. This is only true when the loop height and listening height are the same. As the distance increases, the "zero point" is moved further from the loop. The position of the zero point depends on the loop size. For instance, a 0.4 m × 0.4 m loop with a listening height of 0.65 m has its "zero point" 5–6 m outside the loop, whereas a 10 m × 10 m loop with a listening height of 1.2 m has the "zero point" 2–3 m outside the loop.

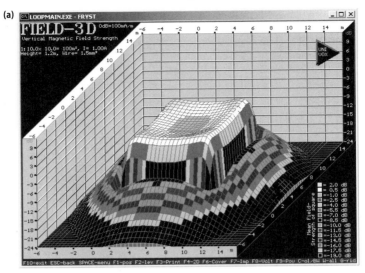

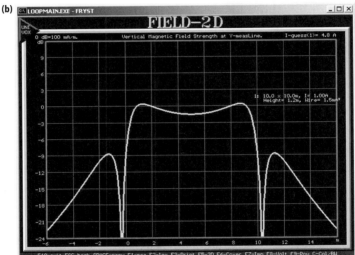

Figure 4.10 (a) Magnetic field strength inside and outside the 10 × 10 m² loop. (b) Cross-section of the magnetic field strength inside and outside the 10 × 10 m² loop.

The magnetic field strength is directly proportional to the current in the loop. The sound pressure in the hearing instrument is directly proportional to the magnetic field strength. The current is dependent on:

- the loop area
- the loop proportions
- the loop height.

Induction-loop Systems

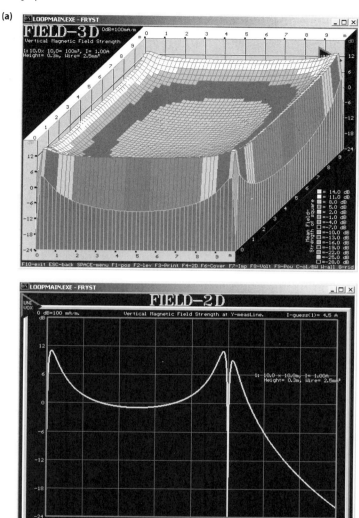

Figure 4.11 Loop heights of (**a**) 0.25 m, (**b**) 0.5 m, (**c**) 1 m, (**d**) 1.5 m and (**e**) 2 m. (*Continued on pp. 128–131*)

Figure 4.13 shows the relationship between current and loop for loop heights of (a) 0 m and (b) 1.2 m and different side proportions, and illustrate the following points:

- For a given area and height, current decreases as the ratio of the sides increases, so that a circular loop requires more current than an oval one.
- In general, for a given height and side proportions, current increases with area.

(b)

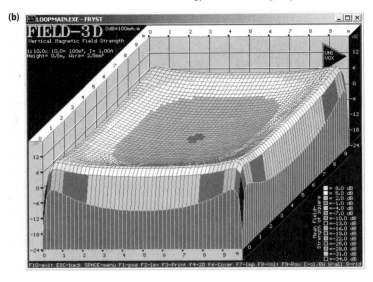

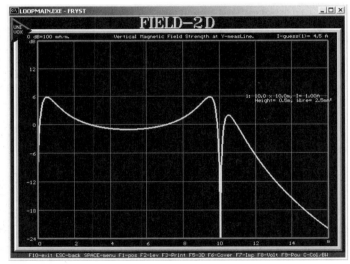

Figure 4.11 (*Continued*)

- Loop height only has a noticeable effect for small-area loops; in this case for non-zero heights, current decreases with area for small loop areas.

4.4.6 Overspill

Overspill occurs when two loop systems are close to each other. The overspill could be considered to be background noise. According to the standard IEC

Induction-loop Systems

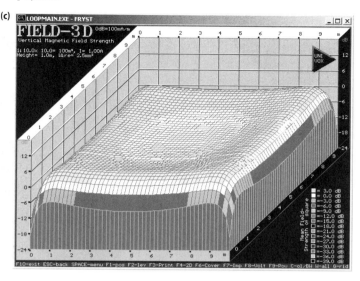

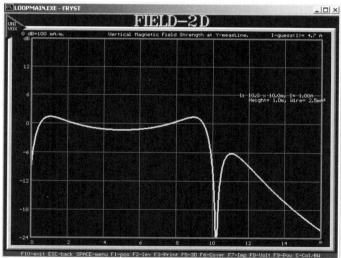

Figure 4.11 (*Continued*)

60118-4 the background noise, measured with a root-mean-square (RMS) detector with time constant 125 ms and an A-weighted filter should be no more than −25 dB.

There are two main methods for minimising overspill:

- Using a smaller loop in a figure-of-eight configuration.
- Placing an anti-phase loop to the side where damping is required.

The amount of overspill with a smaller figure-of-eight loop is decreased to the sides and also above and below the loop plane. However, there are also

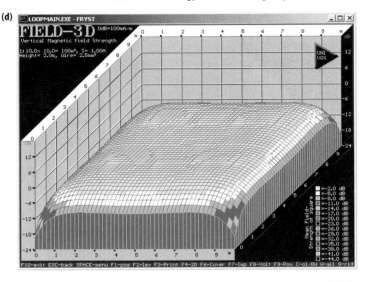
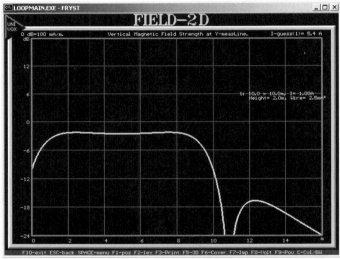

Figure 4.11 (*Continued*)

"zero points" where the loops meet. The "zero points" could be minimised by making the two loops uncorrelated (90° phase shift) and using at least two systems with the same signal source. This replaces the "zero points" with some "filtered sound". The drawback of this method is that reinforced concrete will increase the area of the magnetic field and also increase the overspill and make it more difficult to predict.

It is easier to predict what happens with an anti-phase loop than with uncorrelated loops, particularly when attenuation (damping) is only required at one side. However, hand calculation is difficult, and trial-and-error

(e)

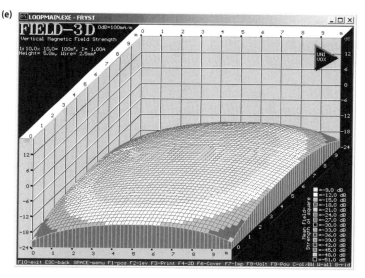

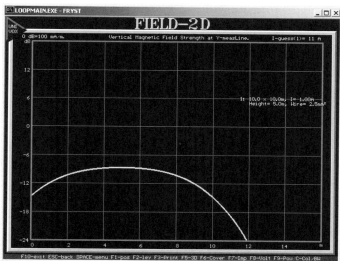

Figure 4.11 (*Continued*)

calculations (iteration) using a computer program are required. The starting point should be a thin anti-phase loop, approximately 1 m wide. The current should be twice that of the main loop, which is a two-turn loop.

Figure 4.14(a) shows the three-dimensional display of the overspill without an anti-phase loop for an 8 m × 19 m loop. It is desired to limit this overspill phenomenon. The solution is to install an anti-phase loop of size 1 m × 10 m to create a wall effect. Figure 4.14(b) shows a three-dimensional display of the overspill with anti-phase loop and Figure 4.14(c) shows the cross-section for main loop–anti-phase loop configuration. Clearly, the region of overspill has been limited.

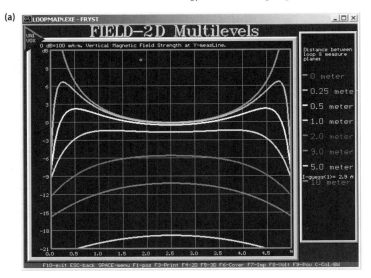

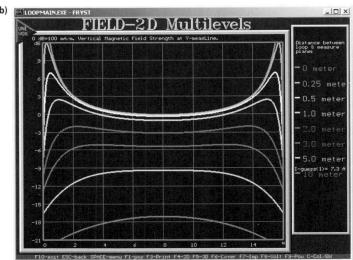

Figure 4.12 Loop size: (a) 5 m × 5 m; (b) 16 m × 16 m.

4.5 Loop Installation

Guidelines for a successful installation include the following:

1. Limit the loop area to avoid wasting energy and to limit overspill.
2. Keep down power requirements by only covering areas required for listening and splitting them into several different loops.
3. Do not cover the stage (when there is one), to avoid wasting energy and to avoid positive feedback between amplifiers and the loop, which can cause

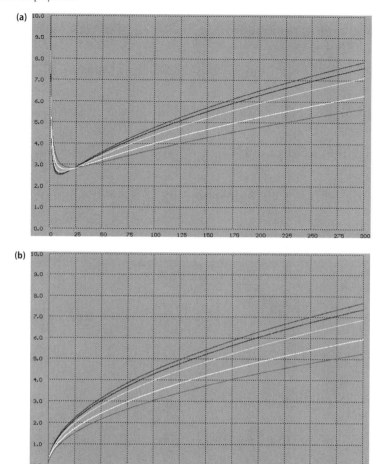

Figure 4.13 Loop height of (a) 0 m and (b) 1.2 m; loop proportions 1:1, 1:2, 1:3, 1:4, and 1:5 in each case.

distortion and limit amplifier power. Particular problems can occur with electric guitars due to positive feedback between the guitar amplifier and the loop system, which can lead to oscillation.

4. When the stage is close to the audience, use an anti-phase loop to minimise overspill to the stage.
5. The connecting wires should be of low resistance, as short as possible, screened and balanced, if possible. The low-level signal wires should not be in parallel with or close to the loop wire.
6. Plan for overspill. A simple approximation for sideways overspill is that the vertical magnetic field will be reduced by 20 dB and by 40 dB respectively at half the loop size (radius) and the loop size from the loop wire.

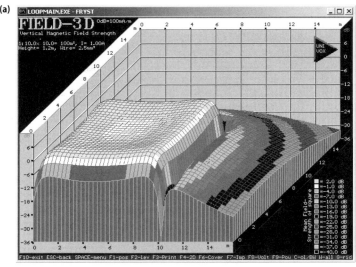

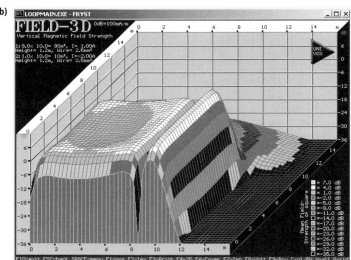

Figure 4.14 Three-dimensional display of the overspill: (a) without anti-phase loop; (b) with anti-phase loop. (c) Cross-section for main loop 8 × 19 m² with anti-phase loop 1 × 10 m².

7. The wire between the loop configuration and the loop amplifier should be closely twisted or tightly parallel to cancel magnetic overspill and reduce inductance. This reduces power consumption and the risk of noise and oscillation problems.
8. Do a quick test of the loop to ensure there is sufficient power and no overspill problems.
9. Use electret or condenser microphones, not dynamic microphones, as they have higher signal output (10–30 dB) and avoid the problems of positive magnetic feedback.

(c)

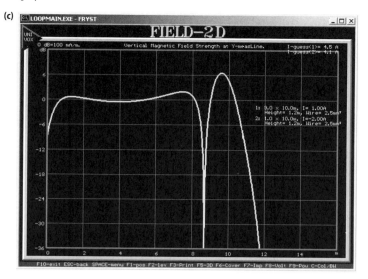

Figure 4.14 (*Continued*)

10. Adjust the loop height to give the best covering area and lowest overspill.
11. Determine where there is metal, particularly if reinforced concrete is used in the room. If there is metal everywhere, then there is likely to be strong attenuation. If there is metal only in the floor or ceiling, then situate the loop as far as possible from the metal. Do not mount the loop wire on a metal frame, as it will absorb the magnetic field. Construct a trial loop.
12. If the amplifier has a built-in monitoring device, then use it to listen to the quality of the sound. Quality will be higher than with a listening device, making it easier to detect problems.
13. Use the tone control for compensating for high-frequency losses with reinforced concrete and be moderate with the bass boost.
14. Follow the instruction manual, which may have calculated values for correct wire thickness and other parameters for an optimal installation.
15. Select the correct cable. The wire should be thick to reduce resistance and losses, but not so thick that output power gain is lower than the maximum saturated output level with limited field strength. This is particularly important with small loops of less than 50–100 m^2.
16. Explain how the loop works to the relevant personnel, including any special functions such as monitoring.
17. Use a field-strength meter that conforms to IEC specifications to measure the signal and noise levels.
18. Find a reference point and decide the listening height, generally 1.2 m above floor level. Carry out detailed measurements at the reference point.
19. Adjust for maximum level by connecting a speech signal and adjust the output current so that the peaks measure 12 dB for 100 mA m^{-1}.
20. Check the area of cover by connecting a sinusoidal signal of 1000 Hz.

21. Use a number of loops in figure-of-eight configurations for large areas where the distance between the smallest sides is more than 10 m.
22. When installing a loop in a large room it can be difficult to judge whether a figure-of-eight or one large loop system is preferable. Therefore, make the fixed basic wire installation first. Then choose the type of loop system, including the number of amplifiers and the loop configuration.

4.5.1 Multi-combination Loop System

When installing a loop system in a large room it is important that the international standards IEC and BSI apply over the largest area possible. The IEC standards are maintained by the International Electrotechnical Commission (http://www.iec.ch), hence the initials IEC, and the British standards are maintained by the British Standards Institute (http://www.bsi-global.com), hence the initials BSI. As well as maximising the area of effectiveness, it is important to achieve this by using as little power and current as possible. It is often difficult to judge if it is best to use a figure-of-eight system, or whether one large loop will suffice. Thus, a multi-combination loop system that could be connected as a single loop or a figure-of-eight and have one or two turns has advantages in terms of flexibility. It can be obtained by using identical loops to cover a larger area, *e.g.* an area of 10 m × 20 m is covered by two 10 m × 10 m loops. Each loop has its own connecting wire to the loop amplifier, and additional amplifiers can easily be added after the wires are installed. The loops can be connected in or out of phase, giving the field distribution of one large loop or a figure-of-eight configuration with a dip between the two loops respectively. In addition, each loop can have one or two turns.

The multi-combination loop method provides the options of using one or two amplifiers, a single- or double-turn loop and in-phase or out-of-phase loops. Decisions on these factors can be made after the wires have been installed. This allows testing to determine the best configuration. The multi-combination loop also has reduced voltage demand and, consequently, increased current, which creates the field strength. As to which combination loop is acceptable in application, this has to be determined by experimentation.

4.6 The Electrical Equivalent of a Loop System

The electrical equivalent to the loop system consists of two passive components: a coil with inductance L and a resistance R in series. This is shown in Figure 4.15.

The load impedance is denoted by Z and is given by

$$Z = R + jX_L(\omega) \tag{4.4}$$

where the resistance R is in ohms, the inductive reactance $X_L(\omega) = \omega L = 2\pi f L$ is in ohms, L the coil inductance in henries and f is the frequency in hertz. In some standards this is referred to as the rated load impedance Z.

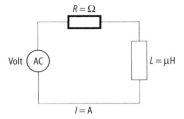

Figure 4.15 The electrical circuit equivalent of a loop system.

4.6.1 Loop Inductance

The main factors that affect the inductance L of the coil are its length and the number of turns. The inductance increases with the square of the number of turns, so that a two-turn loop has four times the inductance of a one-turn loop. The loop inductance increases with length and is assumed to be approximately in the range $1.8 < L < 2\,\mu\text{H m}^{-1}$. The loop inductance (in microhenries) can be calculated from the rated coverage area A in square metres and the specified number of turns N using the approximate formula

$$L\,(\mu\text{H}) = 7.6 N^2 \sqrt{A} \tag{4.5}$$

A more accurate formula, which also takes account of the internal inductance of the wire, is

$$L\,(\mu\text{H}) = 0.2 SN \left\{ 1 + 4N \ln\left[\frac{2S}{r(1+\sqrt{2})}\right] - 2 + \sqrt{2} \right\} \tag{4.6}$$

where $S = \sqrt{A}$ the side of the square in metres, and r is the radius of the loop wire in metres. Then L is the inductance in microhenries.

4.6.2 Loop Resistance

The loop resistance R is directly proportional to the length of the loop wire, so that a two-turn wire has twice the resistance of one turn. Resistance also decreases with wire thickness. The resistance in ohms can be calculated approximately from the following formula:

$$R = \frac{0.0174\,l}{a} \tag{4.7}$$

where l is the wire length in metres and a is the wire cross-sectional area in square millimetres.

4.6.3 Loop Impedance

The total impedance of the loop can be obtained from the inductive reactance and resistance as

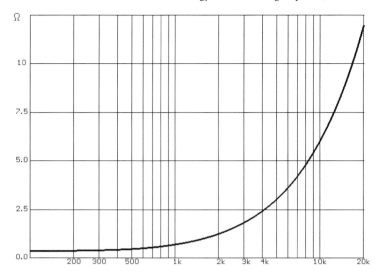

Figure 4.16 Typical impedance curve.

$$Z_T(\omega) = |Z| = \sqrt{R^2 + X_L(\omega)^2} \quad (4.8)$$

where $X_L(\omega) = \omega L = 2\pi f L$ is the coil reactance in ohms. A typical impedance curve is shown in Figure 4.16.

The IEC and BSI standards require the upper frequency to be 5 kHz, which is a compromise between quality and power requirements.

Example

Consider a loop of 10 m × 15 m with the following data:

Variable	Symbol	Value
Loop area	A	150 m²
Resistance	R	0.17 Ω
Inductance	L	96 µH
Wire cross-sectional area	α	5 mm²

The equivalent electrical circuit for this example is shown in Figure 4.17.

A current of 5.43 A in the middle of the loop at 1.2 m above the loop level is required to give the desired magnetic field strength of 400 mA m⁻¹. This requires a voltage of 3.7 V to override the impedance at 1 kHz and give the correct current and magnetic field strength. A normal loudspeaker amplifier will give constant voltage with low output impedance.

The impedance increases with increasing frequency (Figure 4.18) and the current decreases with increasing frequency for constant voltage. In this

Induction-loop Systems

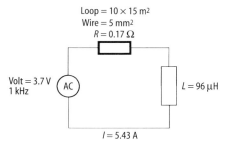

Figure 4.17 The equivalent electrical circuit of the loop-system example.

example, the upper frequency (−3 dB point) is approximately 280 Hz. This occurs when the resistance and inductive reactance are equal, so that

$$R = X_L(\omega) = X_L(2\pi f) = 2\pi f L$$

and

$$f = \frac{R}{2\pi L}$$

Hence

$$f = \frac{R}{2\pi L} = \frac{0.17}{2\pi(96 \times 10^{-6})} = 282 \text{ Hz}$$

The IEC and BS standards require the upper frequency to be 5 kHz, rather than only 282 Hz. The resistance can be changed more easily than the inductance.

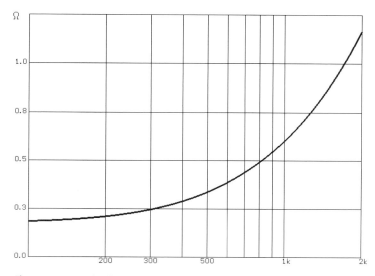

Figure 4.18 Graph of impedance against frequency for sample loop system.

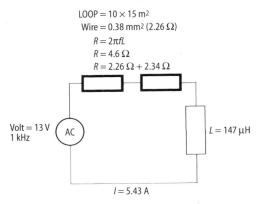

Figure 4.19 The new equivalent electrical circuit of the loop-system example.

Therefore, the inductive reactance $X_L(\omega)$ of the coil at 5 kHz is first calculated, giving

$$X_L(\omega) = X_L(2\pi f) = 2\pi f L = 2\pi \times 5000 \times 96 \times 10^{-6} = 3\,\Omega$$

The resistance can be increased to 3 Ω by using a thinner cable and a serial resistance. However, this will increase the inductance to 147 µH. The new coil inductive reactance can now be obtained as

$$X_L(2\pi f) = 2\pi \times 5000 \times 147 \times 10^{-6} = 4.6\,\Omega$$

The resistance R is then set to 4.6 Ω and obtained from two resistances in series of 2.26 Ω and 2.34 Ω (see Figures 4.19 and 4.20).

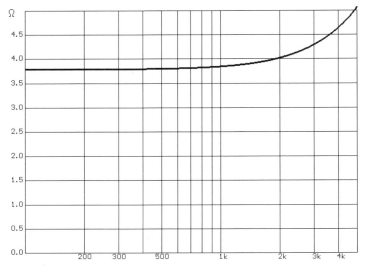

Figure 4.20 The new graph of impedance against frequency for the loop-system example.

Induction-loop Systems

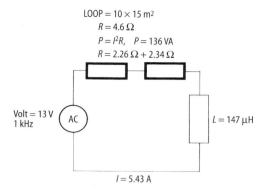

Figure 4.21 The equivalent electrical circuit of the loop system for power calculation.

The impedance will now be fairly stable, giving approximately constant current up to 5 kHz, the −3 dB point. However, there are two disadvantages. The voltage required to maintain the required current of 5.43 A will be increased from 3.7 to 13 V, due to the increased impedance. The power loss across the real part (the resistance) is very high. Figure 4.21 is used in the calculation of the power loss.

From Figure 4.21, the power loss is

$$P = I^2 R = 5.432^2 \times 4.6 = 136 \text{ W}$$

It should be noted that the power loss is frequency independent.

The use of a transformer for impedance matching is sometimes suggested, but the output impedance for a loudspeaker amplifier should be very close to zero. In a good amplifier, the damping factor, namely the connecting impedance divided by the output impedance, could be 1000. In this case, the output impedance corresponding to a loudspeaker impedance of 8 Ω would be 8 mΩ. The loop impedance is in the range 0.2–1.0 Ω. This would make it impossible to do impedance matching with the correct frequency curve. The ideal solution is to have a high impedance output, giving constant current, to a low impedance load, with high current. In this case there is a total impedance mismatch, but then this is how a loop amplifier works.

4.6.4 Two-turn Loop

When the number of loop turns is increased, the current required from the amplifier is decreased. The currents in each turn are in phase and, therefore, each turn adds current and magnetic field strength. The previous example is continued to investigate the use of a two-turn loop.

Example

Following on from the previous example, using a two-turn loop for the same area increases the inductance by a factor of four, to 588 µH, and the resistance

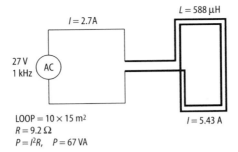

Figure 4.22 Schematic diagram of the two-turn loop system example.

by a factor of two, to 9.2 Ω (Figure 4.22). To give a total current of 5.43 A requires a current of 2.7 A in each wire of the loop. With this increased resistance, a normal loudspeaker can be used as a loop amplifier. However, the problem is still the frequency-dependent impedance, and constant current is the only solution.

To obtain the required voltage at 1 kHz, the impedance Z is first calculated. The new inductance is $L = 588$ μH. The inductive reactance at 5000 Hz is calculated as

$$X_L(2\pi f) = 2\pi \times 5000 \times 588 \times 10^{-6} = 18.5 \, \Omega$$

The new resistance is $R = 9.2 \, \Omega$ and the impedance is calculated as

$$Z_T(\omega) = |Z| = \sqrt{R^2 + X_L(\omega)^2}$$
$$= \sqrt{9.2^2 + 18.5^2} = 20.66 \, \Omega$$

The (frequency-independent) power loss across the resistance is

$$P = I^2 R = 2.7^2 \times 9.2 = 67.1 \text{ W}$$

and the associated voltage is

$$V = IR = 2.7 \times 9.2 = 24.8 \text{ V}$$

In summary, when a two-turn loop is used, compared to a one-turn loop (Table 4.1):

- the required current is halved;
- the inductance is increased by a factor of four;
- the voltage demand is increased, giving a greater risk of voltage clipping;
- there is decreased power loss in the wire.

The installation manual should give sufficient information to determine whether the use of a one- or two-turn loop is more appropriate. A twin cable should always be used, so that the decision on whether to use one or two turns can be made when measuring the field strength. In general, a two-turn loop should be tried first and the impedance decreased by using a one-turn loop if voltage clipping occurs.

Induction-loop Systems

Table 4.1 Comparison of a one-loop and two-loop system.

Variable	One-loop system	Two-loop system	Comments
Inductance L	147 µH	588 µH	Times four for two-loop system
Resistance R	4.6 Ω	9.2 Ω	Times two for two-loop system
Inductive reactance X_L	4.6 Ω	18.5 Ω	Inductive reactance X_L increased
Current	5.43 A	2.7 A	Current halved
Voltage required	13.0 V	24.8 V	Voltage demand up
Power loss	136 W	67.1 W	Power losses fall

Increasing the resistance improves the frequency range, but also increases the voltage required to achieve sufficient current to produce the magnetic field. The theoretical aims in designing a loop system should be to

- reduce the resistance
- reduce the inductance
- minimise power losses.

Unfortunately, it is not possible to achieve these three aims simultaneously for a normal constant-voltage amplifier. In particular, low impedance gives an unsatisfactory frequency response, whereas high impedance gives high power losses. The voltage output varies to compensate for changes in impedance with frequency to maintain constant current and field strength independent of the impedance.

Figure 4.23 shows the frequency-dependent power relationships for loop cables of different cross-sectional areas. It can be seen from Figure 4.23(a) that the power required is approximately 180 W at 400 Hz and 200 W at 1000 Hz for a 0.38 mm² cable area. Whilst it can be seen from Figure 4.23(b) that the power required is approximately 25 W at 400 Hz and 50 W at 1000 Hz for a 5 mm² cable area. These results are presented succinctly in Table 4.2.

4.7 Automatic Gain Control

The international IEC and BSI standards specify that a loop system should have a constant output level at 100 mA m^{-1} independent of the input level. To accomplish this, most loop systems have amplifiers equipped with automatic gain control (AGC) circuitry. The dynamics of AGC operation are defined using the Figure 4.24.

In the figure, the input–output graph defines the AGC knee-point at the lower AGC limit. This is the point at which the AGC mode begins to operate. Below the lower AGC limit the system is in linear mode, and above this point the system compresses the signal. The amount of compression is defined by the compression ratio:

$$\text{Compression ratio} = \frac{\Delta(\text{Input level})}{\Delta(\text{Output level})}$$

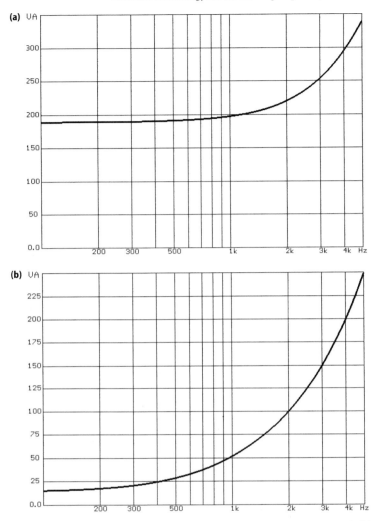

Figure 4.23 Power versus frequency for cables of cross-sectional area: (a) 0.38 mm²; (b) 5 mm².

But this is only the static part of the AGC operation. It takes time for the system to respond to AGC operation, and these response times are termed attack time and decay time. They are defined using Figure 4.25.

Table 4.2 The frequency-dependent power values for cables of different cross-sectional areas.

Cross-sectional area (mm²)	Power (W)	
	At 400 Hz	At 1000 Hz
0.38	180	200
5.0	25	50

Induction-loop Systems

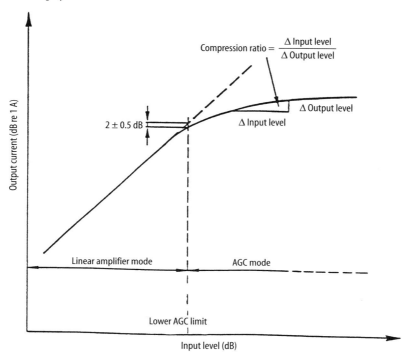

Figure 4.24 Input–output graph defining the AGC knee and degree of compression.

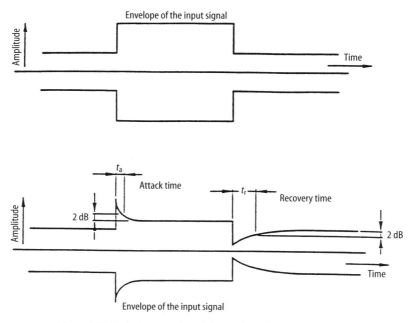

Figure 4.25 Defining attack and decay times for AGC operation.

The top part of Figure 4.25 shows the exterior envelope of a suddenly changing input signal presented to the loop amplifier. The input signal shows a sudden increase in level and then a return to the previous level; in short, a pulse. The amplifier output response can be seen dynamically in the lower part of Figure 4.25. It can be seen that the AGC action takes time to respond to the onset of the change in level, the attack time, and then takes time to recover the original level once normal input levels are resumed, the decay or recovery time.

In practice, AGC is used for automatic volume control. It has a fast attack time of 2–50 ms and a slow decay time of 0.5 dB s^{-1}. It works well with pre-controlled programmes, for instance radio and television, but its performance is not very satisfactory with a microphone or uncontrolled programme materials. In this case, the sound may disappear for a long period in response to high input.

4.8 Loop System Measurements

There are a number of parameters that are measured to determine whether a loop system, *i.e.* the amplifier equipment and the magnetic field generated, meets the requirements of the international technical standards. Also, there is a quality assurance problem of defining whether public and commercial spaces have loop systems that have been calibrated correctly. For these issues, several parameters and measuring instruments are discussed in the following sections.

4.8.1 The Dynamic Range of a Loop System

The international standard IEC 60118-4 requires the long-term average (including peaks and dips) to be 100 mA m^{-1} for speech material. The loop system should also be able to give another 12 dB increase for peaks measured with a true RMS detector with 125 ms integration time. This means that there is only a 12 dB dynamic range between the average value and the peaks. This compromise has been chosen due to the very high power demands of the peaks.

For instance, a magnetic field strength of 100 mA m^{-1} requires only a 2 W amplifier, whereas a magnetic field of 400 mA m^{-1} requires 32 W. In real speech, the 1 ms peaks are often about 20 dB above the long-term average. Therefore, very high peak current is required during short pulses for speech recognition. This is why it is necessary to specify parameters like attack and recovery times in the specification of performance. The dynamic parameter values defined by the various international standards are shown in Table 4.3.

Table 4.3 The dynamic range of a loop system.

Standard	Field strength (mA m^{-1})	Current (A)	Time (ms)	Field strength (dB)	Power (W)
IEC	100	1	–[a]	0	2
IEC	400	4	25	12	32
BS	562	5.62	10	15	63
Real world	1000	10	1	20	200

[a]Continuous.

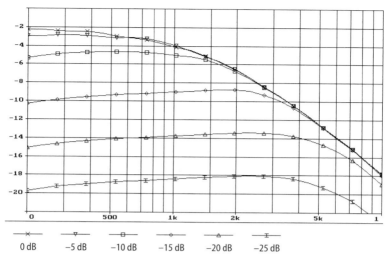

Figure 4.26 Output current from a loop amplifier with a typical inductive load applied.

4.8.2 Magnetic Field Strength as a Function of Level and Frequency

The maximum output of a loop amplifier is dependent on the loop load. In addition, impedance (which is mainly resistance) decreases with frequency. The required power and voltage are low and increase with frequency. Figure 4.26 shows the output current from a loop amplifier with a typical inductive load.

The input increases in 5 dB steps from −25 to 0 dB. The top curve at the input level of 0 dB shows the amplifier saturation at the maximum output level. Amplifier limiting (clipping) is significantly greater at higher than at lower frequencies. Since the spectrum of normal speech and music decreases with frequency, full power is not required at the highest frequencies. Thus, Figure 4.26 indicates that the high-frequency clipping will cause a reduction in speech intelligibility if a loop amplifier is overloaded.

4.8.3 Measurement of the Loop Amplifier

When measuring a loop system, care has to be taken with the connections to avoid damage to the amplifier and the measuring equipment. It should be noted that there is no common earth between the input and output terminals. In particular, incorrect connection of the measurement equipment between the signal earth and the output could lead to a large current through the measurement equipment, as the resistance at one of the inputs is only 10–200 mΩ.

It is normally the voltage that is measured by an oscilloscope as the loop amplifier output, but it is the current that creates the magnetic field, and hence the sound in the hearing aid. The current can be measured if the oscilloscope is connected between the signal earth and the output with the lowest value. The

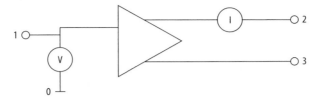

Figure 4.27 Schematic for loop amplifier measurement.

output current from the amplifier will then be shown. It should be noted that there is no common earth on the output terminals.

When taking measurements for frequency-response curves, the loop is connected across terminals 2 and 3 (see Figure 4.27). When measurements are made at these terminals across the loop, the frequency-response curve shows the voltage into the loop, as illustrated in "Plot 2" in Figure 4.28. The output voltage increases with frequency to compensate for higher impedance and maintains a constant current that gives a constant field strength. The current is shown in "Plot 1" in Figure 4.28. The frequency curve is correct for a pure resistive load.

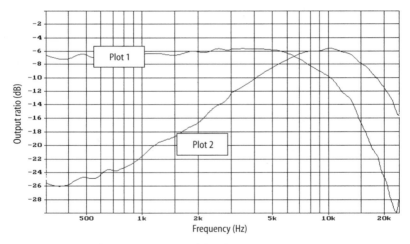

Figure 4.28 Loop amplifier frequency responses.

4.8.4 Field-strength Meters

The only way to verify that a loop is working according to an international standard is to measure it with equipment that conforms to the standard. A field-strength meter is used to measure the field strength and noise level. Standard IEC 60651 for sound-level meters requires the meter to give RMS values with a 125 ms integration time. The instrument is required to be able to measure values correctly up to at least 400 mA m^{-1} (+12 dB), and preferably up to

Induction-loop Systems

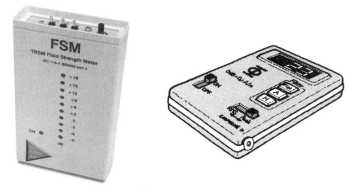

Figure 4.29 Illustrations of field strength meters.

+18 dB using a 125 ms integration time. Illustrations of typical field-strength meters are shown in Figure 4.29.

Noise level is measured using the standard A-curve (also described in IEC 60651) with attenuated bass and treble to produce sounds closer to normal human speech. The basis of the IEC standard comes from the fact that fast peaks (such as +20 dB high peaks relative to the long-term value with 1 ms duration) are included and have an averaged value over 125 ms of about +12 dB with normal conversational speech levels.

4.9 Standards for Loop Systems

Technical standards are important for two main reasons:

- to provide specifications with regards to performance, quality, safety and reliability;
- to give standardisation between the same product produced by different manufacturers.

Safety is always an important part of standards. It covers things like exposure to toxic substances, radiation and loud sounds, as well as electromagnetic compatibility. As new information becomes available, safety regulations in standards often become stricter. Changes in technology also mean that performance specifications are revised upwards.

Most electrical components are standardised. For instance, batteries come in a number of different standard sizes (as well as voltage ratings). Therefore, it is possible to buy a battery with confidence that it will fit in the space available. However, many everyday mechanical components are not often standardised. Therefore, if you break or lose one part, you may have difficulty finding a part that fits and you will probably have to buy the whole component, not just the part you need and carry out a more complicated repair.

There are both national and international standards. Most countries have their own standards. There are now also European standards. The main international standards are maintained by the International Electrotechnical Commission (http://www.iec.ch) and the International Organisation for Standardisation (http://www.isc.ch). UK standards are maintained by the British Standards Institute (http://www.bsi-global.com). The European Committee for Standardization maintains European standards, which are generally available from the national standards bodies of member countries. The American National Standards Institute (http://www.ansi.org/) maintains US standards.

Standards are generally referred to by numbers, preceded by the letters IEC, ISO, BS, EN and ANSI for the different organisations, and often followed by the year they were introduced. Standards are generally updated regularly. When this happens they may be given new numbers.

The international standards for induction loops are as follows:

- IEC 60118-0 (1983-01). Hearing aids – Part 0: Measurement of electroacoustic characteristics.
- IEC 60118-0-am1 (1994-01). Amendment No. 1.
- IEC 60118-1 (1999-0). Hearing aids – Part 1: Hearing aids with induction pick-up coil. The standard specifies a method for determining the electroacoustic performance of hearing aids fitted with an induction pick-up coil and used in an audio-frequency magnetic field. The induction pick-up performance is measured in a loop that simulates conditions of use in a room.
- IEC 60118-3 (1983-01). Hearing aid equipment not entirely worn on the listener.
- IEC 60118-4 (1984-01). Magnetic field strength in audio-frequency induction loops for hearing aid purposes.
- IEC 60118-4-am1 (1998-06). Amendment 1.

IEC 60118-4 requires the frequency response to be linear between 100 and 5000 Hz, with a permitted ±3 dB deviation at 1000 Hz.

4.10 Learning Highlights for the Chapter

The home living environment can be very noisy, person interfaces for public and commercial services are surrounded by noise and competing voices, and entertainment venues have complex sound properties. For the hearing-impaired these are difficult places to access. Induction-loop technology is an assistive technology that can use the telecoil in the hearing aid to make these difficult sound environments accessible once more. The presentation in this chapter gave a good indication of the depth of electrical engineering used by this technology. The induction loop is probably one of the most beneficial applications of electromagnetic principles in our society today.

In this chapter, the basic electrical engineering principles of loop systems were presented. The individual components and physical effects present in a loop system were described. An electrical engineer's appreciation of the factors important to the installation of an induction-loop system was given. As a mature technology, the implication and the need for international induction-loop system standards were explained.

Projects and Investigations

1. Use a field-strength meter to carry out measurements of loop strength of a number of loop systems installed in public buildings. Evaluate the performance of the system by comparing it with the international standard. If performance is found to be unsatisfactory, discuss the findings with the management.
2. Examine how loop systems are used in a commercial environment like a bank. What are the problems of using these installed systems? Consider both the technical and the human-centred problems.
3. Consider the process of designing and installing a single-loop system for a small- to medium-sized room that is to be used as a classroom. All the design guidelines listed in the text should be followed. Draw up an installation procedure. Check the performance of the installed device.
4. Quite often, charitable organisations involved in presenting their work to outlying audiences have to use rooms and locations that do not have permanent induction-loop facilities installed. Such organisations would use a portable induction-loop kit. Draw up a set of guidelines that can be used by lay-personnel to ensure that the temporary installation of a loop system is successful. Contact a local organisation and offer to test out the procedure devised.
5. Simulation tools to demonstrate and investigate induction-loop properties were an important feature of this chapter. Conduct a Web search to identify some of the software tools available for induction loop simulation. Construct a comparison of the features of the software products found. Try out freeware to simulate some of the results presented in this chapter.
6. Using the design guidelines listed in the chapter, design a loop system for a large room. Complete two separate designs using:

    (a) a system with a single loop

    (b) a system configured as a figure-of-eight loop.

    Use the freeware located during project 5 to simulate the two designs. Use the simulations to compare and predict the anticipated performance of the two loop-systems. Give a list of advantages and disadvantages of using simulation tools for design exercises. State practical installation effects not covered by the simulation work.
7. An important device used with induction-loop technology is the hearing-aid telecoil. Investigate the engineering principles of the telecoil. Conduct a survey to see whether the telecoil used with:

    (a) induction-loop facilities in public induction-loop facilities really does satisfy end-users;

    (b) a telephone meets the satisfaction of hearing-aid users.
8. The hearing-aid telecoil is an important transducer used with induction-loop technology. Examine the engineering principles used by a telecoil. Use a simulation package to simulate the extent of the electromagnetic field propagated by a telephone handset. Investigate how the telecoil is calibrated for use with a telephone.

References and Further Reading

Further Reading

Books

Bird, J., 2001. *Electrical Circuit Theory and Technology*, 2nd edition. Newnes Book Publishers.
Edminster, J.A., 1983. *Electric Circuits*. McGraw-Hill Book Company.
Kraus, J.D., Fleisch, D.A., 1999. *Electromagnetics with Applications*, 5th edition. McGraw-Hill, Boston.
Sadiku, M.N.O., 1995. *Elements of Electromagnetics*, 2nd edition. Oxford University Press.

Technical Papers

Aardal, A., 1983. The magnetic field of telephone instruments and their sensitivity to magnetic fields. *Telektronikk* 79 (3-4), 244-249 (in Norwegian).
Anon., 1982. Audio induction loop systems for the hearing impaired. *Audio Engineering Society Preprint, Paper number: REPR 1924 (I-5)*. Bolt Beranek & Newman Inc., Cambridge, MA, USA.
Anon., 1982. Induction loop paging system. *Elektor* 8 (1), 32-37.
Capel, V., 1983. Portable induction loop (hearing aid facility). *Electronics Today International* 12 (7), 52-53.
Kringlebotn, M., Sorsdal, S., 1981. Guidelines for the dimensioning of induction loop systems (hearing aid application). *Scandinavian Audiology* 10 (4), 225-233.
Larbi, K., Johnson, M.A., 2001, Is the tele-coil a successful assistive technology device? *Preprints, First International Conference on Assistive Technologies for the Vision and Hearing Impaired*, CVHI'01, Pisa, Italy.
Laszlo, C.A., 1994. Engineering aspects of assistive device technologies for hard of hearing and deaf people. *Canadian Acoustics* 22 (3), 77-78.
Letowski, T.R., Donahue, A.M., Nabelek, A.K., 1986. Induction loop listening system designed for a classroom. *Journal of Rehabilitation Research & Development* 23 (1), 63-69.
McKinnon, B., 1994. Electromagnetic interference in hearing aid T-coil applications. *Canadian Acoustics* 22 (3), 79-80.
Nabelek, A.K., Donahue, A.M., Letowski, T.R., 1986. Comparison of amplification systems in a classroom. *Journal of Rehabilitation Research & Development* 23 (1), 41-52.

5 Infrared Communication Systems

5.1 Learning Objectives and Introduction

Infrared (IR) light has a number of different applications in the wireless transmission of audio signals, both for hearing-impaired and hearing listeners. In particular, it can be used as an assistive listening device, which allows individuals to control the volume at which they receive auditory signals and to set other parameters depending on the application.

5.1.1 Learning Objectives

The basic aims of this chapter are to give readers an understanding of the properties of IR radiation that allow it to be used to transmit auditory information and to describe some of the resulting applications. Specific learning objectives are:

- to appreciate that IR radiation is part of the electromagnetic spectrum;
- to understand the special propagation properties of near IR radiation;
- to learn the importance of the common properties of IR and radio-frequency design and their effect on the circuit design for the electrical signals;
- to understand the basic principles of the design of IR auditory transmission systems;
- to learn about the range of current applications of IR transmission systems.

5.2 Basic Principles

IR radiation forms part of the spectrum of electromagnetic radiation. IR radiation has wavelengths from less than 1 µm (10^{-6} m) to more than 100 µm, whereas the currently applied electromagnetic spectrum extends over several decades of wavelengths from the submicrometre light region to the radio application region with wavelengths of several kilometres. This is shown in Figure 5.1, where the symbols λ, f and c are used to denote wavelength, frequency and the velocity

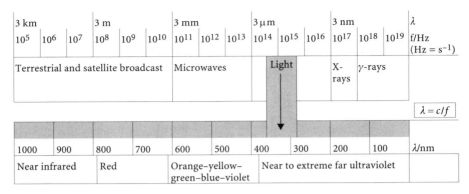

Figure 5.1 Electromagnetic radiation and its applications.

of light respectively. These velocity measures of wave propagation come from the basic formula

$$\text{Velocity} = \text{Frequency} \times \text{Wavelength}$$

The frequency of the wave, denoted f, is usually given in cycles per second, or hertz (Hz). The speed of light is taken to be a constant and denoted by c (m s^{-1}). Thus, using the formula, for waves travelling at the speed of light the wavelength, denoted λ (m), is given by

$$\text{Wavelength} = \frac{\text{Velocity}}{\text{Frequency}} \quad \text{or} \quad \lambda = \frac{c}{f}$$

Early IR systems were based on tungsten lamps with filters or laser sources. Both were unsuitable for consumer audio uses, as neither of them met every requirement of low cost, modulation bandwidth, easy installation with low directivity problems and operation without radiation risk. The introduction of semiconductor emission diodes in the early 1970s allowed the development of IR systems for domestic applications at reasonable cost.

5.2.1 General Technical Requirements for Audio Applications

The use of IR radiation in the wireless transmission of audio signals allows individuals to listen to a distant source at their own chosen volume (or in their chosen language), without requiring either listener or speaker to be connected by a cable to a fixed device. Thus, there are applications for both hearing-impaired and hearing listeners. As this type of transmission is generally required in closed areas, the restricted propagation properties of IR light have an advantage over radio waves, which can penetrate walls and extend to unexpected locations.

When current is flowing through diodes, many of the electrons in the diode material are lifted to higher energy levels. They then release some energy and return to lower levels. The energy released can be transformed into an electromagnetic wave of short duration, in this case in the IR range. Rather than an

Infrared Communication Systems

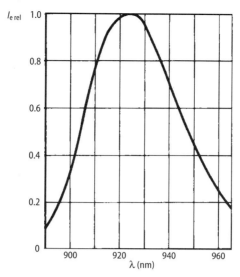

Figure 5.2 Variation of relative emissions with wavelength for a silicon-doped GaAs diode.

exact value for emissions being available, they are expressed in terms of probabilities. The power distributions over a longer period give a power distribution centred on a maximum value. The wavelength of this maximum depends on the properties of the material being used. It was about 930 nm for the first gallium arsenide (GaAs) diodes. Their relative emissions $I_{rel} = I/I_{max}$ decay by half at about 900 and 955 nm. Modern IR light-emitting diodes, commonly referred to as IREDs, use GaAs doped with aluminium (GaAlAs). Figure 5.2 shows the variation of the relative emissions with wavelength for a GaAs diode.

For several reasons, the audio signal controls the diode current indirectly, by means of modulation techniques, rather than directly. High-quality audio channels use frequency modulation (FM) rather than amplitude modulation, giving improved signal-to-noise ratio (SNR). The instantaneous frequency of the carrier $\omega_i(t)$ follows the information signal $s(t)$ as a deviation around the carrier middle frequency ω_c and involving a spreading factor m

$$\omega_i(t) = \omega_c + ms(t) \tag{5.1}$$

The use of the term FM is only correct with regard to the subcarrier used to modulate the intensity of the IR sources. Direct FM of the light frequency is not possible, as emitting diodes are neither monochromatic nor coherent but emit a wide spectral range of uncorrelated light "shots".

5.2.2 Applications

IR systems are used in the following applications:

- amplification of TV, radio and home entertainment audio systems
- amplification of audio signals in theatres, cinemas and concert halls

- multimedia
- one-to-one conversations
- group discussion
- meeting and conference support
- provision of information in museums
- schools
- remote control.

Amplification of TV, radio and home entertainment audio systems, particularly for people with hearing impairments, was the earliest application and still uses the greatest number of IR sets. IR allows a group of people to listen to the TV at different volumes without disturbing other people in the room who do not want to listen to the TV. A one-channel mono transmission system with a 95 kHz subcarrier was developed in 1975 (Griese, 1976). A stereo transmission system for hi-fi use with a second channel on 250 kHz soon followed (Werner, 1976) and 2.3 and 2.8 MHz subcarrier technology was introduced later. Although a well-designed transmitter and headphones for digital CD sound transmission has also been developed, they are not used as much as analogue stereo systems.

To avoid extra audio cabling, mobile loudspeakers with a built-in IR receiver have been developed (Hibbing and Werner, 1985). Many theatres, cinemas and concert halls have installed IR equipment. System standardisation (IEC, 1983) and component miniaturisation allow users to bring their own receivers as an alternative to hiring them for the performance. Theatres and cinemas also use multimedia applications of IR (Werner, 1978). Additional information can be transmitted for blind visitors or visitors from abroad. Cinemas also use IR for music effects that cannot be supplied by loudspeakers due to special effects or, for example, high sound-pressure levels. Even open-air drive-in cinemas have been equipped with IR installations to avoid the need for loudspeaker terminal installation over the whole visitor area. The inclusion of still pictures or video is possible but requires a much wider bandwidth than purely audio transmission.

For one-to-one conversations, adding another microphone input to the transmitter allows people with hearing impairments to have conversations even when the TV receiver is on. A transmitter with microphone input has also been used for speech training for pupils with hearing impairments.

The use of IR for group discussions depends on the particular conditions. When all participants sit in a fixed location with a microphone in front of them, all the contributions can be mixed and transmitted with an IR transmitter. This situation is very similar to conference applications of IR systems.

There is a smooth transition from group discussion to meeting and conference support. In addition, IR systems can be used to allow different groups in a meeting to be addressed individually. Simultaneous translation into a number of languages is a commonly used application of IR systems. A number of different channels are available and there are advantages over induction-loop systems. Most manufacturers offer compatible systems based on a common standard (IEC, 1997a). This makes it easy to rent additional receivers if there are more delegates than expected or available equipment can support. IR systems, rather than loudspeakers, can be used to provide amplification for all participants in lectures and public addresses, including religious services with hearing-impaired participants. They have the advantage of allowing participants to choose their own level of amplification, whereas loudspeaker systems may be too loud for some participants and too quiet for others.

Multichannel IR systems can be used to provide information for museum visitors. Existing technical implementations could not be used due to special fading requirements in overlapping zones. This problem has been resolved by multiplexing several pulse amplitude-modulated channels (Werner, 1985).

In schools, a two-channel system was initially used for supporting pupils with hearing impairments, and a fixed stereo microphone in front of the class picked up the teacher's voice (Griese, 1977). Now teachers wear a small transmitter, including the microphone, round their necks and can move round freely (Griese, 1981).

There are a number of other potential applications. For example, prototype systems for providing information on train arrival and departure and orientation in stations for blind people have been developed. However, there are still a number of unresolved problems, such as temporary obstacles and pre-adjustment for individual hearing, and further developments will be required before such systems can be used.

5.2.3 Technical Features and Application Requirements

As with most other technical devices, many design details are determined by the application and the specifics will differ with the application. The area covered by an IR source for a specified audio quality in the receiver depends mainly on the following:

- the installed IR power
- the location and number of sources
- the modulation scheme
- the strength of interfering sources.

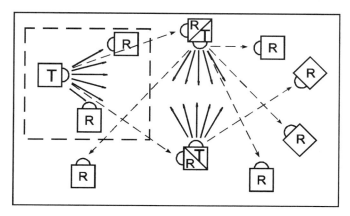

Figure 5.3 Schematic plan of an IR system for a small room (dashed borders) and a large room with a booster/repeater (T: transmitter; R: receiver, R/T: booster/repeater).

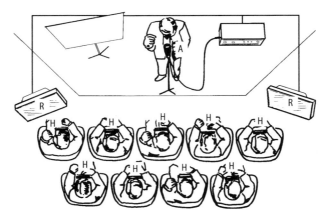

Figure 5.4 Typical application set-up.

Mains-operated transmitter components can provide nearly unlimited IR power for TV and conference listening if cost and safety conditions are met. Performance measurements have shown that:

- one concentrated source near the wall can readily provide the necessary IR power density of approximately 3 mW m^{-2} for room sizes up to about 30 m^2;
- a number of distributed IR emitters are recommended for larger areas to reduce intensity losses, which increase with the square of the distance from the source, as well as losses through transparent areas such as windows.

As shown in Figure 5.3 for a special pulse-modulation system, the transmitter and receiver can either be separate units or even combined in one unit for pulse-repeating purposes; Figure 5.4 illustrates the application of IR transmission in a typical application set-up representing the greatest number of installations. In this set-up the audio source A (microphone), the transmitter T and the radiators are single elements and the participants wear IR headphones H. Such headphones include all the functions from detection to audio reproduction.

5.3 System Components

An IR audio system consists of at least two parts connected by a wireless link:

- a transmitter with a microphone (or other audio signal source), a suitable electrical energy source and the IR emitters;
- a receiver with an optical input device, signal-processing stages, an energy source and an electroacoustic transducer (headphone or loudspeaker).

Each of these parts may be a separate unit connected to other components by cabling or combined into transmitter and receiver units. The main components are illustrated in Figure 5.5.

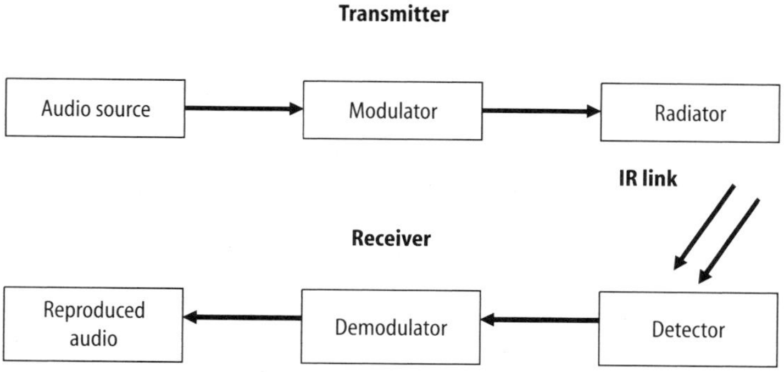

Transmitter

Audio source → Modulator → Radiator

IR link

Receiver

Reproduced audio ← Demodulator ← Detector

Figure 5.5 Main blocks of an IR audio transmission system.

5.3.1 Audio Sources and Signal Processing in the Transmitter

The following signal-processing functions are generally required: amplification, spectral treatment (*e.g.* bandwidth adjustment and equalisation) and modulation. When there is a microphone output the signal level is only in the millivolt range and has to be amplified for the next stage. On the other hand, the level of the audio output of a TV receiver or a CD player can be high enough for direct use. Therefore, the audio input of the IR transmitter has to be designed very carefully, either with restricted level handling capability and electrical or other protection against too high an input signal or with a wide level range including manually or automatically operated gain control.

Only a limited modulation spectrum is available, and it may have to be used for several audio channels in parallel. Multichannel systems, therefore, have to operate with less channel bandwidth than mono or stereo transmission. This leads to an appropriate audio bandwidth limitation, for instance of 8 kHz for conference systems with 40 kHz channel bandwidth.

Most multichannel systems use an electrically multiplexed signal of all channels, rather than separate IR sources for each channel. This has the advantage of allowing the total available IR power to be used, independently of the number of activated audio channels. Precautions are required to avoid non-linear electrical interaction between the channels, particularly at higher amplification. If the resulting non-linear components are in the spectral range of the other channels, audible distortion may result. An equal low-noise floor is also desirable in each audio channel to give good SNR and similar performance in each path.

To improve dynamic efficiency, FM transmission uses an equalisation known as pre-emphasis. This increases the amplitude of the higher audio frequencies. Inverse filtering in the receiver is required to recover the original spectral balance. The replacement of IREDs with, for instance, high-pressure gas discharge lamps or light-emitting polymers has also been investigated. However, factors such as reliability, cost, the current state of the art and efficiency have confirmed the decision to use IREDs for these system applications.

5.3.2 Radiators

Semiconductor devices can emit radiation in several different wavelength bands, including visible light and IR. Light-emitting diodes (LEDs), which produce light in the visible range, are mainly used for displays and illumination, whereas IREDs have their main application in communication technology. The mechanical design is largely dependent on the optical requirements. Therefore, diodes for the visible and IR light range are generally manufactured with the same tools (Figure 5.6).

IRED chips are manufactured by cutting the semiconductor wafer in two perpendicular directions. The chips are small, typically not more than 0.5 mm by 0.5 mm. Emissions come mainly from the edges, and this size gives a good relationship between surface area and total edge length. The complete diodes are soldered into printed circuit boards (PCBs). They include at least the chip, two leads for the power supply and a transparent housing. The housing contains all components and protects the chip. One of the leads normally acts as a chip carrier and can also serve as a reflector. In this way, radiation that would otherwise be absorbed in the rear part of the diode housing or on the circuit board is added to the emissions from the front.

The shape of the reflector, its encapsulation and its optical properties can be varied to produce diodes with different directional radiation characteristics. Wide-angle diodes were often used in the early radiators. The diode with the characteristic shown in Figure 5.7 shows almost cosine dependency on the angle to the reference axis. Its radiation has half the maximum value at an angle of ±60° with the reference axis.

As the number of diodes manufactured increased, so did the market for a wider variety of different types of diodes. In many applications, diodes with medium beam width with a strong on-axis beam are appropriate. Such diodes provide sufficient IR power incident on the walls and sufficient diffuse reflection of IR power. This type of diode has a longer front part, which acts as a

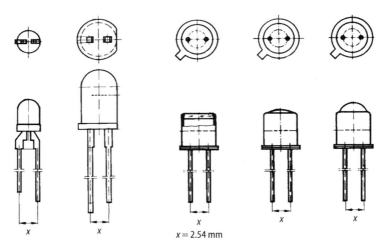

Figure 5.6 LEDs and IREDs.

Infrared Communication Systems

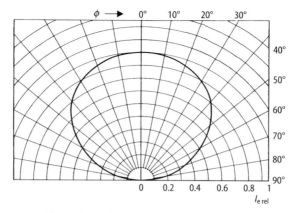

Figure 5.7 Wide-angle diode characteristic.

focusing lens, and a parabolic reflector behind the chip, as illustrated in Figure 5.8. Very narrow beams can be obtained from diodes with a glass lens and an air gap in front of the chip, but they are only useful in point-to-point links.

Direct control of the IR frequency is not possible. Therefore, the source can only be modulated by varying its intensity from zero to the available maximum. One of the simplest ways of doing this is by switching the diodes on and off. This is only possible in single-channel operation, as this modulation causes a high number of harmonics with slow decay. When there are multiple audio channels, all the subcarriers should be sinusoidal. This prevents inter-channel interference from harmonics and non-linearities.

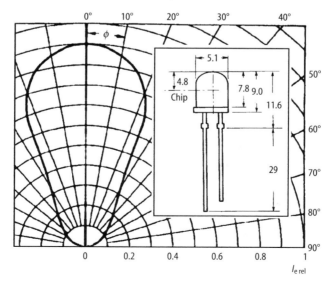

Figure 5.8 Medium-angle diode.

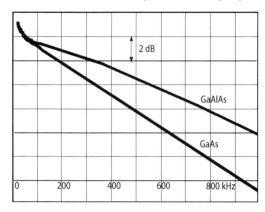

Figure 5.9 Variation of output with frequency.

Relatively low subcarrier frequencies are used, as signal efficiency decreases with rising frequencies. For example, GaAs diodes lose roughly 12 dB between 100 kHz and 1 MHz, as shown in Figure 5.9. Temperature effects also limit the available power from IREDs. Diodes may lose about 50% of their radiant flux when the case temperature is increased from 30 to 85 °C.

Some manufacturers have added aluminium reflectors to diodes to improve cooling and increase radiation towards the front direction. Six of these units are sufficient for a mono transmitter/radiator to provide a normal living room with sufficient IR power (see Figure 5.10). This compact transmitter is generally connected by the jack plug (right) to the headphone output of TV receivers. To keep the transmitter small enough to be placed on top of the TV, the mains transformer and the rectifier diodes are combined with the mains plug (behind the transmitter).

The thermal resistance between the chip and its surround can be reduced by mounting the chips on metal or ceramic backplates with sufficient size and an appropriate heat-sink structure. This design is used in professional equipment, as it has high performance at a reasonable cost. Thin insulating foils with

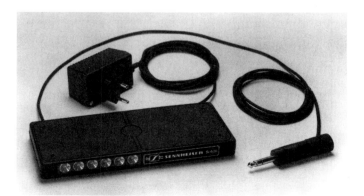

Figure 5.10 Single channel transmitter/radiator for home use.

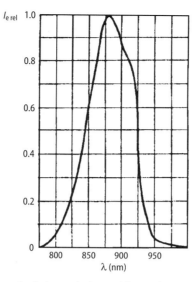

Figure 5.11 Variation of relative emissions with wavelength for GaAlAs diodes.

low thermal resistance between wiring and heat sink can be used for printed wiring. Bonding automates are used to connect the second chip contact. If fans are used to provide additional cooling, care is required to minimise the motor and ventilation noise and also the maintenance requirements due to the limited lifetime of the rotating parts.

The introduction of GaAlAs technology increased the efficiency of the electro-optical conversion and also led to a shift of the spectral maximum from the earlier 930 nm to about 880 nm, as shown in Figure 5.11. There were compatibility problems with earlier units, but the near doubling of efficiency was a convincing reason for change wherever possible.

IR power of a few watts is required for larger rooms and for multiple channels. Most IREDs in use for audio systems have an IR emission of 10 to 20 mW, so that some hundred diodes may be necessary for a congress room with a multichannel interpreter system. In this case, it is best to split up the total power by using separate radiators.

Depending on the room requirements, different radiator models, with about a dozen to several hundred diodes, are available. In larger rooms, radiators should be placed in corners at sufficient height to reduce intensity differences and shadowing effects. Cooling is required to prevent an increase in chip temperature and reduction in IR power, even with the relatively low DC power of less than 2 W from 11 diodes (Figure 5.12). Passive cooling is preferable to the use of ventilators, which may be noisy or have maintenance costs. Smaller radiators can achieve this cooling by using short connections between IREDs and circuit board, a sufficient area of copper on the PCB to provide a heat sink and well-positioned slots in the housing.

Large first-generation radiators had an external DC power supply, but more modern systems have built-in switching supplies for greater flexibility. This does not increase the weight or the power dissipation significantly. Finned profiles are used to increase the heat radiation area without enlarging the housing

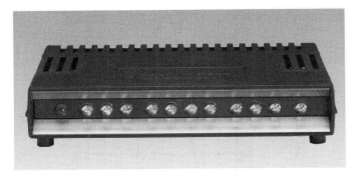

Figure 5.12 IR radiator with 11 emitting diodes.

significantly. These radiators (Figure 5.13) can be used for on-axis distances of more than 100 m. An SNR of about 40 dB can be achieved on-axis at a distance of about 105 m, as shown in Figure 5.14. A high SNR is required for good audio quality, but a lower SNR of 26 dB may be accepted for short time periods or in particular conditions. Signal power becomes reduced off-axis, and the distance for a particular signal power decreases as the angle increases.

IR transmission is generally carried out in rooms with at least partially reflecting walls. This increases the IR intensity in otherwise weakly supplied areas. In free propagation, the intensity decreases with the inverse square of the relative distance to the source. All the optical rules for visible light are valid for the IR range. An ideal reflecting wall acts as a mirror and allows the propagation to draw from a mirror source of the same strength. Beams that hit a transparent window will leave the room. Most materials, including bricks, carpets and wood, absorb some of the incoming IR radiation, and absorption losses of 50% are frequently assumed. However, measurement is required to obtain more exact values.

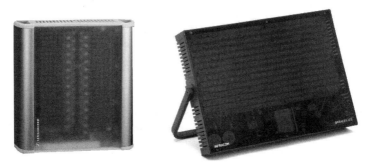

Figure 5.13 IR radiators with some 100 IREDs.

5.3.3 Receivers

The receiver has to obtain sufficient IR power from the radiated signal to reproduce the audio signal with the required quality parameters. These

Infrared Communication Systems

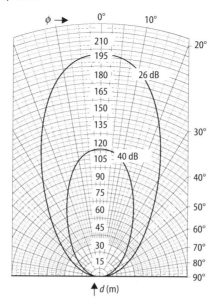

Figure 5.14 Variation of SNR with angle and distance.

include bandwidth, SNR, linearity and channel separation. The receiver can be considered to carry out the following six main operations:

- optical preprocessing
- optoelectrical conversion
- preselection and preamplification
- channel selection
- demodulation and audio amplification
- electroacoustic conversion.

Optical preprocessing can be used to improve the incoming transmitter signal before further processing with regard to level and suppression of unwanted components. The photodiode, and in particular the PIN diode, has been found to give the best option for converting the IR signal to an electrical one. PIN diodes have an intrinsic layer (I) between the P- and N-zones, can be used at higher frequencies and have their maximum sensitivity in the IR range, as shown in Figure 5.15. Their usable range extends from the maximum at about 900 nm by approximately 250 nm in the IR direction and 450 nm towards the visible and ultraviolet spectrum. Thus, bright daylight can produce a higher current in the diode than the carrier of an IR audio system.

A chip size of 3 mm × 3 mm:

- gives low capacitance
- operates at higher frequencies
- has sufficient area for adequate output for incoming IR signals of usual strength.

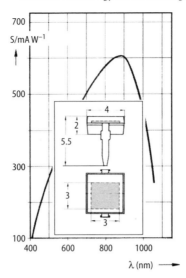

Figure 5.15 PIN diode current as a function of wavelength and radiation perpendicular to chip surface.

The area limitation and the reaction to light components other than those of the corresponding transmitter determine the possibilities for optical preprocessing.

The options for removing unwanted signals depend on their spectral content. The responses to unwanted spectral components can be reduced by an optical filter placed directly in front of the detector chip. Only dye filtering is used, as this is direction independent and IR inputs come from variable directions. Suitable dyes (microscopic colour particles) provide a smooth but soft suppression of the daylight range. They can either be embedded in a separate plastic foil placed on top of the sensitive diode surface or embedded directly in the optically transparent housing. In addition to suppression of unwanted spectral components, the maximum sensitivity of the diode can be shifted to match the spectral output of GaAlAs emitter diodes. For instance wavelengths below 700 nm, where the untreated diode has 70% of its maximum output, can be almost totally removed (see Figure 5.16).

Diodes generally have photosensitive chip areas of less than 10 mm^2. Owing to the high spectral sensitivity, many single-channel applications only require one diode in the receiver. In many cases, increasing the chip area or the number of diodes per input would not be useful due to increased capacitance. Directly covering the chip with a lens-shaped cap gives an increase of the angular sensitivity, going from a maximum on the axis to zero at ±90° and always remaining positive (see Figure 5.17). The front cap acts as a special magnifying glass. The gain increases with the refractive index of the lens material. Highly refractive glass is expensive, heavy and complicated to handle. Therefore, thermoplastic materials are generally used. They provide refraction values of about 1.5 and approximately double the optically sensitive area.

After the IR input signal has been converted by the photodiode into an equivalent electrical signal, further processing mainly involves increasing selectivity and amplification. In the simplest conversion circuit, illustrated in

Infrared Communication Systems

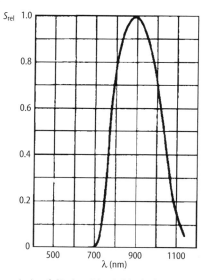

Figure 5.16 Characteristic of diode with visible-light components suppressed.

Figure 5.18, the current through the photodiode D causes a corresponding voltage at a resistor R_2. Most unwanted spectral components can be removed if the transmitter signal bandwidth is limited, as is the case for FM systems. In one-channel audio transmission systems low-frequency components of the room illumination, including harmonics of 50 or 60 Hz fluorescent lamps, can be removed by a capacitor C between the diode load resistor and the first preamplifier transistor T. Resonant or other complex filter circuits instead of a simple RC combination can further reduce unwanted spectral components.

After preselection and preamplification of the complete signal, the appropriate number of channels, *e.g.* two for stereo, is chosen. In single-channel transmission with a 95 kHz subcarrier only the illumination and other interfering signals have to be suppressed. Stereo transmission on 95 and 250 kHz subcarriers can be separated in the receiver with two band-pass circuits (see

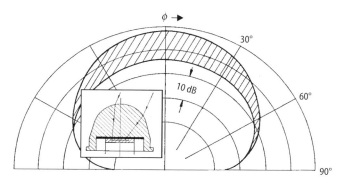

Figure 5.17 Diode with a lens-shaped cap.

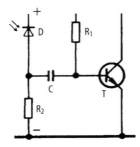

Figure 5.18 Simple conversion circuit.

Figure 5.19). Even higher selectivity is needed for multichannel conference systems than for stereo operation, as they use a channel grid of 40 kHz with each channel occupied by a signal composed of 8 kHz audio bandwidth and 7 kHz maximum deviation. Mechanical resonators generally perform better, with less loss and better long-term stability, than filters based on discrete capacitors and inductors. Alternatives to very expensive crystal filters are ceramic resonators. They are also available as multiple resonator combinations in one package and may either be used for direct channel selection or in an intermediate frequency (IF) stage. The latter approach is generally used in multichannel devices, as it allows the tuning oscillator frequency to be derived from only one crystal reference frequency and standard synthesiser semiconductor circuits to be used.

Demodulation is used to reconstruct the audio content of the signal in the selected channel. Custom-designed circuits are used in special cases, but most applications use integrated circuits manufactured for FM radio. This is possible because radio and IR transmission are very similar at the electrical level and there is, for instance, minimal difference between IR single-channel and FM broadcast mono systems.

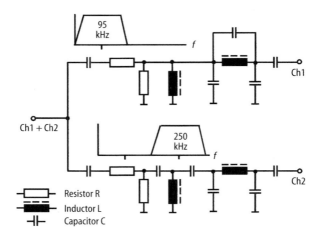

Figure 5.19 Channel selection with band-pass circuits in a 95/250 kHz system.

Infrared Communication Systems

Some integrated circuits already include audio amplifiers; these provide sufficient power for the operation of small electroacoustic transducers, such as earphones or pocket loudspeakers operating at about 100 mW. Higher acoustic power for the transmission of speech or music into large rooms or open-air arenas can be generated by separate amplifiers or a combination of amplifiers and loudspeakers.

5.4 Compatibility and Use with Hearing Aids

Hearing aids with a standardised audio input socket can be connected to IR receivers with audio output by a cable using the appropriate connectors. Some receivers have been designed to supply an adjustable level for hearing-aid use. Connecting cables with fixed or adjustable attenuators can be used.

If the hearing aid can only pick up external signals by induction, there are two types of transmitter loops that conform with the standardised interface (IEC, 1981, 1998, 1999a,b). A loop around the neck can be used with one audio channel and also provides users of binaural hearing aids with mono programmes. Stereo transmission requires two separated magnetic fields, each of which transmits to the corresponding hearing aid. Very small, flat coils have been developed for this purpose. They can be worn behind the ear together with the hearing aid (see Figure 5.20).

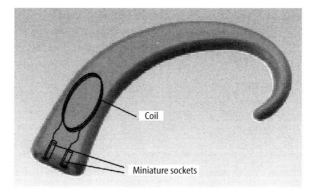

Figure 5.20 Small flat coil to be worn behind the ear ("X-ray" view).

5.5 Design Issues

Design issues for IR systems include the following:

- system placement
- interfering environments
- ergonomic, social and psychological factors.

5.5.1 System Placement

System placement depends on the application. For watching TV and theatre or cinema performances, most people face forward. Therefore, radiators should be installed facing the audience and receivers have diodes pointing in the radiator direction, *i.e.* in the same direction as the observer's eyes. Quality may be reduced slightly if the listeners move their head or body, but should remain good. In pure acoustic situations, such as listening to the radio or CD, the signal from the radiator to the receiver can come from any direction. The similarities between visible light and IR should be used to position the radiator, so that the listener receives as much reflected radiation as possible. Therefore, radiators should not face transparent or highly absorbing areas, such as windows or dark curtains. In conferences where the desks and chairs are not arranged in parallel rows facing the speaker, a diffuse IR level should be provided by distributed radiators.

5.5.2 Interference Issues

The original design of IR systems took account of the IR component from daylight and artificial light, including fluorescent lamps at mains frequency. However, fluorescent lamps with ballast circuits at higher frequencies were then introduced. They have unexpected modulation components up to some hundred kilohertz on spectral lines from mercury, quite near to the emission maximum of the GaAs diodes in use. Some IR applications that use higher subcarrier frequencies do not experience interference from these sources. For other applications, the users of fluorescent lamps and IR systems are informed of the possibility of interference.

IR audio systems can also experience interference from IR remote control systems and IR computer wireless data exchanges (IEC, 1993). Avoiding interference with out-of-band radio sources is easier. Redesigning the connections on PCBs, introduction of selective electronic traps and shielding can be effective in preventing interference.

5.5.3 Ergonomic and Operational Issues

Basic rules for ergonomic design include easy handling, low weight, a one-piece solution (to avoid additional components that can be lost) and adequate operating cycles. In addition, large controls may be required, particularly as many users will be in older age groups and may have reduced vision or manual dexterity.

The first stethoscope format TV sound receivers met these requirements and worked very well. Sound is transported from a central receiver to both ears by acoustic tubes. Modern IR receivers have two channels and the headphone transducers are connected directly to the ears. The circuit and power supply can be placed in the middle of the unit on a very compact circuit board (see Figure 5.21). Current headphone receivers weigh about 45 g.

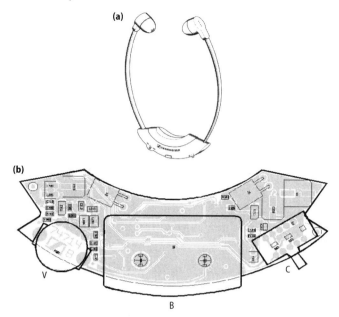

Figure 5.21 (a) IR receiver; (b) cross-section of IR receiver.

The on–off switch is combined with the volume control V for a "silent start". Although tiny metal-hydride button cells are now used, the battery B still takes up most of the space. The switch C allows the selection of stereo and single-channel operation on two different signals. The built-in headphone transducers provide a maximum sound-pressure level of 110 dB and up to 130 dB on a special version. This allows most users with moderate or medium hearing loss (20 to 40 dB) to use the IR system on its own without a hearing aid. However, the high output level of the special version means that advice from audiologists on handling and adjustment is required.

A power consumption of about 20 mW allows operation for about 5 h without recharging the batteries. Most IR headphones have charging units that can be plugged into the mains. For recharging, either the whole headphone system is placed on the charging unit, which is often included in the transmitter, or the box containing the rechargeable cells is removed and placed on the charging unit. Regular charging is desirable to avoid the system cutting out unexpectedly.

IR systems have a range of applications for hearing people. This may make them more acceptable for some people with hearing impairments, as they are not so obviously a technical aid for people with hearing losses. The extended use of portable audio sources, generally called "Walkman", particularly at high volume, is leading to hearing loss. So far, IR systems are not implicated in causing hearing loss, due to user habits. However, further observation will be required to identify those products that do not have any deteriorating effects on hearing, provided that they are used properly.

5.6 Technical Standards and Regulations

All IR audio transmission equipment has to follow the design requirements for good engineering in the relevant application areas. Several general regulations, including directives of the European Community (EC), exist or are being developed.

An important issue for all electronic equipment is electromagnetic compatibility. The EC has published requirements for emissions and immunity for a wide range of radio frequencies (EC, 1989). Following these requirements is legally required in EC countries. Regulations for the visible and invisible light wavelengths are still under discussion.

Another important area covered by standards and regulations is safety (EC, 1992). This includes mechanical safety (sharp edges, weight, *etc.*), electrical safety (for mains-operated equipment) and radiation risk (EC, 1999; IEC, 2000). However, particular care is required in following the manufacturer's instructions carefully before carrying out maintenance or repairs on high-power radiators.

The main technical documents that affect IR audio transmission devices are the following:

- Technical Report IEC 1147 (IEC, 1993)
- International Standard IEC 60118 (IEC, 1998, 1999a)
- International Standard IEC/TS 60825 (IEC, 2000)
- International Standard IEC 61603 (IEC, 1997a–d)
- International Standard IEC 61920 (IEC, 2002).

5.7 Advantages and Disadvantages of Infrared Systems

IR systems have a number of advantages, largely derived from the fact that IR does not penetrate opaque surfaces, such as walls. Therefore, IR systems with different information content can be used in optically separated rooms. Users do not need to change or adjust the receiver when going into another room with different IR information content. IR audio transmission does not require an official licence in most countries, as it is generally confined in a (closed) room. IR transmission equipment can be made totally immune to out-of-band electromagnetic fields and does not suffer from multipath interferences.

The disadvantages and limitations of IR systems are largely the opposites to the advantages. In general, they cannot be used outside in daylight and for long distances. Unlike analogue audio application, which has a large number of channels, IR emitters can only be used for a small number of digital audio links because of the limited modulation range. As IR is an unprotected band, careful investigation is required before installation to exclude other IR sources, which could cause interference. The very small active detector area of IR systems in unidirectional operation means that they require more transmitting energy than radio-frequency equipment. Therefore, portable transmitters require special modulation techniques. However, no system is all-purpose. IR systems have a wide range of applications, but no system can be used to support all listening situations. As with other products, it is important to decide when the use of IR systems is appropriate and when the choice of another technology would be preferable.

5.8 Conclusions and Learning Highlights

There have been very significant developments in sound transmission with IR radiation over the last 25 years. Single and multichannel devices for pure audio and multimedia applications are now available. In principle IR transmission can be applied to all sound sources and used wherever wireless audio is required.

As well as the extension of existing IR technologies to new applications, there are also possibilities for the enhancement of these technologies. This includes the use of a digital format, as well as the development of new materials and components. The information rate at a given location could be increased by the use of extremely selective elements, which split the usable range of IR wavelengths into several bands which can operate independently of each other.

5.8.1 Learning Highlights of the Chapter

IR systems play a useful role in assistive technologies for the hearing impaired. Thus, they are valuable systems allowing accessibility to entertainment for those with age-related deafness. We also learned how these systems extended to broader applications for hearing listeners. We learned how IR radiation can be generated by emitter diodes and received by receptor diodes, and that these basic properties can be engineered as a communication system.

In particular, we learned something of the following:

- how the medium of transmission was seen to be part of the electromagnetic spectrum;
- how diode construction was configured to form and receive a beam of IR radiation;
- how the basic principles of the IR communication system lead to design and construction constraints for the design of the components of the transmission and receiver systems;
- about the range of applications of IR transmission systems and discussed the advantages and disadvantages of this type of assistive technology.

Acknowledgements

The author thanks the companies Braehler and Sennheiser for their permission to use product photographs and diagrams in preparing some of the figures for this chapter. The author and the editors would also like to remember the contributions of Helmut Braehler to this technological area. Helmut Braehler was originally asked to write this chapter but, owing to a severe illness, could not take on the task and sadly passed away while this chapter was being written.

Projects and Investigations

1. Obtain spectral data for daylight, tungsten lamps and fluorescent lamps. Determine the spectral power density (mW m^{-2}) of these sources at a wavelength window of 750 to 1050 nm under the assumption that every source is providing an illumination of 1 klx.
2. The relative emission characteristic of an IRED is given in the following table:

Angle α (deg)	0	10	20	30	40	50	60	70	80	90
Relative intensity	1	0.96	0.86	0.5	0.18	0.1	0.05	0.02	0.01	0

Obtain an approximate expression for this characteristic by determining the appropriate integer value for n in the proposed formula

$$I_{rel} = (1 - |\alpha|/90)^n \cos\alpha$$

where I_{rel} is the relative radiant intensity and α is the angle measured to the vertical axis of the diode.
3. Apply the method of mean-square-error to calculate the accuracy of the approximation determined in project 2.
4. The radiant intensity of an IRED in the axial direction is given by $I_E = 8$ mW sr^{-1}. Calculate the total radiant flux Φ_e by using the approximation

$$I_{rel} = (1 - |\alpha|/90)^n \cos\alpha$$

for the relative intensity and then solving the resulting integral for the semi-sphere of radiation.
5. A radiator with 20 diodes has a total IR power of 400 mW at a characteristic given by the equation in project 4. How many of these radiators will be required to give at least 3 mW m^{-2} at all points in a room 10 m × 20 m. Consider the following two cases:
   (a) no reflection at all;
   (b) total reflection from any surface including users.
   The different possible positions of the radiators should be considered in the solution.
6. By tracing selected light beams, demonstrate that the application of a semi-spherical lens directly combined with a receiver diode chip will never lead to a negative gain.
7. Calculate the on-axis gain of the combination of a semi-spherical lens with a receiver diode chip as a function of the relative dimensions and the

refraction index n of the lens material. Simplify the resulting expression by assuming that the chip is of circular shape.

8. Consider a photo diode with a sensitive area of 7 mm^2, a sensitivity at 950 nm of 0.6 A W^{-1} and a dark current of typically 2 nA (with a maximum 30 nA). Calculate the signal current when the diode is exposed to 3 mW m^{-2} IR radiation and compare this current with the dark current.
9. A photo diode has noise equivalent power of 4.3×10^{-14} W Hz$^{-0.5}$. Calculate the SNR ratio when the diode generates a signal output of 60 nA at a load resistor of 10 kΩ and the signal is filtered to 300 kHz bandwidth.
10. Investigate the literature on the properties of modulation characteristics to explain why the carrier or IF SNR is not directly transferable to the audio SNR.

References and Further Reading

References

EC, 1989. Council Directive of 3 May 1989 on the approximation of the laws of the Member States relating to electromagnetic compatibility (89/336/EEC). *Official Journal of the European Communities* 23.5.89, pp. 19–23.

EC, 1992. Council Directive of 29 June 1992 on general product safety (92/59/EEC). *Official Journal of the European Communities* 11.08.92, pp. 24–32.

EC, 1999. Council Recommendation of 12 July 1999 on the limitation of exposure of the general public to electromagnetic fields (0 Hz to 300 GHz), (1999/519/E). *Official Journal of the European Communities* 30.07.1999, pp. 59–70.

Griese, H.-J., 1976. Audio auf Infrarot, Möglichkeiten und Standards. *Radio-mentor-electronic* (11), 440–442.

Griese, H.-J., 1977. Mehrkanalanlagen mit Infrarot-Übertragung. *Radio-mentor-electronic* 43 (7).

Griese, H.-J., 1981. Sound transmission with infrared light for the hearing impaired, part 3. *Audiologische Akustik* (2), 34–41.

Hibbing, M., Werner, E., 1985. Ton aus der Luft gegriffen, Lautsprecherzeilen drahtlos. *Funkschau* (2), 55–56.

IEC, 1981. *International Standard IEC 60118-4, (1981-01) Hearing aids. Part 4: Magnetic field strength in audio-frequency induction loops for hearing aid purposes*. International Electrotechnical Commission, Geneva.

IEC, 1983. *International Standard IEC 764, Sound transmission using infra-red radiation, first edition*. International Electrotechnical Commission, Geneva. [Replaced by actual standard IEC 61603 and subparts for different applications.]

IEC, 1993. *Technical Report IEC 1147, Uses of infra-red transmission and the prevention or control of interference between systems, first edition*. International Electrotechnical Commission, Geneva.

IEC, 1997a. *International Standard IEC 61603-3 (1997-10) Transmission of audio and/or video and related signals using infra-red radiation – Part 3: Transmission systems for audio signals for conference and similar systems*. International Electrotechnical Commission, Geneva.

IEC, 1997b. *International Standard IEC 61603-1 (1997-01), Transmission of audio and/or video and related signals using infra-red radiation – Part 1: General, IEC 61603-1 Corr.1 (1997-05) Corrigendum 1*. International Electrotechnical Commission, Geneva.

IEC, 1997c. *International Standard IEC 61603-2 (1997-03), Transmission of audio and/or video and related signals using infra-red radiation – Part 2: Transmission systems for audio wide band and related signals*. International Electrotechnical Commission, Geneva.

IEC, 1997d. *International Standard IEC 61603-6, Transmission of audio and/or video and related signals using infra-red radiation – Part 6: Video and audio-visual signals, 100C199/CDV*. International Electrotechnical Commission, Geneva.

IEC, 1998. *International Standard IEC 60118-4-am1, Hearing aids. Part 4: Magnetic field strength in audio-frequency induction loops for hearing aid purposes, Amendment 1.* International Electrotechnical Commission, Geneva.

IEC, 1999a. *International Standard IEC 60118-1, Hearing aids – Part 1: Hearing aids with induction pick-up coil input, Ed. 3.1 Consolidated edition.* International Electrotechnical Commission, Geneva.

IEC, 1999b. *International Standard IEC 60118-6 Hearing aids – Part 6: Characteristics of electrical input circuits for hearing aids.* International Electrotechnical Commission, Geneva.

IEC, 2000. *International Standard IEC/TS 60825-7, Safety of laser products – Part 7 (2000-06): Safety of products emitting infrared optical radiation, exclusively used for wireless 'free air' data transmission and surveillance.* International Electrotechnical Commission, Geneva.

IEC, 2002. *International Standard IEC 61920, Infrared transmission systems – free air applications.* International Electrotechnical Commission, Geneva. Work in progress.

Werner, E., 1976 Wireless audio transmission with infrared light for studio applications. In *53rd Convention of the Acoustical Engineering Society*, Zürich, preprint D-7.

Werner, E., 1978. Drahtlose Kommunikationstechnik im Theaterbetrieb. *Bühnentechnische Rundschau* (Oktober), 8–13.

Werner, E., 1985. Sprechende Bilder, Drahtloser Museumsführer. *Funkschau* (2), 44–46.

Further Reading

Books

Bergh, A.A., Dean, P.J., 1976. *Light-emitting Diodes.* Monographs in Electrical and Electronic Engineering. Clarendon Press, Oxford.

Gayford, M. (Ed.), 1994. Radio microphones and infra-red systems. In *Microphone Engineering Handbook*, Butterworth-Heinemann, chapter 5.

Ueda, O., 1996. *Reliability and Degradation of III–V Optical Devices.* Artech House Optoelectronics Library, Artech House.

Technical Papers

Griese, H.-J., 1978. Sound transmission with infrared light for the hearing impaired, part 1. *Zeitschrift für Hörgeräteakustik* (4).

Griese, H.-J., 1978. Sound transmission with infrared light for the hearing impaired, part 2. *Zeitschrift für Hörgeräteakustik* (5).

Griese, H.-J., 1982. Sound transmission with free propagating infrared light, part 2: Discontinuous modulation techniques. In *71st AES Convention*, preprint 1880 (D-2).

Werner, E., 1982, Sound transmission with free propagating infrared light, part 1: Continuous modulation techniques. In *71st AES Convention*, preprint 1879 (D-1).

6 Telephone Technology

6.1 Introducing Telephony and Learning Objectives

 Electrical technology has been used to support telephony access for hearing-impaired people by both telephone handset manufactures and public network operators. Features such as amplification, sockets for additional earpieces, control of ringer pitch, and coupling to hearing aids can be provided to make telephones more accessible for hearing-impaired people. Where audio communication is not viable, alternatives such as text or signing can be used over telephone systems. Within public telephone networks, relay centres can now enable a hearing person to talk to a deaf person by providing an operator who can translate speech in real time into text.

User involvement in the design of modern telecommunications products is a key issue if the technical complexity of their underlying technologies is to be made accessible to a broad public customer base. There are simple straightforward methods, drawn from ergonomics, human factors or engineering psychology, that can be used to include user issues within the design of products and services. These can range from simple discussion groups, through to laboratory studies and field trials of prototype terminal equipment or network services.

In this chapter, the key ways in which electrical technology can be used to meet the needs of hearing-impaired people for access to telephony products and services within the terminal will be identified. The way that these features have been implemented in telephony terminals to improve access for hearing-impaired people will be explained. Where relevant use of circuit elements will be made, but the chapter does not go into detailed circuit design or the calculation of circuit parameters.

The learning objectives for this chapter are to give the reader an introduction to:

- the basic concepts of user-centred telephone design;
- simple methods for involving the user;
- key support features and how they can be integrated into a telephone terminal;
- designing a simple text telephone terminal;
- engineering videophones for hearing-impaired people.

6.2 User-centred Telephone Design

Simple low-cost features can have a major impact on the ease of use of telecommunications products or services. Designing user-friendly systems needs sensitivity to the users' characteristics, limitations and requirements and the application of user-centred methods. We all find it difficult to use a product or service if the user interface fails to take our human limitations into account. A motor, sensory, or mental impairment only becomes a handicap if it prevents a product from being used. Good industrial design can prevent this interaction and drive up the ease of use to enable all customers to benefit from the product.

People with hearing impairments are simply part of the broad range of human variation that a product needs to be able to cater for. People vary significantly in many ways, including variations due to impairments. A tall person has a different reach from a short person or someone in a wheelchair. A young engineer may have very different mental skills from an artist, accountant or senior citizen.

6.2.1 Designing for Hearing Impairment

Identifying user requirements and then implementing the resulting design improvements is more expensive the further down the design life cycle it is carried out. The full range of users should be considered at the earliest possible stage in a project. The processes are similar whatever the user group.

It's Good to Talk

There is no substitute for talking to customers, and people with hearing impairments are no exception to this good practice. It is relatively easy to do. Government departments and non-government organisations that provide services for hearing-impaired people will often help. They can often identify people to take part in requirements capture, usability testing or field trials of new services or products. They may also be able advise on how to contact people with a specific impairment, and they may have facilities, such as clubs or day centres, where it is possible to hold group discussions or try out new prototypes.

Conceptual Design

The requirements of potential customers should be considered when the concepts of a new product or system are being developed. Here, the designers should aim to define what a product will offer and what usability targets it should meet. Interviewing existing users, analysing ways in which people use similar products and investigating how they currently cope without the proposed product are all useful approaches to gathering information relevant to usage and usability. This can also help in the task of identifying and interpreting existing recommendations and guidelines.

Capturing user requirements provides the foundations for a successful design, though several iterations and the stimulus of early prototypes may be needed. If the intention is to include an accessibility feature into a mass market product it may simply be necessary to ensure that people with hearing impairments are included in the marketing, testing and field trials of the product.

Iterative Improvement

Trying out a simulation or prototype with potential users reveals ways of improving ease of use and allows user performance to be compared with targets. Improvements can be made to the prototype system and supporting documentation, followed by another cycle of improvement. The flexibility of personal computers often enables sophisticated prototypes to be taken out of the laboratory to wherever is most convenient for the potential customers, such as a club or day centre.

Laboratory testing enables usability to be measured scientifically. Potential users carry out representative tasks with the prototype under controlled conditions and performance and opinion data are gathered. The effects of unwanted variables are eliminated by careful planning and statistical techniques. In addition, valuable insights into improvements come from people's informal comments about the system.

Laboratory trials take place in a rather artificial situation. Field trials forego the rigorous control of the laboratory, but they have the advantage of exposing a new product to potential customers in much more natural circumstances. This is a useful way to find out how a new product fits into the lives of real customers. Self-reporting diaries, discussion groups of users and most other ways of monitoring a trial will be applicable to participants with a hearing impairment. It may be necessary to tailor trial support or monitor arrangements to the specific abilities of the participants, *e.g.* it may be necessary to arrange for sign language interpretation for deaf participants or manual language interpretation for deaf–blind participants.

A key aspect of setting up any field trial is to ensure that the system being tested has real value to the participants so that they are motivated to use it. With a communications service this means selecting participants who have a clear reason for wanting to communicate with each other.

Benchmarking

Comparisons between products make it possible to identify which are strongest and where there are opportunities for improvement. A checklist of important system parameters makes it easy to compare products. Wherever possible, the comparison should include evaluation and consultation with the disabled people who will be using the product. Simply checking against recommendations that are based on current practice is not always adequate, owing to the rate of change of telephony technology at the moment.

6.2.2 Putting It All Together

People with motor, sensory or mental impairments are part of a broad population who can benefit from telecommunications services. Designing for all potential users, not just a theoretical average, reduces costs, improves ease of use for everyone and ensures that people with special needs are not handicapped by unfriendly technology. When designing telephony products and services, don't just think about the technology. Know what it will be used for, what the product will do, who the users are and in what situations they will be using it.

In an ideal world a design team will:

1. Consult potential users about their ideas for the product in order to build a requirements specification and identify performance targets.
2. Build a prototype and keep going through cycles of test and modification in the laboratory until it meets the minimum performance identified in 1.
3. Field-trial prototypes or early products in a realistic setting and modify the design to deal with the issues raised by the participants.

This may not be possible owing to practical constraints of the availability of prototypes, access to skilled human resources, time, *etc*. However, simple consultation with a few users before staring out on a project, then testing early prototypes with a few more users, can go along way to identifying any major usability issues and suggest ways of designing them out of a product in a cost-effective manner.

6.3 Design of an Electronic Telephone

Whilst computing networks and, in particular, the Internet, are experiencing explosive growth in terms of the size and numbers of end-users today, it is very easy to forget that "communication networks" or systems have been around for well over a 100 years. To begin with, these systems were based on telegraphy and were used for very low-speed character-based communications. By about 1876, as a result of experiments by Alexander Graham Bell to send multiple telegraph signals over one wire, the concept of the telephone as a speech apparatus was born. This was then further refined into a practical and usable instrument, such that by the turn of the 20th century a sizeable telephone network was beginning to grow in the UK and elsewhere in the world.

It was obvious almost from the start that, for speech communication by the telephone to really grow and become accessible to everyone, rather than just the rich, the system itself would require high levels of automation. Initially, connecting a call was carried out manually by the operator at the local exchange by physically plugging a particular cord into the appropriate socket on a manual switchboard. This was, of course, a labour-intensive method of switching calls and not suitable for large-scale deployment. For this and other commercial reasons, a Kansas City undertaker, called Almon B. Strowger, designed an automatic mechanical substitute in 1889. His main motivation for doing so was simply that he had a suspicion that the local telephone operator was favouring a competitor of his whenever anyone lifted the receiver and

Telephone Technology

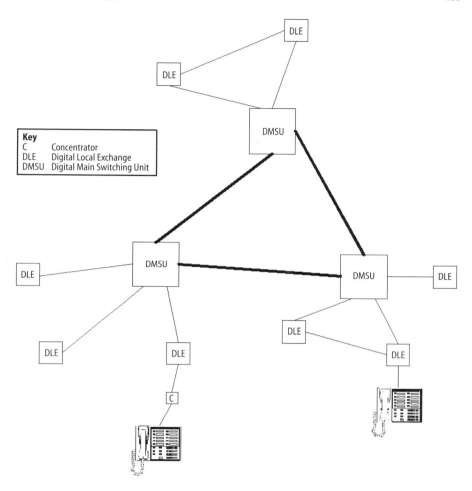

Figure 6.1 Hierarchy of the UK telephone network.

asked for a local undertaker. This was further reinforced when he found out that the operator concerned was the wife of the rival funeral directors! Strowger's design was immensely successful and formed the foundation for switching technology in telephone systems and was only significantly replaced by more modern electronic and digital technology in the UK by the start of the 1980s.

Today, the UK network is entirely switched using digital technology. Figure 6.1 shows the hierarchical structure of the telephone system. To maximise the utilisation of the actual interconnection paths between switching centres, calls are handled by various "tiers" according to where the call originates, where it is destined and whether there are locally more direct links that may exist if there is sufficient call traffic to justify them.

Each customer or subscriber (as they used to be referred to) is physically connected to their local exchange by a pair of wires. Currently, for standard voice services (*i.e.* not digital services), communication over these wires is still using the same basic analogue electrical representation as originally pioneered by Bell. As is described in more detail in the following sections, speech is converted into electrical signals whose amplitude and frequency are a direct analogue of the actual speech itself. At this stage there is no signal encoding, and the only signal conditioning applied is as a result of the performance of the transducers in the handset and circuitry in the telephone. These characteristics combine to restrict the signal frequencies, typically to the range 300 Hz to 3.4 kHz, and gives rise to the slightly "flat" sound of speech when heard on the telephone. In the future, all communication, whether it is voice, data, video, music, *etc.*, will be handled using digital encoding; thus, potentially, one type of network could be used for all forms of communication.

It is at the local exchange that the analogue signals are converted into a digital representation, and this point marks the boundary between analogue and digital communication. Since this applies in both directions, *i.e.* transmitting and receiving speech, the conversion from analogue to digital and back again is required in both directions. Other signals, such as dial tone or call arrival indication (ringing signal to ring the bell), similarly require conversion from a digital to an analogue domain. For this reason, a dedicated circuit (usually a single integrated circuit) called a subscriber's line interface circuit (SLIC) is used to provide the necessary circuit functions to interface the analogue line with the digital domain of the switching and ongoing communication systems.

Having converted the incoming speech into a digital bit stream (typically at 64 kbit s^{-1}), the call can then be switched via the selected digital path over the network to the far end. Clearly, if the calling and called parties are both connected to the same exchange, then it is matter of simply passing the incoming data on one port or connection to the destination port, and *vice versa*, on the same exchange. Alternatively, if, as shown in Figure 6.1, the two digital local exchanges (DLEs) share a common connection, then the traffic may well be sent that way. For longer distance calls, however, it is usual to pass the call up to the next level of hierarchy, usually the digital main switching unit (DMSU). All the DMSUs in the network are fully interconnected, so that a direct path will exist to the destination DMSU that hosts the required distant DLE. From here the call is passed directly to the required customer via his line connection, again using the SLIC, this time to provide the reverse digital to analogue conversion.

Where the concentration of customers on a particular exchange is low, it may be more cost effective or efficient not to bother to provide any switching at the local exchange. Instead, one can pass all the telephony traffic up to a neighbouring local exchange and handle it there as if it were directly connected to that exchange. This is the function of a concentrator, which again converts the analogue calls to digital telephony but simply passes this traffic though to another exchange for actual switching.

6.3.1 Introducing the Modern Telephone

The design of the modern telephone is now quite different to that of, say, 30 years ago. In the past, telephones were designed using virtually no electronic components, and instead used the same basic principles of telephony developed during the early 20th century. For a long time, telephone design had been based on moving-coil receivers, carbon granule transmitters and anti-sidetone induction coil (ASTIC) circuits, *i.e.* electromagnetic components. Nowadays, the benefit of modern semiconductor electronics allows the design to perform better, to be more flexible (so that it can be made for more than one country) and also to be cheaper to manufacture.

In spite of this, however, the basic functions that a telephone has to provide are still the same. These may be summarised as transmission (which also includes a two- to four-wire conversion) and signalling. These two basic functions are separated by the two modes in which the telephone is used. Firstly, it is used either to initiate or answer a call. For both cases some form of network signalling is required. In the case of initiating a call, the telephone is first required to indicate to the network the user's intention to make a call (the user simply lifts the handset to begin the call) and then the telephone is required to transmit the dialled digits that the user enters in a form that the exchange can detect and decode at the far end of the line. Secondly, having set up (or answered an incoming call for that matter), the telephone is required to provide a suitable transmission medium in which the user's voice is converted to suitable electrical signals for transmission down the telephone line and equally provide the receive path to enable the distant end to be heard.

Although these basic telephony functions have not changed during the development of the public switched telephone network (PSTN), they have evolved in the manner in which they are carried out. A good example of this is the way in which the telephone is connected to the network, *e.g.* a single pair of wires is still used to carry out all the communications functions required. Whilst the main part of the network has been updated to digital transmission systems, the communication from the telephone to the exchange is still carried over a single pair of wires that has to provide both the transmit and receive paths for the call. The reason for this has always been to keep the cost of the expensive cabling from the numerous customers to the exchange to a minimum. Providing separate pairs of wires for the transmit and receive paths would be wasteful and inefficient.

Whilst this clearly keeps the number of wires required and, therefore, the size of the cable to a minimum, it does mean extra complexity in the design of the telephone. Over a single pair it is necessary to indicate the initiation or reception of a call and carry the speech associated with the call itself. The speech normally involves both ends and, therefore, must be in both directions over the same pair of wires. Thus, a means must be devised where the simultaneous send and receive signals are split at the user's telephone back into separate paths to be passed to the microphone and receiver in the handset respectively. This is the function of the two- to four-wire conversion that is implicit in the operation of all telephone transmission systems and is a key area of the design process.

Hence, from these rudimentary requirements, certain functional units of the telephone become clear, *viz.*

- it must provide a method of indicating the start of a call to the network;
- it is required to encode and transmit the telephone number dialled by the user;

- it must provide two-way communications for the duration of the call;
- it must indicate to the network the cessation of the call;

and in the case of an incoming call

- it must provide a method of alerting the user of an incoming call.

The way in which these functions are implemented in the modern telephone will now be examined.

6.3.2 Indication of the Start of the Call

Even with only two wires there are several ways in which a telephone could potentially signal the start of the call to the exchange. For example, the circuitry could apply certain voltage signals to the line to indicate different states in a manner used by other communications systems (*e.g.* RS232 serial interface on a personal computer (PC)). In reality a much simpler system is used, mainly because of historic reasons; the principal one being that the exchange essentially provides all the power necessary for the telephone to function. Even in the case of telephones with batteries and power supplies, it is still a design aim that the telephone should provide basic functions even when not locally powered, *i.e.* exchange power should be sufficient to provide the functions listed above. Therefore, to initiate a call, the telephone simply "loops the line" with a low-resistance DC path whose value is chosen to ensure sufficient power for the telephone, but high enough not to affect significantly the AC impedance of the telephone, which is critical for good transmission performance.

Thus, once again, a simple signalling system is used; but even this has more than one function. Not only does the low-resistance termination provide the means to indicate the start of the call, but also the ongoing loop is then interpreted as an indication of the continuing requirement by the user to maintain the call for the period the loop is applied. The current and voltage (*i.e.* power) that is then derived from this state is thus also providing the power the telephone requires for the duration of the call.

The indication of the desire to cease the call is thus simply a matter of removing the loop and the exchange then clears the call by removing the transmission path that had been established for the duration of the call.

6.3.3 Transmission of Signalling Information

As with all transmission systems, it is necessary to encode or translate the information to be transmitted into a form appropriate for the communications medium. In the past, the simplest method to pass signalling information (*i.e.* the required far-end telephone number) was to signal over the telephone pair by breaking and remaking the terminating loop. It could be argued that this signal is open to misinterpretation by the exchange, since, as described before, such a signal is used to indicate the start and end of a call. This is overcome by ensuring that such "make" and "break" periods of the terminating loop are of such a duration that they can be both understood but equally are not to be confused with the start and end of the call.

For this reason, the make period (which occurs between two break periods) should be nominally 33 ms and the break period should be nominally 66 ms, thus making a total of 100 ms to signal a single digit. Now, if one such event (*i.e.* make–break) is defined to be the digit "1", and two events in succession are defined to be the digit "2", *etc.*, then it is clear how the digits "1" through "9" can be signalled. Clearly, it is nonsensical to have the digit "0" encoded as no such event so instead this is defined to be 10 make–breaks periods in succession. Thus, the time required to send a single digit varies from 100 ms for "1" though to 1 s for "0". The signalling rate is a maximum of 10 pulses (in the case of digit "0") per second or 10 pps as it is often written.

Further, it can be seen that it is quite a straightforward process to design a mechanical rotary dialler for the telephone such that the user inserts their finger in the hole for the appropriate digit and rotates the dial until it stops, winding up a spring in the process; see Figure 6.2. The dial is then released and, via a governor system used to regulate the speed, then transmits the digits required as it returns to its rest position. The mechanical dialler (or electronic equivalent for that matter) must also ensure that no more than 10 successive pulses are sent, as this would cause confusion at the exchange.

As the rotary dialler returns to its rest position, a period of about 800 ms is naturally inserted between successive digits dialled; this provides a convenient interlude between the dialled numbers. This period was originally intended to be of sufficient duration to give the exchange equipment time to receive and process the dialled digit (*i.e.* switch the call via a mechanical selection device call a "selector"). This period is therefore referred to as the "interdigital pause" (IDP).

This method of signalling, because it relies on short periods of making and breaking the loop termination, is referred to as loop-disconnect (LD) signalling. It is still supported on the modern digital exchanges in use today, but its use is decreasing as people replace their old telephones. One of the main reasons for changing this method of signalling was the time taken to dial and switch a call. Users are used to entering numbers on keypads, such as calculators, keyboards, *etc.*, and expect to do so with telephones. As telephone numbers have increased in length over the years, the time taken to dial a call using LD signalling has become significant (typically 10–20 s for modern numbers).

(a)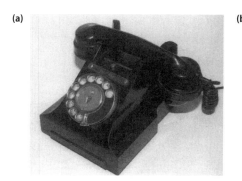

(b)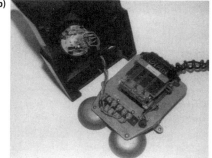

Figure 6.2 A rotary telephone dial: (a) external view; (b) internal view.

Table 6.1 Potential DTMF characters and their corresponding frequency pairs.

	Column 1 – 1209 Hz	Column 2 – 1336 Hz	Column 3 – 1477 Hz	Column 4[a] – 1633 Hz
Row 1 – 697 Hz	1	2	3	A
Row 2 – 770 Hz	4	5	6	B
Row 3 – 852 Hz	7	8	9	C
Row 4 – 941 Hz	* (star)	0	# (hash)	D

[a] Characters A, B, C and D do not form part of the standard telephone keypad and are reserved for special signalling modes.

For this reason, a newer system, known as dual-tone multi-frequency (DTMF) signalling, was introduced about 20 years ago and is now the standard in-band (audible) way call set-up information is encoded and transmitted across the network. As its name suggests, the signalling method uses tones rather than make–break pulses. These tones have been carefully selected to occupy the centre part of the normal audio transmission range of a telephone, which is typically 300 Hz to 3.4 kHz. As can be seen from Table 6.1, these frequencies range from 697 to 1633 Hz and are arranged in two groups: a low-tone group (697, 770, 852 and 941 Hz) and a high-tone group (1209, 1336, 1477 and 1633 Hz). Each digit is then sent using one tone from the low group and one tone from the high group, the particular tone pair being used defining the digit being sent. Using a row/column matrix arrangement in this way gives two advantages. Firstly, it requires only eight separate frequencies to convey the 16 possible combinations available, rather than the 16 required if separate frequencies are used. Secondly, it is much easier for the far end (exchange) to decode the two frequencies together in the face of any other noise or signals (*e.g.* speech) on the line. This is because the frequencies have been carefully selected so that the likelihood of them appearing together in normal speech signals is statistically very low. This ensures that the chance of a wrongly interpreted digit is minimised (as this would lead to a wrong number).

On a standard telephone, the duration that the DTMF tone is applied for is normally a function of how long the user chooses to press the appropriate keypad button. Since the tone is also coupled into the handset receiver as an audible feedback to the user, they normally release the key once they have heard the tone. This makes the period that the tone is sent typically between 50 and 200 ms. Since most exchange DTMF receivers can decode the signal providing it persists for about 30 ms then this is normally adequate. Equipment that dials automatically is normally programmed to have a tone ON period (*i.e.* the time when the tone is heard) of 100 ms followed by a tone OFF period (or inter-digital pause) also of about 100 ms. Thus, even at this speed, a 12 digit number can be transmitted completely in about 2.4 s (12 × 200 ms), which is about five to ten times quicker than LD signalling.

Notice also in the table of frequencies that there are extra codes available for additional characters, viz. "*" (star), "#" (hash or square as it is called) and special codes "A", "B", "C" and "D". This is another advantage of DTMF over LD signalling: more codes can be sent and, therefore, can used for additional services, such as three-way calling, short-code dialling, *etc*. The codes "A" through "D" do not appear on the normal telephone keypad and are reserved for special signalling equipment.

6.3.4 Design of the Transmission Circuit

The key function of the transmission circuit is to provide the interface function between the actual telephone pair (or wires) and the speech transducers, *i.e.* the microphone and receiver. Since the speech is two-way and only a single pair is used for the conveying of the speech signals in both directions, it is necessary for the telephone to perform a "hybrid" or two- to four-wire conversion process; this is illustrated in Figure 6.3.

Whilst it is desirable for some of the near-end speech to be heard locally in the receiver (this is known as "sidetone"), it is very undesirable for this sidetone level to become too high. The problem is compounded by the varying line conditions that the telephone may encounter. For the hybrid function to work well, it is important that the telephone be designed so that its impedance "matches" the line to which it is connected. Clearly, in practice, it is not possible to ensure that the design will always be right for every line, as the lines themselves vary somewhat in their characteristics, typically their length. Thus, it is always a compromise to design the telephone to work as well as possible on a range of different line types.

In older telephone designs, this hybrid function was carried out by a clever magnetic component called the ASTIC. This is shown in Figure 6.4. It was designed to provide a controlled level of sidetone back to the user by cancelling most of the transmitted signal from that of the receiver. In practice, this worked quite well for most line characteristics and was used widely up and till modern electronic telephones.

Nowadays, an integrated circuit to provide the required transmission functions in one complete transmission circuit is used. Such devices usually require

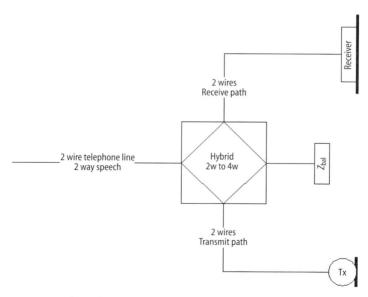

Figure 6.3 Telephone two- to four-wire conversion.

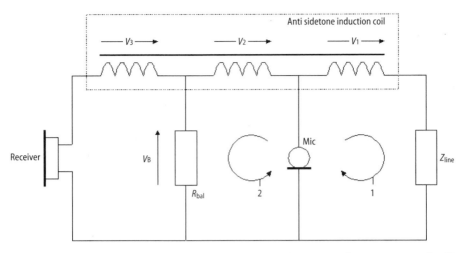

Figure 6.4 ASTIC circuit diagram. The coils are wound so that current flowing in one coil will induce an e.m.f. in the opposite direction in all three coils. When $V_B = V_3$ there will be no sidetone.

only external resistors and capacitors and can be set up for a variety of different countries' transmission requirements. The external components can normally be used to set such characteristics as sending and receiver loudness, terminating impedance and sidetone level. They also normally support different types of transducer, *e.g.* electret (works by varying the charge on a capacitor) or moving-coil (magnetic) microphones.

Besides their use in fully electronic telephones, the transmission circuit can also form the logical link between the telephone line and the electronic dialling circuitry (LD or DTMF). This is made easy by the fact that, often, a direct input is provided by the transmission interface circuit for connection to the DTMF circuit. This obviates the need to design yet more circuitry to couple the signalling tones to line, since the transmission circuit already provides this function. Also, modern transmission circuits often provide a DC power supply (derived from the loop current) that can be used to power peripheral circuitry, such as loudspeaking circuits for hands-free functions or microcontroller devices for additional features such as auto-diallers and displays.

Probably, the main advantage of using a transmission circuit over discrete designs is the control it can provide on setting the key transmission parameters to ensure the telephone performs well for varying line conditions. This is particularly true with the sending and receiving signal levels, since these must be varied to compensate for differing line lengths. In the past, crude devices known as barettors were used. These were little more that enclosed resistive wire (rather like a light bulb) that increased in resistance if the line current was higher (*i.e.* a short line length), and so reduced the potential signal level.

Such control of signal levels is now automatic in the transmission interface circuit, as it can sense varying line current and adjust signal levels more precisely than was ever possible using simple resistive components.

Control of Sidetone Using a Transmission Interface Circuit

Of all the performance characteristics that have to be controlled as part of the design of a telephone, probably setting the telephone impedance and sidetone matching to varying line lengths is perhaps the hardest. Again, using a modern transmission interface circuit makes this easier; but, even so, this is such a sensitive parameter of telephony performance that it will always be a compromise to ensure the best operation for a range of varying line conditions.

The architecture used by most interface circuits is the traditional Wheatstone bridge arrangement shown in Figure 6.5.

In order that the maximum signal from the transmitter amplifier is sent to line (labelled Tx – which effectively modulates the constant-current source driving the line), the signal in the ear, *i.e.* the sidetone, should be minimal. To achieve this using a Wheatstone bridge arrangement, it is essential that the two arms of the bridge should be "balanced" so that the voltages appearing at the inputs to the receiver amplifier due to the handset transmitter are cancelled out. As explained before, it is neither the intention nor is it desirable to make this cancellation 100%, as this leads to no sidetone and the illusion of a "dead" telephone to the user. Instead, it is intended that this sidetone be controlled in such a manner that only a small controlled proportion of the signal transmitted to line is fed back into the receiver as a confidence signal to the user.

Since the line impedance Z_{line} varies according to cable type and length, it is necessary for the sidetone to be minimised across the frequency range (300 Hz–3.4 kHz) and for the variations in Z_{line}. Thus, to achieve a balance of the bridge, the voltage across the inputs to the receiver amplifier in the

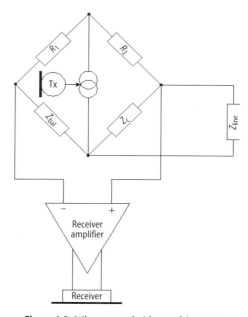

Figure 6.5 Wheatstone bridge architecture.

diagram should be nearly zero, *i.e.* the ratio of the currents and voltages on each side of the bridge should be in the same ratio, such that

$$R_1 Z_t = R_2 Z_{bal} \tag{6.1}$$

where R_1 and R_2 are the ratio arm resistors, and Z_t is given by

$$\frac{1}{Z_t} = \frac{1}{Z_c} + \frac{1}{Z_{line}}$$

Equation 6.1 can be rearranged to give the balance impedance Z_{bal} (which is part of the external components of the telephone transmission circuit):

$$Z_{bal} = \frac{R_1}{R_2} Z_t \tag{6.2}$$

Normally, the target Z_c characteristic is specified for the country for which the telephone is being designed and the ratio arm resistors are normally set to control other factors, such as the required DC characteristic, again as part of the specified requirements of a certain market. Typically, these resistors are set in a given ratio recommended by the vendor of the transmission circuit.

Hence, using Equation 6.2, the balance impedance can be calculated. This will be an ideal value and, in practice, the final value will be adjusted after measurement and testing using simulated line connections to ensure the final sidetone level is acceptable. Similarly, other key parameters such as the telephone's impedance (which should be matched to Z_c), the send and receive loudness and frequency responses are also set by varying the external components of the transmission circuit. This whole process is iterative by nature, requiring several adjustments before the best overall compromise can be achieved. The data sheet on the actual transmission circuit used is often invaluable as a starting point, typically giving suggested values to start with plus guidance on the best order in which to set the circuit components to avoid wasted effort, as many parameters effect each other as they are varied. Such data sheets are usually available from the interface circuit manufacturers and can often be found on their Web sites.

6.3.5 Call Arrival Indication (Ringing)

The design of a telephone must also include some form of call arrival indication. Exchanges still use the same AC signal to indicate an incoming PSTN call as they have done for many years. This voltage is typically 75 V_{rms} 25 Hz AC (usually with a DC offset of 50 V). Traditionally, this high voltage was used so that an AC bell inside the telephone could be driven with sufficient power to ensure a reasonably sound output level even on long lines. Clearly, when idle, *i.e.* waiting for a possible incoming call, the telephone should provide a low-impedance path to AC signals only. When the handset is on-hook, *i.e.* idle, the DC loop is disconnected by the hook-switch and only the ringing circuitry is connected, which is AC coupled via a 1.8 µF capacitor in the wall-socket. This capacitor prevents the exchange from seeing a DC loop when idle so that the called user's telephone can be rang to indicate an incoming call. Any DC loop

Telephone Technology

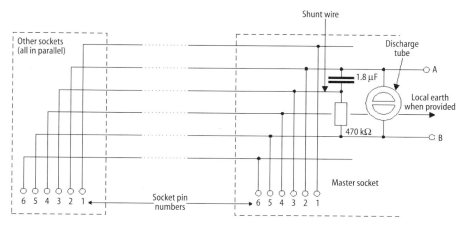

Figure 6.6 Diagram of UK telephone connection.

that is subsequently applied whilst ringing is still present on the line is then interpreted by the exchange as the call answer indication.

For this reason, telephones in the UK are normally connected via three or sometimes four wires. Two wires are used for transmission and signalling ("A" and "B" wires) and a third (known as the "bell shunt" wire) is used to connect the ringing signal, which is AC isolated by the capacitor in the master wall socket to the ringing device as shown in Figure 6.6. Sometimes a fourth wire is used for earth-recall signalling, which is provided for supplementary exchange services, but this function is now mainly indicated by a timed-break recall (TBR) signal. TBR is similar to dialling an LD digit "1"; however, since it is only sensible to use this signal in conjunction with DTMF dialling (where no other short line break signals are used) then its interpretation is not misunderstood by the exchange.

Modern telephones rarely contain bells now, since they are considered old fashioned, cost more to produce and the sound output can be variable, depending on line length, *i.e.* on a longer line the sound output can be reduced. Instead, a modern telephone normally has a tone caller device that drives a low-cost transducer, *e.g.* a piezoelectric resonator or loudspeaker. Whilst the tone caller circuit (often a single interface circuit plus a few resistors/capacitors) is usually still driven directly from the incoming AC signal, the circuit typically only uses this voltage to power the tone caller device itself. It then produces its own signal to drive the transducer to produce the classic "warble" sound. This sound is usually produced by sending short bursts of two or more fixed frequencies in quick succession *e.g.* 900 Hz for 100 ms, followed by 1100 Hz for 100 ms, followed by 900 Hz for 100 ms and so on. The speed at which the frequencies "switch" gives the characteristic "warble" sound, and the actual frequencies used are varied to give different apparent types of pitch to the sounder. Such options are often provided by switches on the phones to allow the user to "personalise" the ringing sound to his or her preference.

As was explained above, once the user lifts the handset to answer the call, the telephone hook-switch operates and connects the DC loop, which is detected by the exchange (due to the DC offset applied as part of the ringing signal), and this ceases the ringing signal. Note, however, the designer of the telephone is advised to ensure that the circuit will withstand ringing voltages applied to the telephone even in the "off-hook" state, *i.e.* when the telephone should be used for standard voice transmission just in case 75 V AC continues to be applied. This is also true of other hazardous voltages that can potentially appear on telephone lines due to fault conditions, *e.g.* overvoltage spikes due to lightning strikes. Whilst it is impossible to design for every possible real-world condition, such good design practices ensure a longer lasting telephone!

6.3.6 Telephone Design Enhancements to Provide Additional Accessibility Features

Since the purpose of the telephone is to enable any user to communicate with whomsoever they choose, it is not very desirable if the actual realisation of the telephone design causes certain users not to be able to use the product. It can be even the simplest of modifications that can make the telephone more attractive to certain groups of users. For example, the size of the keypad buttons can make all the difference between straightforward dialling and possible wrong numbers for an individual whose fingers are not very dextrous, perhaps due to arthritis. Also, the simple addition of a small "pip" or bump in the centre of the keypad digit "5" will help a blind person locate which key is which and, consequently, enable dialling of the required number.

When designing a telephone, even if it is not considered to be a special variant aimed particularly at users with impairments, it is worth considering some or all of the following enhancements to the design. Such an approach will allow the widest possible range of users and may be the final reason why one product is selected over a competitor's design.

Hearing-aid Compatibility

Since the telephone is predominately a voice communications instrument, this would seem to be an obvious enhancement to add so that hearing-impaired users can find using the telephone easier. Since hearing aids are normally equipped with a magnetic pick-up mechanism, it is quite easy to provide this feature by using a receiver in the handset that has an inductive coupler coil included. The inductive coupler is little more than a coil that is mounted inside the receiver and designed to produce the required magnetic field in response to the electrical signals applied to the receiver.

Most transducer manufactures that make receivers for telephone handsets provide inductive coupler versions of their receivers, so including this feature can be as simple as specifying an alternative receiver. It should be noted that an inductive coupler receiver might not be quite as sensitive as a similar receiver that does not contain this additional coil, but it is normally quite straightforward to adjust the design to compensate for this difference.

Amplification

Another feature that is often provided on telephones is receiver amplification. This is often a desirable feature for any user, not just the hearing impaired, as the range of receive signal levels can vary on different connections (particularly international calls) by anything up to 10–20 dB. Whilst this is becoming less significant with more modern digital connections, where transmission losses over digital paths are effectively 0 dB, it is still desirable for users to be able to compensate for far-end users who are very quiet or, equally, very loud!

This feature is normally provided by simply inserting additional gain between the receiver outputs of the transmission circuit and the receiver transducer itself. Small single-chip op-amps have been designed by several interface circuit vendors specifically for this application. When adding such a feature extra care must be taken in the design to ensure that, when used at maximum volume, there is no danger of hearing damage to the user if a very high signal level is applied from the far-end or even locally via the handset microphone. Such a precaution is called acoustic shock protection, and the maximum limits permitted are defined in the relevant safety specifications.

Amplification can also be provided on the microphone path to assist users who have speech impairments, but this is not as common.

Additional Receiver

Some users want the ability to be able to listen to a call when someone else is using the telephone. For example, a sign-language interpreter or support assistant may want to hear a call so he or she can relay the content to a hearing-impaired person who is using the handset to speak the replies. Such a feature can be provided by simply connecting an additional receiver to the handset receiver drive circuit. However, care has to be taken to ensure that the additional receiver is correctly matched to the drive circuit. It is often easier to use an additional amplifier to buffer the normal receive output. This also has the advantage of being an optional extra that is only fitted to telephones requiring this feature.

Ringer Pitch and Volume Control

As was explained in Section 6.3.5, it is considered desirable to allow the user to be able to customise the sound of the telephone ringer. Users often complain that the "ring" of a telephone is often too quiet to be heard at any distance. In the past, when mechanical bells were used, the broad spectrum of sounds made by the bell was quite characteristic and could be heard at some distance.

Providing the ability to control the volume and pitch is usually quite straightforward. Whilst it is possible to design mechanical solutions to reduce the volume, such as a thumb wheel control which gradually covers the holes allowing the acoustic sound out, and even possibly to vary the pitch, it is generally easier and better to do this electrically. This is especially true if a standard tone caller interface circuit is being used, as the pitch is often controlled by an external resistor and the level can be reduced simply by attenuating the voltage applied to the resonator, *e.g.* switch in a series resistance. Thus, by providing a switch or variable resistor, one for pitch selection say, and the other to control volume (which simply provides the ability to select a particular resistor value), the user has the facility to "personalise" their phone with multiple ringing sounds.

Another problem with ringer volume is that some users try and connect too many telephones to their line, such that the "ringer equivalence number" (REN) is exceeded. Typically, an exchange line has the capacity to drive telephone ringers up to REN = 4, meaning that the total of the REN of all instruments connected should not exceed this value. This value is determined as part of the approvals process and the manufacturer is obliged to give the value along with the approvals label. Using this value can sometimes be an oversimplification as, often, the electronic ringer circuits may have a "threshold" effect; *i.e.* they are not simply a resistive load, but require a certain voltage to operate properly. If this voltage is reduced due to several other telephones being connected, then it is conceivable that they will never ring, as the voltage never reaches the required value to operate.

Another feature that is often useful, especially when there may be several telephones on the same desk, is visual indication of incoming ringing. Again, this can be provided quite easily and is often no more than a light-emitting diode (LED) or neon fed via a suitable resistor/capacitor circuit.

Visual Display

In the past, only higher priced telephones had a display to provide visual feedback for the number dialled, recall of a stored number or even the number of an incoming call if Caller Display services are provided. Nowadays, most telephones, apart from the lowest cost ones, provide a display that is usually of the liquid-crystal display (LCD) type so as not to consume much power. Indeed, with the advent of LCD technology and low-power CMOS integrated circuits (ICs; which essentially only consume power when changing logic state), it is possible to include additional features that make the provision of a display even more desirable, *e.g.* clock/calendar function, calculator, call timer, number stores, *etc*. The size, clarity and viewing angle of the display are some of the essential design constraints that must be considered carefully given a target market, since if the characters are too small or barely visible in daylight then the user will quickly find the display of little benefit. Also any "enunciators" or prompts that are used, for example, "BATT LOW", must be as descriptive as possible to the average user.

These displays are now often alphanumeric rather than just numeric to make the storing of numbers by name more user friendly. Name entry is usually achieved by using the standard numeric keypad, such that the number and order of presses indicates particular letters. This is particularly true with mobile phones, where keypad buttons are at a premium, but if care is taken in the design of the user interface this process can work remarkably well.

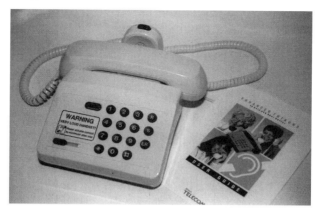

Figure 6.7 Picture of ADC Tribune.

Other Features

There are several other enhancements that can be made to a telephone to make it easier to use. One obvious feature is key press feedback. As mentioned above, most users are now familiar with the DTMF tones associated with tone dialling and would be concerned if they did not hear these tones when dialling. For this reason it is quite desirable to extend this audible feedback to other buttons when pressed if desired as some actions (*e.g.* recall) do not in themselves generate an audible signal.

Other factors that make one telephone better for one person than another are perhaps more subtle, but nonetheless important. The shape of the handset matters to some people; others may complain if the handset "creaks" when used due to poor design of the handset mouldings or method of assembly. Cable routing on the underside of a telephone again shows perhaps a bit more thought in the design, so that excess cordage can be hidden. Being able to wall mount a product is essential for some applications where there is no obvious flat surface in the vicinity of the wall socket. Again, in a situation such as this, handset hook-switch operation must be just as reliable wall mounted or desk mounted, and this can be a very challenging design requirement for the telephone designer.

The Tribune telephone shown in Figure 6.7 was designed with many of these enhancements added to make it appeal to a wider range of users who may have a hearing or visual impairment.

6.4 The Text Telephone

6.4.1 Introduction

A text telephone is a device used by hearing- and speech-impaired people to communicate over networks in typed text rather than speech. A picture of a

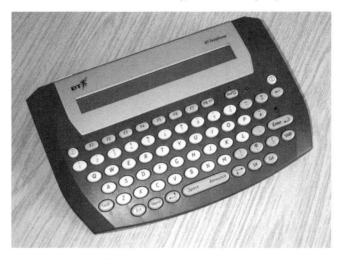

Figure 6.8 A text telephone.

modern text telephone can be seen in Figure 6.8. This section will provide an overview of the electrical design aspects of a text telephone.

In order to reduce development time, it is recommended that, where possible, ICs are used to implement specific functions, *e.g.* a modem.

Modular software development will assist in debugging and provide flexibility in the design.

There are several modem standards that can be adopted. This section will not deal with a specific modem standard but will give an overview of the International Telecommunications Union–Telecommunications (ITU–T) V.18, which the Office for Telecommunications (OFTEL) is recommending for adoption and development of text telephones.

6.4.2 Basic Principles

The basic functions of a text telephone are:

1. Set-up or receive a call with another text telephone.
2. Display and transmit text characters sent to another text telephone.
3. Display text characters received from another text telephone.

Text characters are entered via the keyboard and stored as hexadecimal data in the micro-controller ready for transmission.

A modem is used to convert hexadecimal data to analogue signals for transmission over a telephone line to a receiving modem; see Figure 6.9. The receiving modem converts the analogue signals back to hexadecimal format so that the received data can be displayed as characters for the user to view.

Telephone Technology

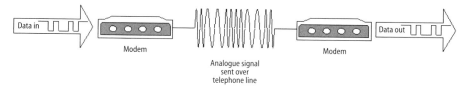

Figure 6.9 Modem principles.

Application Aspects

Using Figure 6.10, the core functions of a text telephone may be listed as:
1. Line interface circuit (incorporating a hook switch)
2. Analogue transmission circuit and line-derived power supply
3. Micro-controller
4. Modem
5. DTMF signalling
6. Keyboard
7. Display
8. Incoming call indicator
9. Line status
10. Talk through.

Line Interface
The line interface design will need to take into account the standards applicable to the telecommunications network it is to be used on. The line interface provides user protection to line-side signals, *e.g.* ringing signal,

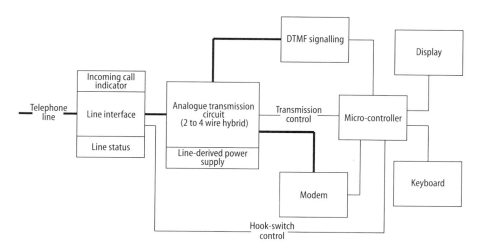

Figure 6.10 Text telephone modules.

lightning protection, *etc*. The primary function of the line interface is the hook-switch to connect the modem function to the telephone line to send and receive data.

The hook-switch can be either a mechanical switch operated by the user or a software-controlled electronic switch. The electronic hook-switch is more complicated to design but offers more degrees of freedom over the mechanical switch, *e.g.* calls could be auto-answered and messages stored with the electronic switch. The mechanical hook-switch design needs to consider user protection from high voltages on the telephone line.

The line interface may need to incorporate a bleed current circuit to maintain the random access memory (RAM) data and power the micro-controller in the off-line state. There is an option to use batteries and/or a mains power supply to simplify the design.

A hardware design that does not require batteries and/or a mains power supply will be more practical to a user with dexterity difficulties and will simplify the user instructions. From a user's point of view, a line-powered text telephone will be easier to operate and maintain.

Analogue Transmission Circuit and Line-derived Power Supply
The primary function of the analogue transmission circuit is to interface the modem function to the telephone line through a defined (characteristic) impedance. The transmission circuit performs the two- to four-wire hybrid function for the send and receive channels. There are many transmission-circuit ICs available with application notes to assist the developer. The reader can look to Section 6.3 for details on transmission circuit design principles.

The power requirements of the micro-controller, modem and display module require a line-derived or external power supply. For reasons mentioned in the *Line Interface* section above, the line-derived power supply is better from the user's point of view.

Line-derived power supply ICs interfaced with the transmission circuit are able to extract the maximum line current and minimise the characteristic impedance changes. Changes in the terminal's characteristic impedance will affect the transmission performance.

The performance of the line-derived power supply will influence the choice of ICs used for the other functions to remain within the available power budget.

Micro-controller
There are micro-controller products that incorporate features that will reduce the component count and simplify the control software. Examples of the features useful to the terminal design include:

1. DTMF generator.
2. Additional memory so that external ICs are not required – RAM and electrically erasable programmable read only memory (EEPROM).
3. Power save modes to reduce power consumption.
4. High number of configurable input/output (I/O) ports.
5. Multiple interrupts to respond to events and generate real time intervals.

A micro-controller to control the different text telephone functions will enable software modules to be developed in isolation, *e.g.* the keyboard scan and display drive.

Modem
Modem is a contraction of the term modulator/demodulator. A modem converts digital signals into analogue signals that can be transmitted over a telephone line and transforms incoming analogue signals into their digital equivalents.

There are ICs available to perform the modem function to published standards, *e.g.* Committée Consultatif International Télégraphique et Téléphonique (CCITT) V.21, which is widely used in the UK.

The advantage of using an IC is that the protocol can be easily changed with minimal effect on the hardware design.

DTMF Signalling
DTMF signalling is used to set up a call to another text telephone. Two simultaneous tones are used to represent digits in the range 0–9, * and #.

Modem ICs and micro-controllers are available with DTMF generators. This is one way of reducing the IC count and power consumption of the hardware design.

Keyboard
A QWERTY keyboard is interfaced with the micro-controller to enable the user to enter alpha/numeric characters. A minimum of 36 keys will be required for a simple alpha/numeric keyboard: A to Z and 0 to 9. Additional keys are required for the terminal operation, *e.g.* hook-switch; see Figure 6.11.

The keyboard is a matrix of rows and columns where a pressed key makes a connection between a row and column.

The keyboard interface with the micro-controller will be dependent on the port configuration. The keyboard interface consumes minimal power since a connection is only made when a key is pressed. The software determines whether single or multiple keys can be pressed simultaneously.

The most efficient use of I/O is when the number of columns equals the number of rows, *e.g.* using eight bi-directional I/O lines: four rows by four columns equals 16 keys, whereas two rows by six columns equals 12 keys.

Display
LCD modules are available in many configurations of lines and characters, *e.g.* one line by 40 characters, two lines by 20 characters, *etc*.

The layout of the display will have an influence on the software design, *e.g.* how characters are scrolled across the display once it is full.

The type of display will be a factor in the power budget for the hardware design. Backlighting may not be possible using line-derived power supplies.

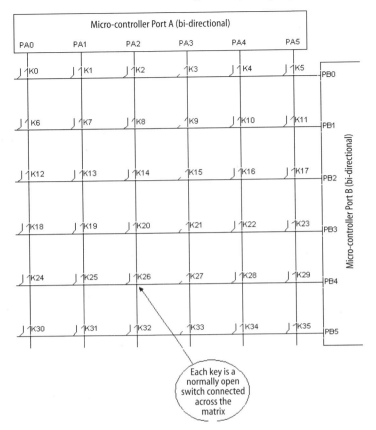

Figure 6.11 Example of a keyboard matrix.

Incoming Call Indicator
The incoming call visual indicator can be as simple as a neon flashing in sympathy with the ringing signal.

Additionally a tone caller IC can be incorporated into the line interface design to provide an audible signal.

Line Status
The line status can be indicated using a low-current, high-efficiency LED.

One LED could be used for hook-switch status, on-line and off-line. It is optional to use a second LED to indicate voice/tone activity.

The voice/tone activity indication can be used by an experienced user to detect when the called number is not a text telephone. The LED can be interfaced with the transmission circuit receiver output to illuminate in sympathy with the speech signals.

Speech signals will light the LED in bursts, whereas the modem carrier tone will be a constant brightness.

Talk Through
The "talk through" feature allows a user to talk to the called number.

Half-duplex modem protocols allow speech to be interleaved with text messages, allowing a user to use speech to respond to text messages. It is a prerequisite that the distant text terminal has a loudspeaker.

Baudot is an example of a half-duplex modem protocol that transmits modem signals only when text needs to be sent. Whilst there are no keyboard entries, the transmission link between the two text telephones can be used for speech signals. Baudot is mentioned in the following section on the V.18 standard.

Note that deaf people who lip-read use speech to communicate with others in "face to face" conversations. It is quicker to reply using speech than it is to type a text message.

Another use of the talk-through feature is when the user suspects a connection to a speech terminal as indicated by the line status LED. The talk-through feature can be used to request the far-end switch over to a text telephone. It is likely that some telephone lines will be shared by text telephone and speech telephone users.

A loud speaker on the Text telephone for incoming speech may not be considered necessary when a conventional telephone can share the same telephone line for speech calls. Adding a loud speaker will impact on the power budget and add complexity to the terminal's operation.

V.18 – an International Standard for Text Telephones

V.18 is a recommendation published by the ITU–T for inter-working between the many variants of text telephones around the world. A problem with text telephones today is that it is difficult to communicate internationally. This is quite apart from the problem of different languages and is due to isolated national or even regional development. For example, many text telephones in the UK use a modem based on ITU–T recommendation V.21 (300 bit s^{-1} FSK). Most deaf people in France use a Minitel, based on V.23, as a text terminal. The two can obviously not communicate directly.

V.18 was developed to allow inter-working between new and existing text telephones and to define an internationally recognised modem and character set for future text telephones. It is not a physical modem definition, it is a protocol for determining the correct modem to use in text telephone communications. The first version was published September 1994. It was not until the third edition in January 1998 that a workable version was finally released. The main reasons for the long delay were variations in existing text telephones and a lack of documented operational procedures.

V.18 Modes
V.18 has two modes of operation: compatibility mode and V.18 mode. Compatibility mode is used for communicating with existing text telephones. The second is a standardised mode for all future text telephones. Compatibility mode will connect to text telephones based on the following modems:

- V.21 (CCITT) – UK, Sweden
- Baudot (45 and 50 bps) – US, Ireland, Australia, UK
- EDT – Italy
- Bell 103 – US
- V.23 – France
- DTMF – Netherlands

V.18 mode is used between two V.18 text telephones. It incorporates a full duplex 300 bit s^{-1} V.21 modem and refers to ITU–T recommendation T.140 (ITU T.140 (02/98) Protocol For Multimedia Application Text Conversation) for the character set and user-interface features. Character conversion tables for the compatibility modes are included in annexes.

T.140 covers the following:

- text conversation protocol;
- global 16 bit character set based on ISO10646 (UNICODE);
- limited set of presentation controls, *e.g.* new line, erase, alert, graphic rendition;
- efficient coding;
- can be used in multi-point environments, *e.g.* conferencing.

V.18 Features

V.18 automatically tries to detect the type of device it is connected to. It has a feature known as automoding that analyses the tones received and sends probes to determine the modem being used, the bit-rate and the character set of the remote device. Automoding includes:

- a cut-down version of ITU–T recommendation V.8 (Procedures for starting sessions of data transmission over the PSTN);
- a "CI" calling tone (see V.8);
- probes with country specific order to provoke a response;
- analysis of tones received to determine valid responses.

The V.18 recommendation also defines a simultaneous speech and text mode for users with partial hearing or deaf-with-speech to hearing user. This is a significant improvement over the alternate mode used in previous text telephones.

Appendices to the recommendation describe a V.18 implementation test specification and options for usage of V.8 and V.8bis. Full V.8 and V.8bis allows V.18 to handshake with and identify itself to the latest multimedia terminals.

V.18 Summary

Although V.18 is a significant step forward from previous text telephone modem technology, there are still few terminals around. This is mainly due to the fact that the major modem manufacturers have not implemented V.18 on their devices due to the cost of design and relatively small market.

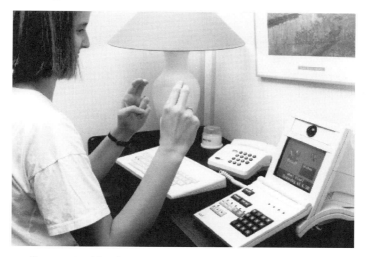

Figure 6.12 Videophone in use for sign-language communication.

6.5 The Videophone

There are two main areas where a videophone could assist a deaf or hearing-impaired person. The one most often considered is to use a videophone to convey sign language (see Figure 6.12); the second is to assist lip-reading by adding visual cues to speech. As will be discussed later, these two applications have somewhat different requirements concerning video quality and camera field of view, but the underlying videophone technology is common to both, and this will be reviewed first.

6.5.1 Basic Principles

The core component of a videophone is the video "codec", derived from the words encoder, or coder, and decoder. The encoder takes in a video signal from a camera, converts it to digital form, and compresses it to a bit-rate suitable for transmission down an available network. The decoder receives this compressed signal from the network and expands it out again to a moving video signal for display.

Compression is necessary, as the original video signal has a far higher data rate than common public networks can support. For example, in Europe, a full studio-quality television signal has 25 frames (pictures) per second, and a spatial resolution of 720 by 576 pels (picture elements) per frame, with each pel requiring 16 bits for full colour. This results in a data rate of 166 Mbit s^{-1}! (Note: other areas of the world use a different television standard of 720 by 480 pels and 30 frames/s, but the overall data rate is similar). Compare this with the data rate available over a modem on the PSTN of 33.6 kbit s^{-1} using V.34bis, or 128 kbit s^{-1} on the integrated services digital network (ISDN) using two "B" channels. The required compression of over 1000 times cannot be achieved without loss of quality; but, if done in a controlled way, then acceptable and usable moving pictures can still be obtained.

The first step in compression is to reduce the spatial resolution. Various world standards bodies, particularly the ITU, have agreed certain standard resolutions for use in videophones, the most commonly used being:

- CIF (common intermediate format) – 352 by 288 pels and 30 frames/s;
- QCIF (quarter common intermediate format) – 176 by 144 pels and 30 frames/s.

Most colour images are normally captured and displayed using red, green and blue (R, G and B) colour components. For transmission or compression purposes, however, these are usually transformed into an equivalent set known as Y, Cr and Cb, where the Y signal contains the most information, and is equivalent to the old "black and white" television pictures, or the effect obtained if the colour control is turned right down on a colour television set. Cr and Cb are known as "colour difference" components, and are essentially the difference between the R and B components and the Y component. The eye has much lower visual acuity for the colour components, so they can be more heavily compressed than the Y signal, typically comprising only 10–20% of the final bit-rate.

The Y, Cr and Cb signals are compressed by eliminating statistical redundancy, and then by further reducing quality in a way that is subjectively as least perceptible as possible (known as perceptual redundancy, in that the eye and brain do not notice the drop in quality too much). The ITU has developed standard video coding algorithms for achieving this; these work well for most types of video content, the key standard being H.261 (in 1990), but being largely superseded by the improved H.263. In both, each frame is divided into a grid of blocks termed "macroblocks", each consisting of a 16 by 16 array of pels. Statistical redundancy is removed by a combination of methods. The first is change detection: if an area of the picture has not changed from one frame to the next, then there is no need to retransmit it, and the decoder can simply repeat the last received information for those areas.

The second compression method is "motion compensation", which attempts to track the motion of objects, or parts of objects, from one frame to the next. Thus, if that part of the image in a given macroblock in the current frame can be matched to a part of the previous transmitted image by, say, moving it 3 pels to the left and 2 pels down, then by just transmitting the "motion vector" as the pair of numbers {–3, 2} the decoder can retrieve the correct part of the last received picture for display at that macroblock position. In practice, objects are rarely so obliging as to travel purely by such spatial translation (they rotate, deform, occlude, *etc.*), but the motion compensation can often form a good first approximation to the motion. By subtracting this approximation from the original signal a residual signal is obtained that is often easier to compress than the original signal.

The residual signal from the motion compensation stage, and any macroblocks where there is no effective approximation at all (*e.g.* newly revealed background), pass to a "transform coding" stage. This takes pels in blocks of eight-by-eight at a time and performs a discrete cosine transform

(DCT) on them. This is a mathematical operation that converts the 64 input numbers into 64 "DCT coefficients", which are similar to Fourier coefficients in that they represent the information as frequency components. These frequencies are effectively spatial frequencies: low frequencies correspond to larger slowly varying brightness variations in the block; high frequencies correspond to rapidly varying brightness patterns across the block. Once in the transform domain, three effects make it easier to compress the data:

- It turns out that, for most images, the higher frequency components are close to zero in value, and can be set to zero with little subjective detriment to the picture.
- The eye is less sensitive to amplitude errors in the higher frequencies, so they can be represented with reduced accuracy (quantisation).
- Considered over many blocks of data, each coefficient has a highly peaked probability distribution, centred on zero. This allows the use of variable-length coding, whereby short codewords of only a few bits are applied to frequently occurring values, and longer codewords are applied to infrequently occurring values. Overall, this uses fewer bits than using a fixed length of codeword to cater for the set of coefficient values.

It is thus in the transform domain that most of the compression takes place. For each frame, the compressed transform coefficients, plus the motion vectors and change detection map from the previous stages, are transmitted to the decoder. The decoder performs an inverse DCT function on each transformed block, combines the results with macroblock information from the locally stored previous decoded image according to the motion vectors received, and combines the results using the change detector map to reconstruct the current image. In fact, it is not a perfect reconstruction due to the approximations applied in the various stages, and particularly the quantisation of DCT coefficients, so there is a certain loss of quality. The more change there is from one frame to the next, then the more information needs to be transmitted; or, looked at another way, the more information needs to be discarded to keep to whatever channel bit-rate is available. Thus, with more motion and visual complexity in the video, more distortion occurs. This loss of quality can be characterised in various dimensions.

- Reduced frame rate: an encoder will often not be able to encode every frame as this would generate too many bits, so "frame dropping" occurs. This may be regular (such that say 15 or 10 frames/s are received) or irregular (such that, at periods of high visual activity, the rate drops erratically to only a few frames per second). The visual effect of reduced frame rate is increasingly jerky and disjointed motion. A low frame rate also results in a perceptible delay.
- Reduced spatial resolution: a certain amount of this is imposed by the chosen working resolution, usually CIF or QCIF. In addition, the effect of setting higher frequency transform coefficients to zero is to reduce resolution further. The visual effect of this is increased fuzziness or blurring of the picture. Again, the effect becomes worse during periods of high activity in the picture, as the codec reacts to increasing output bit-rate by using coarser quantisation of DCT coefficients.
- Visible distortions and blockiness: as above, this occurs due to coarse quantisation of DCT coefficients. The effect is an increasing graininess in

the picture, often most noticeable near the edges of moving objects, or in plain background areas, which in severe cases can appear as distinct square blocks and patterns within blocks.

The extent to which the various degradations above occur is governed in part by the amount of activity and complexity in the video scene to be coded. Inevitably, a scene with a person almost filling the frame and for example gesturing rapidly generates a lot more information, and hence requires higher compression, leading to higher degradation, than one of a person sitting talking quietly. However, the design of the video encoder also has an important part to play, two factors being the motion compensation process and the strategy for controlling frame rate and quantiser levels.

Motion compensation requires the encoder to search the local area near each macroblock for a good match in the previous encoded frame. A full search of the range ±8 pels horizontally and vertically requires $17 \times 17 = 289$ search positions for each macroblock. Increasing this to ±16 pels requires 1089 positions! For rapid movements, such as sign language, a range of ±32 might be desirable, and the processing power required turns out to be many billions of operations per second. Fortunately, there are more efficient ways of searching than a full search of every possible position, and the processing power can be reduced to that available on a good PC (for a software implementation of the codec), or a more specialised IC (a hardware implementation). Generally, specialised hardware will still do a better job, resulting in slightly higher compression, than a purely software implementation.

The other important factor is the strategy the encoder uses to decide when to drop frames or to use a coarser quantiser, to keep the bit-rate generated within the transmission channel constraint. Desirable frame rates for signing and lip-reading are discussed in Section 6.5.2. However, a common approach is to attempt to keep the frame rate up to some target rate, such as 15 frames/s, by judicious adjustment of the quantiser; but, if a very coarse quantiser has to be used, resulting in disturbing picture distortions, then the frame rate will also be further reduced temporarily. Many commercial videophones now include a user control that enables the receiving person to signal to the transmitting end whether their preference is for higher frame rate or higher quality on a continuous scale between the two extremes. The encoder will then try and favour the desired outcome, although it cannot guarantee this.

Note that the design of the video decoder has very little effect on the received picture quality. In effect it receives a series of instructions from the encoder on how to build up each new frame, and makes no decisions itself. It must follow the instructions exactly, or a completely distorted and useless picture will result after a few frames, since one frame is built partly from the preceding one. The only influence a decoder may have is if it has a "post-filter", which attempts to clean up the picture by removing, say, gross blockiness in the images prior to display.

6.5.2 Application Aspects

For any videophone application, there are some practical aspects that apply to most situations.

Lighting is often a significant problem. For evening use, most domestic and much office lighting is insufficiently bright to generate a good clean signal from the camera (unless it is very expensive!). This is exacerbated by the lighting usually coming from overhead, whereas ideally it would come from in front of the person using the videophone. A practical solution is to site a table lamp with a diffusing shade next to the videophone. For daytime use, natural light from a window is beneficial, so the system needs to be sited such that the user faces the window. Backlighting of the user, for example sitting the user with their back to a window, will usually result in just a silhouette!

It is best to avoid a cluttered background behind the user, as this distracts from clear perception of the user by their correspondent, and also wastes valuable transmission bit-rate by having to encode the background detail every time it is revealed by user movements. A plain background is best of all! In practice, there are other practical considerations to siting the videophone as well, including the privacy of the user.

An ideal videophone would have its camera positioned at the point on the display screen where the eyes of the person in the received images appear, ensuring perfect eye contact. In practice, the camera usually has to be mounted at the side or above the display screen, resulting in a subtle but disconcerting lack of eye contact. It is very useful to have a "self-view" picture continuously available, as well as the incoming picture, so that the user can ensure they stay appropriately within camera shot. Typically, the self-view picture will be smaller than the incoming picture, so as to be less distracting.

Sign Language

For sign language use, the videophone picture needs to include the head and shoulders, the body almost down to the waist and an area of space to either side, as signs can encompass this whole area. However, it is also necessary not to "zoom out" too much; this is because, with the limited spatial resolution of the codec, the clarity of detail of finger positions, and also importantly of facial expression (which modifies the meaning of signs), will deteriorate. This is where the self-view picture is important, so that the users can monitor their position. Experiments have shown that to convey sign language freely, a frame rate of at least 15 frames/s is desirable (Sperling *et al.*, 1985). Below this rate, signers have to slow down their rate of signing to avoid becoming unintelligible. In practice, with a two-way videophone conversation, the signers quickly learn to adapt their signing rate and style, and the spatial extent of their signs, to the capabilities of the videophone system (Whybray, 1991).

Early trials of videophones with sign-language users showed that, despite the limited picture quality, the people involved really liked being able to communicate in their preferred visual language, found communication of humour and mood to be more natural than, say, a textphone, and really liked being able to see each other (Whybray, 1991, 1992). For comfortable long-term use it appears that a bit-rate of 128 kbit s^{-1}, as available on an ISDN connection, is quite acceptable.

The majority of people who use sign language as their preferred means of conversation are those who are profoundly deaf from birth. These people also tend to have less well-developed English (or equivalent spoken/written language) skills. Textphones are, nevertheless, the means of telecommunication most commonly used by them, and it is therefore desirable to add some text communication functionality to a videophone. The text facility can be used to enhance a videophone call, *e.g.* to convey precise details, such as numbers/addresses, and to enable enhanced communication with a non-signer. Ideally, the text function could also be invoked without the videophone part, to provide communication with standard text-phone devices such as the V.18 standard.

Lip-reading

Most people who lip-read are not profoundly deaf, but have some residual hearing, which, when combined with the additional stimulus of sight of the speakers lips, is sufficient to enable them to lip-read. It is found that, in perception of speech, the audio and video cues complement each other so that the combined intelligibility, if both are available, is very much higher than if just one or the other is provided. It is, in fact, very difficult to lip-read with complete absence of sound, although, remarkably, some people can do this. So, for a videophone to be of use for lip-reading, it needs to convey not just the video but also the audio signals.

Lip motion can be very rapid; but, as with sign language, it has been found that 15 frame/s is the threshold below which intelligibility falls (Frowein *et al.*, 1991; Vitkovitch and Barber, 1991). For lip-reading, some visibility of the interior of the mouth and the tongue is important; so, a reasonably close camera shot of the face is required, plus adequate frontal lighting to illuminate the mouth interior to some extent. The audio needs to be of good quality, and as near exactly time aligned to the video as possible. Experiments have shown that a delay of audio with respect to video of 40 ms or a lead of 20 ms are desirable limits, and this is very hard to achieve unless the video frame rate is steady and at least 15 frame/s. Even good ISDN videophone systems do not commonly achieve this, suggesting that, although the percentage of people who might benefit from lip-reading using videophones is higher than for sign language, the practical problems of getting the benefit may be greater.

The quality of the audio channel should remain high. Although it might be thought that if a hearing-impaired person cannot hear, say, high frequencies well, savings in bit-rate applied to the audio could be made, in practice hearing impairments vary so widely that there is no simple answer to how one could restrict the bandwidth or quality. Audio signals can be compressed to lower rates than video (typically 8 to 16 kbit s^{-1} is adequate), so it is best to provide normal telephony quality rather than compromise it further. A lip-reader may well use a hearing aid, so direct coupling of the audio signal to this would be beneficial, through an induction loop and use of the hearing-aid "T" setting.

6.5.3 Systems and Standards

Although there is a clear market niche for videophones for sign language and lip-reading, the high technical complexity, and hence cost of videophones, militates against development of specialised ones for this limited market. It is much more likely that ones developed for large-scale commercial or domestic use will be taken as-is, or adapted for use in these areas. Although early videophones were developed by different manufacturers to their own designs, and were incompatible (*i.e.* could not communicate with each other!), fortunately there are now world standards that are very widely adopted, and guarantee inter-working.

H.320 (Integrated Services Digital Network) Videophones

The first completely standardised videophones comply with the ITU H.320 standard, and operate on the ISDN. ISDN connections are available through a large part of the world, and a basic connection provides two independent "B" channels of 64 kbit s^{-1} each, which are often combined to provide 128 kbit s^{-1}. Calls are made by keying in a telephone number as on conventional phones, but of course a videophone call can only be made to another H.320 videophone. Attempting to call a normal phone results in a voice-only call. At the time of writing, in the UK the ISDN is available to domestic users as BT's Home Highway product for example, and call charges per B channel are the same as normal PSTN calls, though the rental charge is significantly higher.

H.320 videophones are available in a range of formats, including compact desktop models, set-top boxes to connect to domestic televisions, PC implementations (which require an ISDN card plus camera at least), and full-size business conferencing systems. All are compatible, however.

H.324 (Public Switched Telephone Network) Videophones

The ITU H.324 standard is designed for use on the normal telephone network (PSTN). The maximum two-way data rate possible at the time of writing was 33.6 kbit s^{-1}, so inevitably the quality is significantly lower than for ISDN. The advantage is that the PSTN is ubiquitous and relatively cheap. As with H.320, various systems are available, though PC-based ones predominate, as many PCs have a suitable modem and sufficient processing power to implement the video coding in software.

H.323 (Internet Protocol) Videophones

The ITU H.323 standard is for videophones that use the Internet protocol (IP) as the means of transmission. For domestic users, this can sometimes be done over a PSTN line through their Internet service provider, although the H.324 standard is really more appropriate and makes more efficient use of the limited capacity. Also, H.324 sets up a direct connection to the other party, thereby resulting in guaranteed bit-rate and low delay. An IP connection over the Internet suffers various packet delay and loss problems. H.323 is, however, feasible on a local-area network, typically used in office environments, or with higher speed Internet access that is now becoming available. There are ongoing issues to do with knowing the "IP address" of the terminal being called though, as many IP addresses are dynamically allocated and change for each new call.

Unfortunately, although the three standards above all use H.261 or H.263 video codecs, many other parts of the system, including the network access, signalling protocols, multiplex (mean of mixing audio and video data) and even the audio codecs, are different, so no direct interconnection is possible. It is possible to connect via gateway devices that translate the various protocols, but these are not yet widely deployed.

6.5.4 Future Systems

There have been attempts to analyse images of sign language to be able to extract the hand and finger motions, and transmit these to enable graphical reconstructions of the sign language at the far end (Downton and Drouet, 1991). Unfortunately, the difficulty of doing this 100% reliably, given the complex motions, occlusions, and effects of lighting involved, has proved impossible except for simple signs. As machine vision techniques advance, this situation may improve, but it is likely that conventional video coding and transmission speeds will advance faster, rendering such an approach unnecessary for most uses. There is still a place for this work, though, in terms of automatic understanding of sign language, and transmitting over mobile links where bandwidth will lag behind that available on the fixed networks.

Broadband IP connections are just starting to become available to domestic users at the time of writing, and it is anticipated that this will lead to a general increase in use of videophones and higher quality pictures, both to the benefit of hearing-impaired people.

6.6 Conclusions and Learning Highlights

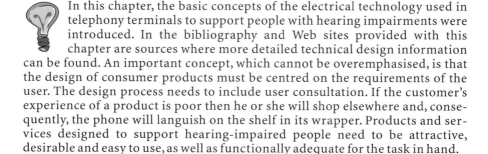

In this chapter, the basic concepts of the electrical technology used in telephony terminals to support people with hearing impairments were introduced. In the bibliography and Web sites provided with this chapter are sources where more detailed technical design information can be found. An important concept, which cannot be overemphasised, is that the design of consumer products must be centred on the requirements of the user. The design process needs to include user consultation. If the customer's experience of a product is poor then he or she will shop elsewhere and, consequently, the phone will languish on the shelf in its wrapper. Products and services designed to support hearing-impaired people need to be attractive, desirable and easy to use, as well as functionally adequate for the task in hand.

6.6.1 Learning Highlights of the Chapter

The chapter surveyed the structure and technology of the modern telephone network. The reader was introduced to the basic concepts of user-centred telephone design. In this topic, the importance of designing the telephone interface to suit a range of human users was outlined. Simple methods for involving the user and key support features were surveyed. The key question of how they should and are integrated into a telephone terminal was discussed. Two specialist applications were then investigated. The first was the technology and design of a simple text-telephone terminal, and the second was how to engineer videophones for use by hearing-impaired people.

Although electromagnetic compatibility performance is an important concept and property for telephone design and usage, it is beyond the scope of this chapter and is a separate topic. There are specialist test houses that provide consultancy on this topic.

Projects and Investigations

Telephone Electronics

The following project work assumes that the student has access to calibrated transmission performance measuring equipment, *e.g.* the ability to measure the send, the receive and the sidetone levels, including impedance measurement. The measuring equipment may be automated or manually operated.

The following list is a suggested sequence to develop the electronics for a telephone.

1. Identify and acquire a copy of the transmission performance standards/ specification to conform to.
2. Select a transmission-circuit IC and calculate component values using the application notes. At this stage, a simple line interface using a diode bridge is acceptable. Use a telephone handset with known transducers to reduce the development effort. The handset influences the transmission levels and frequency responses.
3. Adjust the DC characteristic to comply with the transmission specification.
4. Adjust the input (characteristic) impedance (600 Ω or complex) to give an acceptable return loss.
5. Adjust the send level and frequency response to comply with the transmission specification.
6. Adjust the receive level and frequency response to comply with the transmission specification.
7. Adjust the sidetone balance impedance to give good sidetone performance. Note that it may also be necessary to adjust the send and receive levels.
8. Design and implement a receiver acoustic-shock protection circuit. Measure and adjust the acoustic shock and receive levels to comply with the transmission standard.
9. Measure the maximum signal level that can be sent to line. Design and implement a send signal limiting circuit.

10. Measure the send and receive noise levels.
11. Design and develop a line interface circuit controlled by either a mechanical or electronic hook-switch. The electronic hook-switch will require software control.
12. Extend the transmission circuit design to include DTMF signalling and microphone MUTE control.

Text-phone Electronics

The following list is a suggested sequence to develop the electronics for a textphone.

1. Develop a technical specification to identify the technical features and standards that will be implemented. Where it is possible, refer to national and international standards rather than reproduce the text.
2. Develop a line interface and analogue transmission circuit incorporating an electronic hook-switch, modem and micro-controller.
3. Extend the hardware to incorporate a display module and keyboard.
4. Develop application software to:
   4.1. Scan a keyboard and display the characters on a display module.
   4.2. Transmit modem data to a proprietary text terminal.
   4.3. Receive modem data from a proprietary text terminal.
   4.4. DTMF signalling to line to set up a call to another textphone.

For learning purposes, it will be technically easier to use an approved mains-powered DC supply to power the micro-controller and modem IC. The mains power supply should be double insulated for user protection. The use of a mains power supply will ease the technical design constraints on the line interface and transmission circuit.

References and Further Reading

 References

Downton, A.C., Drouet, H., 1991. Image analysis for model-based sign language coding. In: *Proceedings of 6th International Conference on Image Analysis and Processing*, Como, Italy, 4–6 September.
Frowein, H.W., Smoorenburg, G.F., Pyfers, L., Schinkel, D., 1991. Videotelephony and speech reading: the effect of picture quality. In: von Tetzchner, S. (ed.), *Issues in Telecommunications and Disability*. COST219 Luxembourg Office for Official Publications of the European Communities. ISBN 92-826-3128-1.
Sperling, G., Landy, M.S., Cohen, Y., Pavel, M., 1985. Intelligible encoding of ASL image sequences at extremely low information rates. *Computer Vision, Graphics, and Image Processing* 31, 335-391
Vitkovitch, M., Barber, P., 1991. Facial speech at varying frame rates. In: *Annual Meeting of the Applied Vision Association*, April, Manchester, UK.
Whybray, M.W., 1991. Visual telecommunications for deaf people at 14.4Kbit/s on the public switched telephone network. In: von Tetzchner, S. (ed.), *Issues in Telecommunications and*

Disability. COST219 Luxembourg Office for Official Publications of the European Communities. ISBN 92-826-3128-1.

Whybray, M.W., 1992. Moving picture transmission at low bitrates for sign language communication. In: *IEE Colloquium on "Image Processing for Disabled People*, Heriot-Watt University, 2 October.

Further Reading

Books

Bigelow, S.J., 1997. *Understanding Telephone Electronics*, 3rd edition. Butterworth-Heinemann (ISBN: 0750699442).

Brandt, A., 1995. *Telephones for All: Nordic Design Guidelines*. Danish Centre for Technical Aids, Department of Technology, Communication and Special Education, Arhus, Denmark.

Gill, J., Shipley, T., 1999. *Telephones – What Features do Disabled People Need?* PhoneAbility, RNIB, 244 Great Portland Street, London W1N 6AA (ISBN 1-86048-0209).

Lazzaro, J.J., 1993. *Adaptive Technologies for Learning and Work Environments*. American Library Association, 50 East Huron Street, Chicago, IL 60611, USA.

Roe, R.W., 1995. *Telecommunications for All*. Office for Official Publications of the European Communities. Catalogue number: CD-90-95-712-EN-C.

Technical Papers

Tetzchner, S., 1991. Issues in telecommunications and disability. Office for Official Publications of the European Communities. Catalogue number: CD-NA-13845-EN-C (ISBN 92-826-3128-1).

Web Sites

British Standards Institution (BSI)	www.bsi.org.uk/
CCITT list of modem standards	webopedia.internet.com/Standards/Standards_Organizations/CCITT.html
COST219bis Telecommunications: Access for disabled people and elderly	www.stakes.fi/COST219/
DIEL home page – Advisory Committee on Telecommunications for Disabled and Elderly People	www.acts.org.uk/diel/
European Telecommunications Standards Institute	www.etsi.org/
International Standards Organisation (ISO)	www.iso.ch/
ITU–T home page	www.itu.int/ITU-T/index.html
Oftel home page	www.oftel.gov.uk/
Telecommunication services for people with disabilities	www.oftel.gov.uk/publications/1995_98/consumer/dis998.htm
TRACE: Designing more usable telecommunications	www.trace.wisc.edu/world/telecomm/

7 Alarm and Alerting Systems for Hearing-impaired and Deaf People

7.1 Learning Objectives

The aim of this chapter is to discuss and describe alarm and alerting systems for deaf and hearing-impaired people. Particular emphasis will be placed on understanding the technical principles on which these devices and systems are based. Specific learning objectives are as follows:

- understanding the main functional blocks of an alarm or alerting system;
- knowledge of the specific components or devices that can be used practically to implement these functional blocks;
- understanding the technical principles on which these components or devices are based;
- understanding the design principles involved in the development of alarm and alerting systems for deaf and hearing-impaired people.

7.2 The Engineering Principles of Alarm and Alerting Devices

Both hearing and deaf people will generally require or want to be aware of the following in both the home and workplace:

- a fire
- someone trying to telephone them
- a person at the door
- an intruder trying to break in
- the presence of carbon monoxide
- a baby or small child crying (if they have children)
- a person being cared for, either voluntarily or professionally, requiring attention
- equipment (or domestic appliances) malfunctioning.

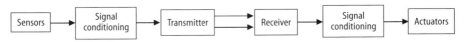

Figure 7.1 Generic block diagram of an alarm or alerting system.

These different functions are generally carried out (for hearing people) by a fire alarm, a telephone ringer, a door bell, a burglar alarm, a carbon monoxide alarm, a baby monitor, a "nurse call" alarm and an equipment control panel, often with an audible alarm. These devices may seem very different from each other, but they are all alarm and alerting devices and contain basic components that perform the same types of function. However, the details of how these functions are implemented vary with the different devices.

The generic structure of an alarm and alerting device is illustrated in Figure 7.1 and consists of the following four main components:

- sensors or input transducers, which receive the input signal and convert it to an electrical signal;
- signal-conditioning or -processing components, such as amplifiers;
- output transducers or actuators, which convert an electrical signal to an appropriate form and output it to the user;
- a transmission system, generally consisting of a radio frequency transmitter and receiver, for transmitting the electrical signal output by the sensor(s) to the output transducer.

Figure 7.1 illustrates the generic structure, though not all alarm and alerting devices will include a transmission system and in some cases the input transducer(s) will be connected to the output transducer(s) either directly or via signal-conditioning components. However, signal transmission is required more frequently in alarm and alerting devices for deaf and hearing-impaired people than those for hearing people. This is because many of the output transducers used to convey the alert to a deaf user need to be in direct contact or in relatively close proximity to the user and, consequently, at a distance from the input transducers, so that signal transmission is required to close the gap. In the case of hearing people, the output transducers can transmit information over a greater distance and, therefore, are often in close proximity to the input transducers. With regard to implementation, a number of additional components, such as user controls, a power supply and, in some cases, a microprocessor, are also important, but these components will not be discussed here.

The structure of this chapter follows the generic structure of alarm and alerting systems. The various sensors, signal conditioning components, transmission systems and output transducers used in alarm and alerting systems for deaf and hearing-impaired people are discussed in Sections 7.3, 7.4, 7.5 and 7.6 respectively. First, design issues are discussed in Section 7.2.1 and a categorisation of different types of alarm and alerting system is given in Section 7.2.2.

7.2.1 Design Issues

A number of approaches can be taken to designing alarm and alerting systems for deaf and hearing-impaired people. The three main approaches are:

- design for all
- design specifically for deaf and hearing-impaired people
- modification of devices designed for hearing people to be used by deaf and hearing-impaired people.

Design for all, which is also called universal design, has a number of advantages and should be the preferred approach. However, few alarm and alerting systems are based on *design for all* principles. design for all principles require alarm and alerting systems to be designed to be used by everyone; this includes both deaf and hearing people, as well as the wider group of disabled people. At the simplest level this would require the availability of output signals produced by different types of transducer, including visual, *e.g.* flashing lights, tactile, *e.g.* a vibrator, and aural, *e.g.* a loud bell. Different types of actuator, which provide the output signal, are discussed in Section 7.6. However, the provision of a wide range of different types of actuator and the other features required by the design for all approach may require the whole design concept to be re-examined. It should be noted that, although inclusive design to meet the needs of disabled people is an important component of design for all, the concept also includes, for instance, design to take into account different needs based on age, strength and body proportions.

The other two approaches are likely to have cost implications, due to the smaller market provided by deaf people than by the hearing population and the modifications and/or additional devices required in the third approach. They both have the further disadvantages of giving deaf people a narrower choice of products than hearing people and limiting the outlets from which they available, often to specialist suppliers of products for deaf people.

When the third approach is used, there are issues of the relative advantages and disadvantages of modifying a single device, for instance by addition of an appropriate output transducer or (additional) amplification stage(s), or developing a unified system for all the alarm and alerting devices in the building. The inclusion of an additional output transducer will be easiest if the original device has been designed with additional output ports, but this could be considered as an aspect of the design for all approach.

When a unified system is developed, it may be necessary to have a technique for distinguishing the different signals from each other, as well as for ensuring that the output signals received by the user can be clearly distinguished from each other. This is the approach taken in the alarm and alerting system developed for a particular deafblind person described in Chapter 8. The development of a general sensing, signal recognition, transmission and output device, as shown in Figure 7.2, could have some potential. However, it may be difficult to develop the signal-recognition component to be sufficiently general purpose and the device contains the majority of the components of a standard alarm or alerting device. Therefore, this approach will not be considered further here.

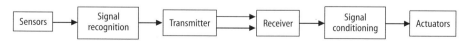

Figure 7.2 Sensing, interface, transmission and output device.

7.2.2 Categorisation of Alarm and Alerting Systems

There are a number of different ways to categorise devices, including according to function, design principles and the underlying technologies. It is probably most useful to categorise alarm and alerting devices according to design principles and function, using the following five categories:

- design principles
- single or multifunctional
- type of output transducer
- function (for single-function devices)
- with or without signal transmission.

It should be noted that these different categories cannot be arranged in a strict hierarchical order.

As has already been stated, the following three types of design principles can be used in alarm and alerting systems:

- design for all
- design specifically for deaf and hearing-impaired people
- modification of devices designed for hearing people to be used by deaf and hearing-impaired people.

Alarm and alerting devices for hearing people are generally single function. However, a number of multifunction alarm and alerting devices for deaf and hearing-impaired people have been developed. For instance, there are multifunction radio-pager systems with fire and intruder alarm and door and telephone alert functions, as well as baby monitors to which alarm clocks can be attached. Devices designed using design for all principles are generally single function, whereas devices designed specifically for deaf and hearing-impaired people can be either single function or multifunction. Single-function devices for hearing people can be modified for deaf and hearing-impaired people and, in addition, multifunction devices can be constructed by combining a number of single-function devices, changing the output transducer and adding a signal-recognition stage.

Classification according to the type of output transducer used gives the following categories:

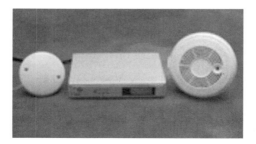

Figure 7.3 Smoke alarm with vibrating pad (courtesy of RNID).

Alarm and Alerting Systems for Hearing-impaired and Deaf People

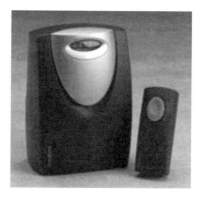

Figure 7.4 Libra flashing light door chime (courtesy of RNID).

- loud buzzers or bells
- loudspeaker
- flashing or strobe lights
- television signal
- light emitting diodes (leds)
- vibro-tactile devices
- electro-tactile devices.

Single-function devices can be classified by function as follows:

- fire alarm
- carbon monoxide alarm
- baby monitor
- intruder alarm
- "nurse" call for a person being cared for to attract attention
- telephone ringer
- doorbell
- alarm clock.

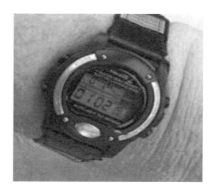

Figure 7.5 Vibralite 2 wristwatch with vibrating alarm (courtesy of RNID).

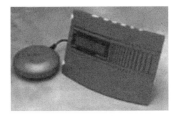

Figure 7.6 Vibrasound digital alarm clock with vibrating pad and very loud alarm (courtesy of RNID).

Examples of single-function devices, namely a smoke detector, a door chime, a wristwatch alarm and a digital alarm clock are given in Figures 7.3 to 7.6. An example of a multifunction device, the Walkabout Classic, is given in Figure 7.7. This uses radio frequency transmission (see Section 7.5) to transmit the sound of the telephone, doorbell, baby or other sound source over a range of up to 100 m. The transmitter with a built-in microphone is placed near the sound source and the user carries the receiver on their person. The built-in volume control allows the sound received to be amplified.

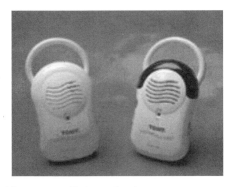

Figure 7.7 Walkabout Classic (courtesy of RNID).

7.3 Sensors, Transducers and Actuators

This first stage in an alarm or alerting device is a transducer that detects or is triggered by the signal of concern. A transducer is defined as a device that accepts energy from one part of a system and emits it in a different form in another part of the system. If the transducer energy is supplied by the input signal then it is called passive, whereas transducers that have an external source of energy are active.

Transducers can be divided into two classes: sensors and actuators (Bannister and Whitehead, 1991). Sensors accept an input signal, generally in analogue form (as most real variables are continuous functions), and transform the signal to another type of energy, generally an electrical signal, which is output to the system. Actuators (Usher and Keating, 1996) transform an electrical or other signal to an appropriate form to be perceived and then output it. Therefore, sensors or input transducers include piezoelectric pressure sensors, and output transducers or actuators include vibrators and flashing lights. Before the output of a sensor is transmitted further, it may require signal processing or conditioning, for instance by conversion to digital form and/or amplification.

However, the distinction is sometimes made between sensors and input transducers, with the term sensor used purely for the sensing element and the term transducer to denote the sensing element plus the components for transforming the input signal to an electrical signal (Usher and Keating, 1996). The detection of an event of interest by a sensor requires an associated measurable property or the existence of another measurable variable from which the event of interest can be deduced. For instance, the sensor in a fire alarm may detect temperature, temperature changes or smoke. The measurable variable that is detected by a sensor is called a measurand.

Sensors are most commonly classified according to the main forms of energy that carry the signal (Gardner, 1994), giving the categories of thermal, radiation, mechanical, magnetic, chemical, biological and electrical sensors. However, since one of the main themes in this chapter is the relationship between design and function, the sensors used in this chapter will be categorised according to function rather than energy type. Therefore, some sections include several different types of sensors that use different types of energy to fulfil the same basic function. Sections 7.3.1–7.3.3 discuss the sensors used in fire alarms, carbon monoxide alarms and intruder alarms respectively. Sections 7.3.4 and 7.3.5 discuss piezoelectric sensors and microphones; the former can be used as both a pressure sensor and to detect auditory signals, such as a baby crying or a telephone ringing, and the latter is only used to detect auditory signals.

7.3.1 The Sensors in Fire Alarms

To function effectively, the sensor in a fire alarm needs to detect a fire rapidly and not be subject to false alerts. Since "fire", as such, cannot be detected, a measurable variable is required, and fire sensors can be categorised according to the measurand used into heat and smoke detectors. Heat detectors can be further categorised into fixed temperature, differential temperature and compensator types. A fixed-temperature sensor (Figure 7.8) is triggered when the surrounding temperature exceeds a fixed value, generally 65 to 75 °C (Ohba, 1992).

Fixed-temperature sensors work on a variety of principles, and the most common type is based on a bimetallic element in which the different metals have different rates of expansion as temperature increases. Strips of two different metals are welded together to form a laminated structure. This is straight at the welding temperature and is deformed into a circular arc as the temperature changes due to the differential expansion of the two metals. The radius of curvature is inversely proportional to the change in temperature and,

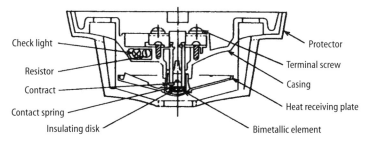

Figure 7.8 Fixed-temperature, single-location sensor (from Ohba (1992), courtesy of John Wiley and Sons).

therefore, deformation increases with temperature. When used as part of a sensor in a fire alarm, the bimetallic element carries one of the contacts for closing a switch. When a sufficiently high ambient temperature, generally 65 to 75 °C, is reached, deformation of the bimetallic element closes the switch, generating an electrical signal and activating the other components of the alarm system.

A differential-temperature sensor is triggered when the rate of temperature increase in a room exceeds a set value. Differential-temperature sensors can detect fires at lower temperatures than fixed-temperature devices, but will not be triggered even at high temperatures if the rate of temperature change is low. Single-location types are actuated by temperature change at a fixed location and are most commonly used, whereas dispersed types are actuated by the change in temperature over a wider area. The heat-sensing element can be bimetallic or monometallic, a semiconductor thermocouple or air expansion.

Smoke detectors can be further categorised into photoelectric and ionisation types. They are triggered by combustion products, such as smoke, reaching a predetermined density. Smoke consists of the solid and liquid particles emitted when an object is burned or decomposes under heat. It generally remains in the air. Ionisation detectors are good at detecting fires burning with a flame, where the smoke particles are small (0.01 to 10 μm) and dark in colour, whereas photoelectric detectors are better suited to detecting smouldering fires, where the smoke particles are larger and lighter in colour (Ohba, 1992).

An ionisation smoke detector (Figure 7.9) consists of a source of americium-241 placed between two electrodes. It emits alpha particles, which ionise the air molecules in the space between the electrodes, making it conductive. Therefore, applying a voltage will give an ion current. When there are smoke particles between the electrodes, the ionised air molecules are adsorbed onto them. This leads to an increase in particle weight and a reduction in the speed of charge transfer between the electrodes and, consequently, a reduction in current flow. The magnitude of the current can, therefore, be (inversely) related to the concentration of smoke particles. The alarm system will then be triggered when the current drops to a certain level. Photoelectric detectors can be divided into optical dispersion detectors, which detect light scattered by smoke particles, and optical attenuation detectors, which detect the attenuation of light by smoke.

The heat and smoke detectors discussed so far can be used to detect the start of a fire and trigger a fire alarm. If more detailed information about the

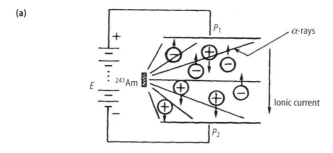

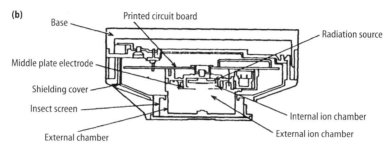

Figure 7.9 Ionisation smoke detector (from Ohba (1992), courtesy of John Wiley and Sons): (a) principle; (b) structure.

progress of the fire is required, a high-sensitivity particle sensor (see Figure 7.10) can be used. The air stream containing combustion products passes through the return duct and is pumped out for sampling by the vacuum pump. Any smoke particles in the air stream appearing in the laser beam in the chamber are detected by the light dispersed. The optical signal from the photodiode is amplified in the high-gain multistage amplifier and processed in a sensing processor before being transmitted to a central unit, where it is decoded to give information about the progress of the fire (Ohba, 1992).

7.3.2 Carbon Monoxide Sensors

Carbon monoxide sensors can be used, for instance, to detect a gas leak from a malfunctioning gas fire. Carbon monoxide is a highly toxic colourless and odourless gas that can cause death in very low concentrations. Many commercial carbon monoxide gas alarms use tin dioxide as the gas sensor (Figure 7.11). These sensors are based on the principle that adsorption of a gas onto a semiconducting material, such as a metal oxide, can produce a large change in electrical resistivity. A number of different metal oxides, including zinc oxide and titanium dioxide, show this effect, but tin dioxide is most commonly used in gas sensors.

Under certain conditions, tin dioxide behaves like an n-type semiconductor due to the initial reversible reaction of atmospheric oxygen with lattice

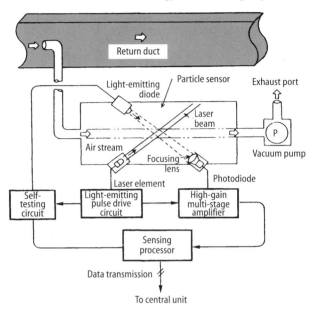

Figure 7.10 Particle sensor (from Ohba (1992), courtesy of John Wiley and Sons).

vacancies in the tin dioxide and the resulting reduction in electron concentration (Gardner, 1994). This reaction produces oxygen ions, which can react irreversibly with the gas to be measured. The theory predicts an increase in the electrical conductivity of the material. This increase in conductivity can be related to the increase in carrier concentration and, using the reaction kinetics, to a fractional power of the concentration of the gas being measured. This explains the increase in surface conductivity in thin single-crystal films. However, an extension of the theory to include a concentration-dependent mobility term is required to explain the large effect observed in thick metal-oxide layers.

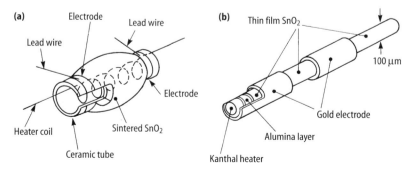

Figure 7.11 Commercial tin dioxide gas sensors: (a) thick-film device; (b) microdevice (from Gardner (1994), courtesy of John Wiley and Sons).

Alarm and Alerting Systems for Hearing-impaired and Deaf People 225

The response time of carbon monoxide sensors generally decreases with increasing carbon monoxide concentration. Typical parameters are as follows:

- no alarm at concentration levels below 30 ppm
- an alarm in 60–240 min for 70 ppm concentration
- an alarm in 10–50 min at 150 ppm concentration
- an alarm in 4–15 min at 400 ppm concentration.

7.3.3 Intruder Detectors

Intruder detectors are used to detect when an individual enters a warning zone either around or within a building. Therefore, they are generally only used when the building is not occupied or when occupants are asleep, to avoid being triggered by legitimate activities. They are known as terminal sensors and have the following three states (Ohba, 1992):

- normal or secure state
- detection of broken wires and activation of the sensor due to an intruder
- short circuits in the sensors and wiring.

There is always a small current in the terminal sensors and the wiring to allow a warning to be given immediately a broken wire or short circuit occurs.

Infrared sensors are often used outdoors for intruder detection, as they have low power consumption and are easy to use. However, they have the disadvantage of being easily triggered by falling leaves, rain and fog. Heat sensors are often used in indoor security. They act by detecting changes in the background heat radiation due to the presence of an intruder. They are passive and provide several sensitive zones or regions receiving heat radiation.

Intruder sensors on windows and doors use a combination of a permanent magnet and a reed switch. The permanent magnet is set in the moving part of the window or door and the reed switch is embedded in the frame. The reed switch consists of two slivers or reeds of ferromagnetic material, such as nickel–iron, hermetically sealed into a tube (Bannister and Whitehead, 1991). The ends of the reeds are sealed and there is a small gap between them. The whole assembly is inserted into a coil. Current flow in the coil sets up a magnetic field and attracts the reeds, closing the switch. When there is no field the reeds move apart, opening the switch. The reeds have low inertia, giving operating speeds of less than 1 ms for some reed switches. The main limit on operating speed is contact bounce, illustrated in Figure 7.12. The contact ends of the reeds are plated with rhodium or another precious metal to provide contact resistance and extend their life, which is measured in millions of operations. The use of mercury-wetted contacts gives the fastest and most reliable switches. The surface tension of the mercury film between the contacts ensures immediate, unbroken contact, thereby often eliminating contact bounce. This arrangement is inexpensive, but the switches need to be fitted where they cannot be detected and will not affect the operation of the window or door.

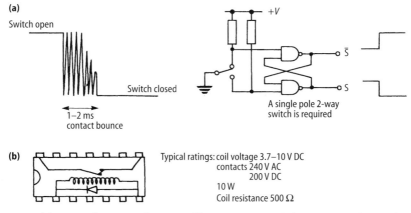

Figure 7.12 (a) Contact bounce and its control by two cross-coupled NAND gates. (b) Reed switch dual-in-line package (from Bannister and Whitehead (1991), courtesy of Chapman and Hall).

7.3.4 Piezoelectric Sensors: Sound and Pressure

The piezoelectric effect involves the generation of an electric charge when a force is applied to a suitable material, such as certain crystals (Usher, 1985; Bannister and Whitehead, 1991; Dally *et al.*, 1993; Morris, 1993). Naturally occurring crystals, such as quartz and Rochelle salt, have a very strong piezoelectric effect. There are two types of synthetic material that exhibit the effect: crystalline structures, such as lithium sulphate and ammonium dihydrogen phosphate, and polarised ferroelectric ceramics, such as barium titanate. Polarisation of the ferroelectric ceramics is achieved by heating to a temperature above the Curie point, at which the ferroelectric properties break down, and then cooling slowly in a strong electric field. This results in a redistribution of molecular charge in a preferred direction determined by the applied field. The crystal surfaces are coated with metal electrodes to effectively form a parallel-plate capacitor.

When a piezoelectric crystal is deformed by applied pressure (Figure 7.13), the positive and negative charges in the crystal are displaced relative to each other, producing external charges of opposite signs on the external faces of the

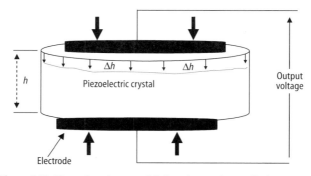

Figure 7.13 Piezoelectric crystal deforming under applied pressure.

crystal and a potential difference across the crystal faces. The charge q that develops is related to the output voltage v_o by (Dally et al., 1993)

$$q = v_o C \tag{7.1}$$

where C ($=kKA/h$) is the capacitance of the crystal, and to the applied pressure p by

$$q = S_q A p \tag{7.2}$$

where A is the area of the electrode and S_q is the charge sensitivity of the crystal. The charge sensitivity depends on the type of crystal and the orientation of the sensor, which is generally a cylinder, relative to the crystal axes. The output voltage v_o developed by the piezoelectric sensor is given by

$$v_o = S_v h p \tag{7.3}$$

where S_v ($= S_q/kK$) is the voltage sensitivity of the sensor, K is the relative dielectric constant of the crystal and h is the width of the crystal. The voltage sensitivity is also related to the orientation of the axes of the sensor cylinder relative to the crystal axes. Typical values of the charge and voltage sensitivity are given in Table 7.1 (Dally et al., 1993).

Most piezoelectric transducers are made from single-crystal quartz, as it is the most stable piezoelectric material, and is nearly loss free both mechanically and electrically. It can be operated up to 550 °C. Its low charge sensitivity relative to barium titanate is not a serious disadvantage, due to the availability of high-gain charge amplifiers for processing the output signal. Unlike other transducers, which have fairly low output impedance, piezoelectric crystals have very high, but variable, impedance. Since a piezoelectric sensor acts as a capacitor, the output impedance is given by (Dally et al., 1993)

$$Z_c = \frac{1}{j\omega C} \tag{7.4}$$

giving impedances of 10 kΩ for high-frequency applications.

Piezoelectric sensors are used in force and pressure sensors. Since sound waves give rise to air-pressure changes, piezoelectric sensors can be used to detect sound, and piezoelectric sound sensors are therefore used in a number of alarm and alerting systems. Piezoelectric sensors have very high natural frequencies, low weight, small size and very good sensitivity. Owing to their high output impedance, they have to be combined with signal-conditioning components, such as voltage followers and charge amplifiers, to convert the charge to a measurable voltage. Miniature voltage-follower amplifiers, such as a p-channel metal oxide semiconductor field effect transistor (MOSFET) unity

Table 7.1 Charge and voltage sensitivities of piezoelectric crystals.

Material	Orientation	S_q (pC N^{-1})	S_v (V m N^{-1})
Quartz, SiO$_2$	X-cut, length longitudinal	2.2	0.055
Single crystal	X-cut, thickness longitudinal	−2.0	−0.050
	Y-cut, thickness shear	4.4	0.110
Barium titanate	Parallel to polarisation	130.0	0.011
Ceramic, poled	Perpendicular to polarisation	−56.0	−0.004

gain amplifier or voltage follower, can now be incorporated into the transducer housing.

7.3.5 Microphones: Sound Sensors

Microphones are used to receive sound energy and transform it into electrical energy. They can therefore act as sensors for audio signals, such as a telephone ringing or a baby crying. Most microphones contain a thin flat piece of metal or plastic called a diaphragm. The changes in pressure due to the acoustic waveform are transmitted to the diaphragm and make it move. This movement is then converted to voltage changes. Pressure microphones respond to the difference in atmospheric pressure and pressure of a sound wave, whereas pressure-gradient microphones are sensitive to pressure differences on either side of the diaphragm (Figure 7.14). Pressure-gradient microphones are directional in operation, as they respond best when there are opposing pressure differences on the two sides of the microphone, whereas pressure microphones are omnidirectional and respond equally to pressure changes from any direction (Bannister and Whitehead, 1991; Noll, 1995; Decker, 1996).

The differences in frequency-response properties of the different types of microphone are generally not critical when they are used as sensors in alarm and alerting devices, where they are usually only required to detect an auditory signal rather than give a high-quality reproduction of it. In a crystal microphone, the diaphragm is attached to piezoelectric crystals, such as quartz, so that movement of the diaphragm bends the crystals and gives rise to a small electric current. Crystal microphones can be either directional or omnidirectional and have a frequency response from about 80 to 6500 Hz, so they are useful in situations involving the human voice. However, the piezoelectric effect gives rise to a very small voltage. This means that the microphone should not be separated by more than 16 to 20 m from the amplifiers to avoid amplifying internal noise. This is not a problem in alarm and alerting devices, where the amplifiers and microphone are likely to be combined into one package.

In the dynamic microphone, as shown in Figure 7.15, a small core of wire fitted round the core of a permanent magnet is attached to the diaphragm

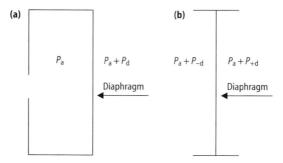

Figure 7.14 (a) Pressure microphone; (b) pressure-gradient microphone (from Decker (1996), courtesy of Lawrence Erlbaum Associates).

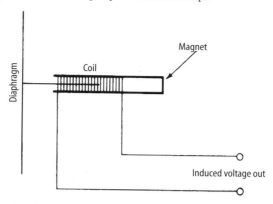

Figure 7.15 Dynamic microphone (from Decker (1996), courtesy of Lawrence Erlbaum Associates).

(Decker, 1996). The coil is moved in and out of the magnetic field by movements of the diaphragm. This changes the field and gives rise to current in the field windings of the coil. As the dynamic microphone has a larger output voltage and less internal noise than the crystal microphone, it can be operated further from the source of amplification. However, it is less sensitive and can be affected by neon lights, dimmer switches and ungrounded power cables.

Condenser microphones have good performance, though the impedance is high and the output consequently small, but they are very expensive and are therefore not used in alarm and alerting devices. In the capacitance microphone, changes in air pressure in the sound wave lead to a variation in microphone capacitance. This variation in capacitance gives rise to small charge and discharge currents, which can be measured as changes in voltage across a resistance, which generally has a value of 1 MΩ.

The electret microphone has similar construction and performance to a condenser microphone, but it is much cheaper. The surfaces of the diaphragm and the back plate are close together and form a capacitor, which has a permanent charge rather than being charged by the power supply applied. Changes in air pressure produced by the sound lead to a change in the spacing between the two places. Electret microphones can be made relatively small, which can be useful in alarm and alerting devices. The main disadvantage of electret microphones is the fact that they require disconnecting from other equipment when not in use so that the battery used to power the microphone does not discharge (Decker, 1996).

7.4 Signal Conditioning

Amplification is the main type of signal conditioning or processing used in alarm and alerting devices, and the only one that will be discussed in this chapter. An amplifier is a device that receives a signal from a sensor or other input device and outputs a magnified version of this signal to an actuator or other output device, a transmitter or another amplifier. The signals from sensors are generally small, on the order of a few milli- or micro-volts, and have to be amplified sufficiently to be transmitted and/or operate an output device.

In general, amplifiers are required to be distortionless, *i.e.* to preserve the shape of the input waveform. A distortionless amplifier is linear and has the following relationship between the input $v_i(t)$ and output $v_o(t)$ signals

$$v_o(t) = A v_i(t) \tag{7.5}$$

where A is the amplifier gain. If the relationship between $v_i(t)$ and $v_o(t)$ contains higher powers of v_i, then the output will have a different shape from the input and the amplifier will show non-linear distortion.

An amplifier with a non-linear characteristic that is not centred round the origin can be made to operate linearly by first biasing it to operate at a point near the centre of the load line or characteristic (Sedra and Smith, 1991). This is done by applying a DC bias voltage V_i at the operating point or quiescent point Q.

The instantaneous operating point will be in an almost linear segment of the curve centred about Q if the amplitude of the signal to be amplified, $v_i(t)$, is sufficiently small. The time-varying portion of the output $v_o(t)$ will then be proportional to this signal $v_i(t)$. The output voltage will be an undistorted reproduction of the input voltage when the transistor is operated in the linear region between saturation and cut-off.

7.4.1 Voltage and Power Amplifiers

Amplifiers can be divided into two classes: small signal or voltage and large signal or power amplifiers. A small-signal amplifier generally uses only a small portion of its load. A power amplifier has low internal impedance and can consequently produce a large current, whereas a voltage amplifier has a high internal current and can develop large voltages. In voltage amplifiers, the main factors of concern are amplification linearity and gain, whereas power efficiency and power handling capacity are important in power amplifiers. A DC power supply is required to supply the additional power drawn from the load over that delivered to it, as well as make up any power dissipated as heat.

Power amplifiers can be divided into five classes, called A, B, AC, C and D, according to the transistor conduction angle, which gives the angle of variation of the output over one cycle of operation for a full cycle of the input signal (Sedra and Smith, 1991; Boylestad and Nashelsky, 2002; Floyd, 2002). Of these five classes, it is classes AB and C that are mainly used in alarm and alerting systems.

In class AB, the conduction angle is slightly greater than 180° and the DC bias is non-zero and much smaller than the peak current of the sine wave signal.

In class C, the output is biased for operation at less than 180° of the cycle and the output current is a periodic pulse.

Both voltage and power amplifiers are used in alarm and alerting systems, as shown in Figure 7.16. Voltage amplifiers and class AB power amplifiers are used in signal conditioning of the signal received from the sensor or to be

Alarm and Alerting Systems for Hearing-impaired and Deaf People

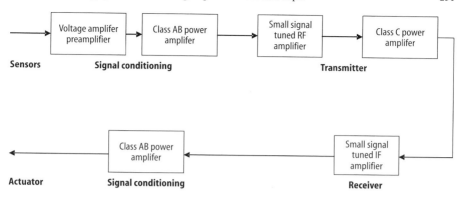

Figure 7.16 The use of different types of amplifier in alarm and alerting systems.

transmitted to the actuator, whereas small-signal tuned amplifiers and class C power amplifiers are used in the radio transmission systems of pagers and other alarm and alerting systems that require signal transmission.

Voltage amplifiers are used as preamplifiers to condition the signal received from the sensor before it is passed on to a power amplifier. This will include amplification to increase the signal amplitude to a level suitable for further amplification by power amplifiers and, possibly, a change of the input impedance characteristics. There may be more than one preamplifier stage. Class AB power amplifiers are used to amplify the signal before it is output to the output transducer or actuator, and sometimes also before signal transmission. Therefore it is a class AB power amplifier that would be used, for instance, to make a bell or buzzer louder.

Small-signal tuned amplifiers are used in the frequency modulated transmitter to increase the amplitude of the oscillator output and increase the transmitted frequency. Class C power amplifiers are used to boost the final power from the transmitter to the aerial tuning unit and antenna and as frequency amplifiers if the carrier frequency is too low. They are also used to give radio frequency power boosting and frequency multiplication in the frequency modulated superheterodyne receiver.

7.4.2 Transistor

Transistors are the main components of most of the amplifiers used in alarm and alerting systems. A transistor is a three-layer three-terminal semiconductor device. The basic principle is the use of the voltage between two terminals to control the current in the third terminal. Therefore, a transistor can be used to realise a controlled source, which is the basis of amplifier design. Alternatively, the transistor can act as a switch by using the control signal to make the current in the third terminal change from zero to a large value. There are two main types of transistor, both of which are used in amplifiers: the bipolar junction transistor (BJT) and the field effect transistor (FET) (Sedra and Smith, 1991; Boylestad and Nashelsky, 2002; Floyd, 2002).

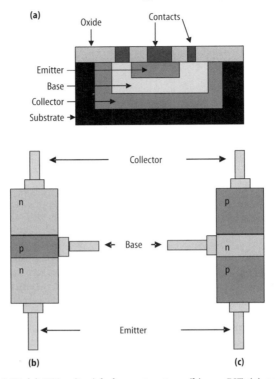

Figure 7.17 (a) BJT, epitaxial planar structure; (b) npn BJT; (c) pnp BJT.

A bipolar junction (Figure 7.17) consists of three doped semiconductor regions, in either an npn or pnp arrangement. A terminal is connected to each of these regions and the three terminals are labelled emitter (E), base (B) and collector (C). The emitter layer is heavily doped and the base and collector layers are lightly doped. The widths of the outer layers are much greater than those of the inner p- and n-type layers. Different modes of operation are obtained according to the bias (forward or reverse) of the three junctions. The transistor operates as an amplifier in active mode with the emitter–base junction forward biased and the collector–base junction reverse biased. The bias conditions for active-mode operation are given by two external voltage sources. In the npn transformer the forward bias voltage produces a current in the collector terminal, which is an exponential function of the forward bias voltage. Its value is independent of the value of the collector voltage as long as the collector–base junction remains reverse biased. The emitter current is equal to the sum of the collector and base currents. Operation of the pnp transistor is similar.

In the FET (Sedra and Smith, 1991; Boylestad and Nashelsky, 2002; Floyd, 2002) the current is controlled by the electric field established by the voltage applied to the control terminal. Unlike the BJT, where current is carried by both electrons and holes, the FET is a unipolar transistor with current carried by either electrons or holes, giving n channel and p channel FETs respectively.

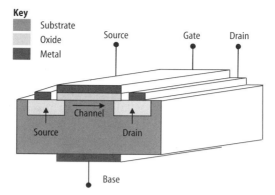

Figure 7.18 Enhancement-type n-channel MOSFET.

The enhancement metal oxide semiconductor field effect transistor or MOSFET (Figure 7.18) is the most commonly used type of FET. It occupies a smaller silicon area on an IC (Integrated Circuit) chip than a BJT. There are three terminals: the gate (G), source (S) and drain (D) terminals. The current in the third terminal is determined by the voltage between the two terminals. Therefore, like the BJT, the FET can be used both as an amplifier and a switch.

7.4.3 Voltage Amplifiers

Voltage amplifiers are used in alarm and alerting systems as preamplifiers to condition the signal before it is passed on to a power amplifier. There may be more than one preamplifier stage. Voltage amplifiers can be implemented using either BJTs or MOSFETs. In general, FET amplifiers do not achieve such high voltage gains as BJT amplifiers. There are three different basic configurations for BJTs, the common emitter, the common base and the common collector (Sedra and Smith, 1991; Boylestad and Nashelsky, 2002; Floyd, 2002). All three configurations have a voltage divider bias, driven by an AC voltage source with internal resistance R_s, as shown in Figure 7.19.

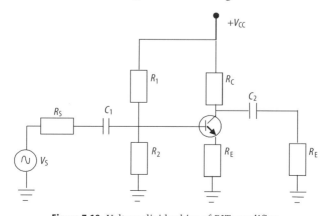

Figure 7.19 Voltage divider bias of BJT amplifier.

Just as there are three BJT amplifier configurations, so there are also three FET amplifier configurations, with the common-drain, common-source and common-gate FET configurations analogous to the common-collector, common-emitter and common-base BJT configurations respectively. Single-stage BJT or FET amplifiers can be connected in sequence with various coupling methods to produce multistage amplifiers. The total gain of a multistage amplifier is the product of the individuals gains or the sum of the gains in decibels.

7.4.4 Small-signal Tuned Amplifiers

Tuned amplifiers operate over a small band of frequencies centred on a resonant frequency and are required to provide high gain and good selectivity. Their applications in alarm and alerting systems with signal transmission include the intermediate-frequency amplifier in a superheterodyne receiver and the radio frequency amplifier in a frequency modulated transmitter. The frequency response is characterised by a peak at a particular frequency, called the centre frequency, 3 dB bandwidth and skirt selectivity. The skirt selectivity is generally given by the ratio of the 30 dB bandwidth to the 3 dB bandwidth. Tuned amplifiers (Leven, 2000) use a parallel LCR circuit as the load or input to a BJT or MOSFET amplifier, as shown in Figure 7.20 for a MOSFET amplifier. This circuit is a single tuned amplifer as it uses one tuning circuit.

A multiple tuned amplifier with additional tuning stages is used in the intermediate-frequency receiver of a radio receiver, as the single tuned amplifier does not provide sufficient selectivity. A radio frequency choke is often used in series with each resistor of the bias circuit to prevent the bias resistors affecting the tuning circuit.

The multiple stages can be either synchronous or stagger tuned (Sedra and Smith, 1991). Synchronous tuning involves the use of N identical resonant circuits and gives a reduction in bandwidth by a factor of $(2^{1/n} -1)^{1/2}$. Stagger tuning is illustrated in Figure 7.21, and generally results in a much flatter overall response than with synchronous tuning.

Crystal and ceramic tuned amplifiers are increasingly used in modern communications systems to give stability and high sensitivity (Q factor). Both types work on the piezoelectric effect, which gives electric charges on opposite

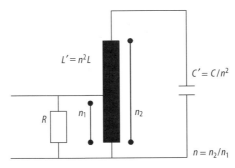

Figure 7.20 Parallel LCR circuit with MOSFET amplifier.

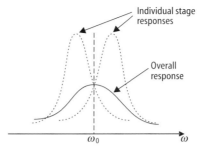

Figure 7.21 Stagger tuning.

faces of a properly cut slice of crystal when it is bent. The ceramic filter is cheaper than the crystal one and does not require a series or parallel tuning capacitor for fine tuning, but it has poorer selectivity and is more sensitive to temperature variations. Therefore, crystal filters are used in communications receivers and ceramic filters in domestic ones. However, improvements in fabrication mean that ceramic filters are also used in communications receivers, for instance in wide-band intermediate-frequency receivers (Leven, 2000).

7.4.5 Class C Power Amplifiers

radio frequency amplifiers generally operate under class C bias conditions. They are used in alarm and alerting systems to boost the power from the transmitter to the aerial tuning unit and antenna and as frequency amplifiers if the carrier frequency is too low. They are also used to give frequency multiplication and radio frequency power boosting in the frequency modulated superheterodyne receiver (used in the transmission system of an alarm or alerting device), as shown in Figure 7.22.

Class C power amplifiers can be constructed with either bipolar junction or FETs. A common-emitter Class C amplifier with a resistive load is shown in Figure 7.23. The negative V_{BB} voltage biases the amplifier below cut-off. At the positive peak of each cycle the base voltage is briefly greater than the barrier potential of the base–emitter junction. The transistor is turned on during this

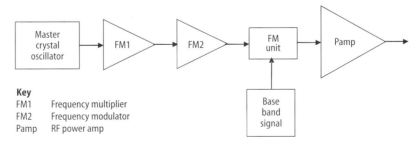

Figure 7.22 Frequency modulated receiver.

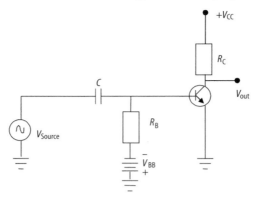

Figure 7.23 Class C power amplifier circuit.

brief interval. Since class C amplifiers are only on for a small percentage of the input cycle, they have low power dissipation.

A class C amplifier is used together with a parallel resonant circuit (tank) (Floyd, 2002), shown in Figure 7.24. The oscillation of the tank circuit is initiated and sustained by the short pulse of collector current on each cycle of the input. The current is passed through a parallel LC circuit tuned to the frequency of the input sinusoid to provide a full cycle of operation for the resonant frequency. This gives a sinusoidal output voltage with decreasing amplitude over successive cycles, due to energy losses in the resistance of the tank circuit. However, the collector current pulse re-energises the resonant circuit and prevents the oscillation amplitude from decreasing. When the tank circuit is tuned to the second harmonic of the input signal, the class C amplifier acts as a frequency multiple (×2), as re-energising occurs on alternate cycles. Higher frequency multiplication factors can be obtained by tuning the tank circuit to higher harmonics of the input frequency.

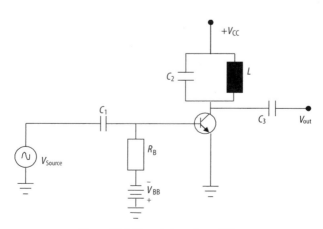

Figure 7.24 Tuned class C amplifier.

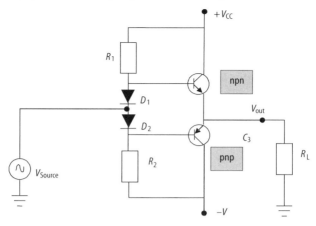

Figure 7.25 Class AB amplifier.

7.4.6 Class AB Power Amplifiers

Class AB amplifiers are the most commonly used audio power amplifiers, as they have much higher efficiency than class A and eliminate the crossover distortion that occurs in class B. It is class AB power amplifiers, therefore, that are used, for instance, to make a bell or buzzer louder. More generally, they are used to amplify the signal before it is output to the output transducer of an alarm or alerting system and sometimes to amplify the signal before transmission. Like class B, class AB combines two transistors in push–pull operation, either using transformer coupling or two complementary symmetry transistors, *i.e.* a matching pair of npn–pnp bipolar junction or n-channel–p-channel FETs.

Crossover distortion occurs in class B amplifiers, as both transistors are cut off for a small range of input voltages centred round zero, giving zero output voltage. It is removed in a class AB amplifier by adjusting the bias to just overcome the base–emitter voltage of the transistors. This gives a small nonzero current on the complementary output transistors even in the absence of an input signal (Sedra and Smith, 1991; Floyd, 2002). This bias can be achieved by using a voltage divider and diode arrangement in combination with the two amplifier transistors, as shown in Figure 7.25.

7.5 Radio Frequency Transmission

A transmission system, consisting of a transmitter and a receiver, is one of the main components of the generic structure of an alarm and alerting device. However, as discussed in Section 7.2, unlike input and output transducers, not all alarm and alerting systems require signal transmission.

Frequency modulated, radio frequency waves are most commonly used to transmit the signal in alarm and alerting devices. The basic structures of a radio frequency transmitter and a receiver are discussed in Sections 7.5.1 and 7.5.2 respectively. Since, as discussed below, frequency modulation and demodulation play an important role in signal transmission and reception, the principles of frequency modulation are introduced in Section 7.5.3 and the structures of a modulator and a demodulator are described in Sections 7.5.4 and 7.5.5 respectively.

7.5.1 Transmitter

The main components of a transmitter are shown in Figure 7.26. A transmitter modulates the information signal onto a carrier, amplifies the waveform to the desired power level and outputs it to the transmitting antenna (Smith, 1986). It includes a radio frequency oscillator that is modulated by the information signal. The modulated signal is then multiplied in frequency up to the desired transmitting frequency and amplified to the required power level in the power amplifier. In some cases, modulation takes place in the power amplifier. The transmitters used in alarm and alerting systems are generally narrowband and use frequency modulation.

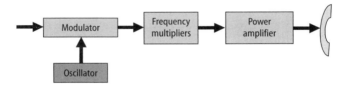

Figure 7.26 Block diagram of a transmitter.

There are a number of commercially available transmitter modules, such as the ABACOM Technologies (http://www.abacom-tech.com) TXM series of FM transmitter modules (Figure 7.27), which can be used in paging, fire alarms and "nurse call" transmitters. For operation they require power to be connected to the module supply pin, serial data to the data input and an appropriate antenna. The different modules in the series have frequencies of 418 or 433.92 MHz, serial data transmission rates up to either 10 or 20 kbytes per second and effective radiated power (ERP) of 0.25 or (in one case) 10 mW. They all draw less than 10 mA current and have supply voltages in the range 2.7–3.6, 3.5–5 and 6–9 V. The modules are small in size and can be mounted on a printed

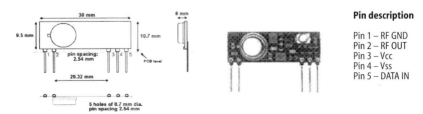

Figure 7.27 ABACOM Technologies TXM FM transmitter module (courtesy of ABACOM).

circuit board (PCB). They do not require further tuning and can take analogue or digital data input.

These transmitter modules can be combined with a number of different platforms, including the 1-6CH-TXM one- to six-channel FM remote control platform. In combination with the HT-12E encoder integrated circuit, this platform is compatible with the 1-, 2- and 4-CH-SRX receiver platforms and provides a radio frequency link to control up to six remote devices in either latched or pulse modes and at distances of up to 200 m. The assembled PCB is supplied with an enclosure that includes a PP3 9 V battery compartment with access door.

7.5.2 Superheterodyne Receiver

The main components of a superheterodyne receiver are illustrated in Figure 7.28. The superheterodyne receiver has the advantage of allowing high-quality fixed-frequency filters and amplifiers to be used. The frequency of the input signal is shifted to the fixed frequency of the receiver filter, so that the radio frequency amplifiers do not need to follow a varying input frequency, and variable-frequency filters, which are generally of lower quality, are not required.

The receiver has two main stages (Smith, 1986; Carson, 1990). In the first, called the mixer or first detector, the incoming radio frequency signal is combined with the sinusoidal output of a local oscillator. In the second stage, called the demodulator or second detector, the signal is amplified by the intermediate-frequency amplifier and then demodulated. After demodulation, the signal is further amplified to the level of the desired output.

The mixer output circuit is generally tuned to the difference between the frequencies of the oscillator and the incoming signal, though it is sometimes tuned to their sum (Smith, 1986). The receiver is designed so that the frequency of the local oscillator is varied to track the incoming frequency. When the input signal consists of a carrier signal of frequency f_c and an information signal of frequency f_m and the first local oscillator frequency is f_o, then the mixer outputs signals with the two frequencies $f_c + f_m + f_o$ and $f_c + f_m - f_o$. The local oscillator frequency f_o is chosen so that one of these frequencies, generally the difference, is equal to the centre frequency f_{if} of the intermediate frequency filter, so that

$$f_{if} = f_c + f_m - f_o \qquad (7.6)$$

Since an information signal is generally modulated onto a high frequency carrier, the carrier signal frequency is usually much higher than the information-signal frequency, so that f_m can be ignored in Equation 7.6, giving

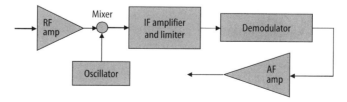

Figure 7.28 Block diagram of a superheterodyne receiver.

$$f_{if} = f_c - f_o \quad \text{or} \quad f_o = f_{if} + f_c \tag{7.7}$$

The intermediate-frequency filter output $f_{if} + f_m$ is then reduced in frequency to the relatively low frequency of the information signal f_m in the demodulator, where it is mixed with the second oscillator frequency, fixed at f_{if} (Smith, 1986). Problems can occur when there are several signals of different frequencies in the input. There is another signal frequency, known as the image frequency f_{im}, which will give a signal at the intermediate frequency when mixed with the local oscillator frequency f_o.

Using Equation 7.7:

$$f_{im} = f_{if} - f_o = 2f_{if} + f_c \tag{7.8}$$

The image frequency should be filtered out by an image suppression filter, called a preselector, before it enters the mixer, as it cannot be separated from the desired signal after leaving the mixer. The preselector should be tuneable if the receiver is designed to cover a band of frequencies. However, this is generally not a problem in the transmission systems occurring in alarm and alerting systems. The tuned circuit is often replaced by crystal, ceramic or mechanical filters.

The receiver is the weakest link in any radio communications system. The very large number of radio frequency signals transmitted at diverse frequencies and power levels makes it difficult for a receiver to receive the desired signal and no others. Local oscillators in the receiver will also act as transmitters. A weak signal may be radiated from the antenna at the frequency of these local oscillators. The radio and intermediate frequency circuits may also radiate weak signals directly. This radiation can be minimised by, for instance, shielding the local oscillator/mixer circuits using double-balanced mixers, keeping oscillator power low, and by using buffer amplifiers between the antenna and the mixer/oscillator circuits.

There are a number of commercially produced frequency modulated superheterodyne receiver modules, which are suitable for use in pager receivers and wire free security, amongst other applications. These include the ABACOM Technologies (http://www.abacom-tech.com) SILRX series of modules, which is shown in Figure 7.29. All these receivers operate on a supply voltage of 4.5–9 V and have a maximum serial data reception rate of either 10 or 20 kbytes per second. The operational frequency is 403, 418 or 433.92 MHz. All the receivers in the series have both digital and audio logic level data output. They are small in size, can be connected to a PCB and can be placed horizontally or vertically. For operation the receiver requires a clean power supply, an antenna and an appropriate data decoding circuit. Careful use of the receiver carrier detect output

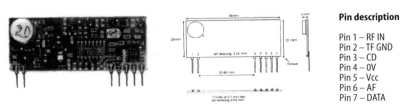

Pin description

Pin 1 – RF IN
Pin 2 – TF GND
Pin 3 – CD
Pin 4 – 0V
Pin 5 – Vcc
Pin 6 – AF
Pin 7 – DATA

Figure 7.29 SILRX FM superheterodyne receiver module (courtesy of ABACOM).

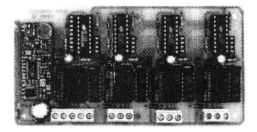

Figure 7.30 4CH-SRX receiver platform (courtesy of ABACOM).

allows long-term battery operation. For instance, an SILRX receiver on a 3 ms on, 800 ms standby cycle draws a current of less than 100 µA.

The SILRX receivers can be used together with the 1-, 2-, and 4-CH-SRX platforms to provide one, two or four independently binary coded output channels (Figure 7.30). The user can configure each relay output for either latched or pulsed mode, as well as the four-bit address for each output channel. Screw-terminal connector blocks are used for the power supply input and channel output connections to external equipment. An LED gives the status of each channel. There are 256 possible addresses, which can be set with an eight-position SIP switch. Either a quarter-wave wire antenna or a 50 Ω coaxial feed to a suitable external antenna connection can be made via a PCB pad.

7.5.3 Modulation

The term modulation is used to refer to the modification of an information signal so that it can be transmitted more easily over long distances. This is normally achieved by modifying a high frequency carrier signal by the low frequency signal being transmitted (Stremler, 1982). The carrier wave is a pure sinusoid

$$f_c(t) = A(t)\cos[\omega_c t + \phi(t)] \quad (7.9)$$

Therefore, the carrier wave has three parameters that can be modified by the information signal:

- the amplitude $A(t)$
- the frequency ω_c
- the phase $\phi(t)$.

This gives amplitude, frequency and phase modulation respectively. Frequency modulation is generally used in radio frequency transmission. Since a sinusoidal signal has constant phase and frequency, frequency modulation is based on the generalised angle $\theta(t)$.

In frequency modulation, the instantaneous frequency ω_i of the carrier signal linearly follows the information signal as

$$\omega_i(t) = \omega_c + k_f f_m(t) \quad (7.10)$$

where k_f is a constant, called the sensitivity of the modulation. If the signal f_m is a voltage, then k_f has dimensions of radians/seconds/volts. The constant ω_c is added on, as the signal frequency should be shifted up to ω_c before it is modulated for efficient transmission. The generalised angle $\theta(t)$ is given by (Lathi, 1983)

$$\theta(t) = \int_0^t [\omega_c + k_f f_m(\alpha)] \, d\alpha \qquad (7.11)$$
$$= \omega_c t + k_f \int_0^t f_m(\alpha) \, d\alpha$$

and the frequency modulated wave is

$$f_{sfm} = \cos\left[\omega_c t + k_f \int_0^t f_m(\alpha) \, d\alpha\right] \qquad (7.12)$$

There are two types of frequency modulation:

- narrowband frequency modulation has $k_f \ll 1$
- wideband frequency modulation has $k_f \gg 1$

The spectrum for narrowband frequency modulation can be shown to be similar to that for amplitude modulation double sideband (DSB). However, the spectrum for the modulated signal $F_s(\omega)$ is antisymmetric when the spectrum for the information signal $F_m(\omega)$ is symmetric.

Wideband frequency modulation has an infinite number of sidebands and, therefore, an infinite bandwidth. However, it can be band-limited by filtering to remove insignificant sidebands. Wideband frequency modulation has better signal/noise ratio than narrowband frequency modulation.

7.5.4 Modulator

Most frequency modulators are based on a combination of an oscillator and a device that varies the capacitance or inductance of the oscillator circuit. One of the simplest approaches uses a capacitor microphone to vary the capacitance of an LC oscillator. The capacitance, and hence the frequency of oscillation, changes as the sound waves impinge on the microphone diaphragm. The change in frequency increases with sound volume.

Another approach, which is more practical in some cases, is based on a variable reactance reversed biased diode or varactor, in which the capacitance is a function of the applied voltage (Leven, 2000). The varactor diode is connected across the tuned LC circuit of the oscillator. The frequency of oscillation can be varied by varying the reverse voltage applied to the diode and the system is therefore known as a voltage-controlled oscillator. The controlling voltage is the sum of the DC reverse voltage and a smaller amplitude modulating voltage (Figure 7.31).

There are a number of different LC oscillators that can be used in frequency modulators. The Colpitts oscillator is often used when the circuit capacitance is varied. It consists of a basic amplifier and an LC feedback circuit with split capacitance, as shown in Figure 7.32. The approximate frequency of the circuit is given by

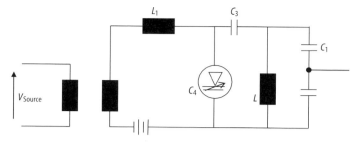

Figure 7.31 Diode frequency modulator.

$$f = \frac{1}{2\pi} \frac{1}{LC_T} \quad (7.13)$$

where C_T is the total capacitance, which can be obtained by treating the two capacitors as effectively in series and combining them. The feedback factor β is the ratio of the two voltages V_f and V_o and, using Figure 7.32, can be shown to be equal to

$$\beta = C_2/C_1 \quad (7.14)$$

The loop gain is the product of all the gains travelling round the loop from the amplifier input. It is the product of the feedback factor and the open loop gain A. For oscillation the loop gain should be zero and the loop phase shift should be zero. This gives

$$A = C_1/C_2 \quad (7.15)$$

However, in practice start-up conditions require that $A > C_1/C_2$. A practical circuit is shown in Figure 7.33. The Q factor determines the selectivity of the circuit, which is a measure of how well it can be tuned to a desired frequency and exclude other frequencies. Increasing Q increases circuit selectivity and gives a sharper response. The Q factor is affected by the input and output resistances.

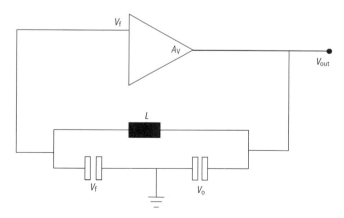

Figure 7.32 Colpitts oscillator.

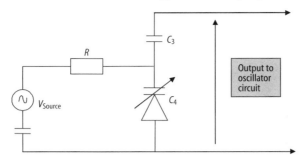

Figure 7.33 Circuit for Colpitts oscillator.

The effects of input loading can be minimised by using an FET or operational amplifier. In this case, the reactance of C_2 should be at least ten times the output resistance of 10–100 Ω, which will be in parallel with it, so that the signal voltage is mainly across the capacitance rather than across the output resistance (Leven, 2000).

7.5.5 Demodulator

An FM modulator converts variations in amplitude to variations in frequency, whereas an FM demodulator converts variations in frequency to variations in amplitude. There are a number of different types of demodulator. The phase-locked loop (PLL) demodulator is the simplest type of demodulator and one of the most commonly used (Carson, 1990; Leven, 2000). It consists of a phase detector, a low-pass filter, an amplifier and a voltage controlled oscillator, as shown in Figure 7.34. The components can be assembled discretely or on an IC chip.

The frequency modulated signal f_1 and the signal f_2 from the voltage controlled oscillator are input to the phase detector, which is a DC coupled mixer that takes two AC input signals. The detector combines the two signals to give an output consisting of the sum and difference frequencies, as well as a number

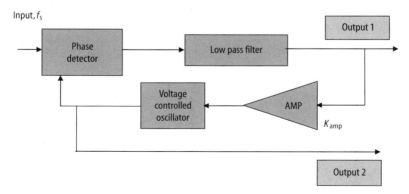

Figure 7.34 Phase-locked loop demodulator.

of harmonics. This output signal is then passed through a low-pass filter to filter out all the other components, leaving the difference term. The filter also improves the frequency response. Either a lag compensation or lead lag compensation filter can be used. The filter output is used to control the frequency of the voltage-controlled oscillator and lock this frequency to the frequency of the incoming frequency modulated signal within the frequency deviation of the system. The error voltage output from the low-pass filter is used to obtain the demodulated output, which will be linear if the voltage-controller oscillator is linear.

The amplifier is a DC amplifier that amplifies the output of the phase detector and low-pass filter. Either an operational amplifier or a transistor-type amplifier can be used. The amplifier gain can be varied with external resistors in the case of a discrete system or by a single external resistor when a chip is used.

The voltage-controlled oscillator (Leven, 2000) acts as a voltage-to-frequency converter in which the phase-error voltage gives the output frequency. It generally contains two varactor diodes in a multivibrator configuration. Its conversion gain can be obtained as the slope of the plot of the free running frequency against the phase-error voltage. The free running frequency is the output frequency when a constant DC correction voltage is applied.

The voltage-controlled oscillator can be implemented on a chip and a configuration circuit is given in Figure 7.35. The resistances and voltages in this circuit should satisfy the following conditions:

- the resistance R_1 should be between 2 and 20 kΩ;
- the supply voltage V_s should be between 10 and 24 V and also between +0.75 V and +V;
- the free running frequency should be less than 1 MHz. This is given by

$$f_o = \frac{2}{R_1 C_1} \frac{V - V_s}{V} \qquad (7.16)$$

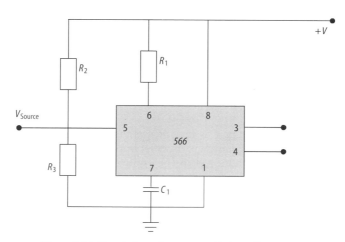

Figure 7.35 Circuit for voltage-controlled oscillator chip.

7.6 Actuators

As discussed in Section 7.2, actuators transform an electrical or other signal to an appropriate form to be perceived and then output it. In the case of alarm and alerting devices for deaf and hearing-impaired people, actuators transform an electrical signal to visual or tactile form and only to sound if it can be amplified sufficiently to be audible. Actuators that are used in alarm and alerting devices for deaf people include:

- loud buzzers or bells
- flashing or strobe lights
- LEDs
- television signals
- vibro-tactile devices
- electro-tactile devices.

7.6.1 Auditory Signals: Loud Bells and Buzzers

An auditory signal will only be effective in alerting people with hearing losses if it satisfies the following conditions:

- the intensity of the signal is sufficiently great;
- the frequency of the signal is in the range of audibility;
- the distance between the person and the signalling device is not so great that the sound is inaudible or too soft to be effective;
- sound transmission is not blocked by doors, walls or other obstacles.

An additional stage of amplification can generally make auditory signals sufficiently loud to be effective as alarms or alerting devices for at least some hearing-impaired people. Pulsing, high-frequency "beeps" are commonly used in signalling devices used with computers, microwave ovens, alarm clocks, and telephones. However, replacing the high-frequency signal with a lower frequency sound may increase audibility for many people with a hearing loss. For instance, substituting a gong-type bell for a high-pitched one may increase the range of people who can hear it. The frequency of a system depends on its mass, length and tension, or stiffness, as follows:

$$f = \tfrac{1}{2} L \sqrt{t/m} \qquad (7.17)$$

where f represents frequency, L is length, t is tension and m is the cross-sectional mass. Therefore, frequency is inversely proportional to the square root of mass and directly proportional to the square root of tension or stiffness. Consequently, a lower frequency can be obtained by increasing the mass of the system and/or reducing the stiffness and frequency decreases as the mass increases. In practical applications, bells of greater mass are often used to provide a lower frequency signal.

Audibility of a sound is also effected by its distance from the alarm or alerting device, as sound energy or intensity decreases in accordance with the inverse square law, *i.e.* if the distance doubles then the sound intensity is reduced by a factor of four on a linear scale. However, sound is generally measured on a logarithmic scale in decibels, so doubling the distance changes the intensity by $10\log_{10}(0.5)^2 = -6$ dB. Therefore, if the sound at a particular distance from the source is 50 dB, then at twice the distance the intensity will be 44 dB and at four times the distance it will be 38 dB.

This means, for instance, that some people with a hearing loss will be able to hear a telephone when they are sitting next to it, but not from across the room or in another room. However, it should be noted that the problem of hearing alarm and alerting devices at a distance is also experienced by people with "normal" hearing. This problem cannot be solved purely by amplification, as amplifying the signal sufficiently to make it audible at a distance would make it uncomfortably loud from close by. However, a number of appropriately placed amplified signal sources and/or a portable receiver or pager can be used to give a telephone ringer or other alerting alarm signal that is audible for at least some people with a hearing loss without being excessively loud throughout even a large building.

Obstacles, such as a closed door or a wall, between the signal and the person impede the flow of sound. In this case, the mass of the door, or other obstacles, produces an impedance to the flow of sound energy. Impedance has two components: resistance and reactance, and reactance consists of mass reactance X_m and compliance reactance X_c. The total reactance (both X_m and X_c) leads to storage of sound energy and, consequently, reduces the intensity of the auditory signal. This problem can again be resolved by the use of several remote-signalling devices or a portable receiver or pager.

7.6.2 Lights

Visual signals in the form of (a flashing) light are the most commonly used non-audible alarm signals. For instance, the traditional door bell or telephone ringer can be replaced or supplemented by a flashing light. Although an appropriate light source could be substituted for the more commonly used bell or buzzer, it is often more efficient to purchase and install a commercially available device.

Some alarm and alerting systems use an ordinary 60 W bulb as the output transducer, whereas others are connected to the house lighting circuit(s) and make the lights in all the rooms connected to the given lighting circuit flash on and off. The use of the main house lights is likely to be more effective than the use of a flashing bulb or LED in alerting the user and will be able to wake light sleepers. This approach also has the advantage of avoiding the need for a radio frequency transmitter and receiver. Some systems have the option of the alert, generally a doorbell, making the lights flash during the day and dim at night. In principle, different patterns of flashing lights could be used to indicate different alarm or alert signals, but there are few multifunction alerting systems with the house lights as the output transducer.

Flashing lights are inexpensive, easily available and have a number of applications. However, they are not suitable for deafblind people with little usable vision or people with epilepsy. In addition, a flashing light or LED may not be effective in waking heavy sleepers.

7.6.3 Light-emitting Diodes

LEDs are very reliable and have low power consumption. They can be combined with a suitable circuit to make them flash. A number of products for general use, such as some smoke alarms, have both audible and LED alarm signals. However, LEDs are generally not visible from as great a distance as radiant light in daylight conditions and they are unlikely to wake most sleepers. Therefore, they are unsuitable for use as the output transducer in an alarm clock and require to be supplemented by another output transducer for use at night if used, for instance, in fire or carbon monoxide alarms.

LEDs work on the same principles as the infrared diodes discussed in Chapter 5, but have a peak of power output in the visible spectrum rather than in the infrared spectrum. This peak emission wavelength determines the colour of the LED. It is related to the band gap (the energy gap between the two outer electron levels in the atom) according to the following equation (Cooke, 1990):

$$E_p = hc/\lambda = hf \qquad (7.18)$$

where E_p (J) is the energy of a photon of light and λ its wavelength, f the frequency of the electromagnetic radiation, c the speed of light (3×10^8 m s^{-1}) and h Planck's constant (6.62×10^{-34} J s). This gives wavelengths of 635 nm for red, 585 nm for yellow and 656 nm for green LEDs.

A variety of circuits can be constructed using switches, such as transistors and timing devices, to make radiant lights or LEDs flash. An example of a circuit to make LEDs flash is given in Figure 7.36.

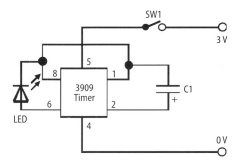

Figure 7.36 Circuit to make LED flash (courtesy of Samuel Goldwasser, from Strobe Lights and Design Guidelines, Useful Circuits, and Schematics, http://www.repairfaq.org/REPAIR/F_strbfaq.html).

7.6.4 Television

Several baby-monitors for deaf people use the users' television as the output transducer. When the baby cries the system will interrupt viewing and transmit a picture of the baby. The television loudspeaker will generally also transmit the sound the baby makes. A time delay is generally incorporated into baby monitors for deaf people so that the system only responds to a sound that lasts more than a certain minimum time to avoid false alerts, such as a door slamming. However, the output transmitted by the vibrating output transducer only indicates that the baby is making a noise, whereas hearing parents are able to hear the baby through the baby monitor and consequently have more information about what the baby is doing. Therefore, visual output through the television is very useful in supplementing this limited information. However, the picture of the baby on television is unlikely to wake sleeping parents, and the associated loudspeaker output will only wake people with a mild hearing loss. Consequently, the television output should be replaced or supplemented by a vibrating pad at night.

7.6.5 Vibro-tactile Devices

Vibro-tactile output devices for deaf and deafblind people use a small electric motor with an eccentric out-of-balance weight on its shaft to produce vibration (Figure 7.37). Different patterns of vibration can be used to indicate the nature of the alert, for instance to denote whether there is a fire or whether the telephone is ringing. Alternatively, a vibrator could be combined with a visual signal, such as an LED of a particular colour or a written message on a small screen, to indicate the nature of the alert.

A sound indicator is an electronic device that gives out a vibratory signal when it picks up an audio signal (*e.g.* a telephone bell) above a pre-set level. Usually, the vibratory signal lasts for a fixed minimum length of time, and the amplitude of the vibration is usually constant (*i.e.* independent of the amplitude of the input signal). With some devices it is possible to tune the device to pick up only audio signals at or about a fixed frequency. This is useful in minimising the number of times the device is activated by picking up the wrong audio signal.

Vibratory signals have the advantage over visual signals in that they can be used by deafblind and deaf people. They have the further advantage of being relatively quiet in use (with any noise being due to the operation of the device, particularly if it is powerful). Therefore, pagers and cell phones often have a vibration in addition to an audible signalling mode, so as to alert the user without disturbing other people in the vicinity.

Unlike audible and visual signals, which can be perceived at some distance (by people with sufficient hearing or vision), vibro-tactile alarm and alerting signals can only function when they are in either direct or indirect contact with the body, for instance under a pillow, through which the vibrations can be felt. However, the vibro-tactile transducer does not have to make direct contact with the original source of the alarm signal. This may, therefore, require the use of a vibrating pager device to allow users to move about, but still receive the alarm or alerting signal.

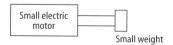

Figure 7.37 Block diagram of vibrating pad.

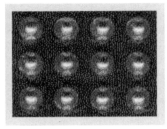

Figure 7.38 An array of tactors (courtesy of ForeThought Developments).

7.6.6 Electro-tactile Devices

An electro-tactile device applies electrical energy to the skin to give a vibratory sensation by stimulating the nerve axons of mechano-receptors. An array of electro-tactile output transducers or tactors is shown in Figure 7.38. Devices based on electro-tactile technology are being developed, for instance to improve access to computer graphical interfaces for blind people and communication of speech to deaf and deafblind people. However, electro-tactile devices are unlikely to have any advantages over vibro-tactile devices in the communicator of alarm and alerting signals to deaf people, and there could be health risks for some users.

7.6.7 Paging Systems

Pager systems (Figure 7.39) are generally worn on the body. The alarm or alerting signal is transmitted from the original source to the pager receiver by a very low-power radio frequency transmitter. The pager communicates the signal to the user through a vibrator (or an audible signal in the case of a hearing user).

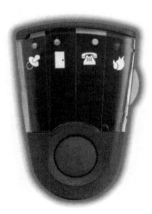

Figure 7.39 Pager (courtesy of Bellman).

The following factors have led to the development of vibrating radio pager devices that are useful for deaf and deafblind people:

- the decreasing cost and size of radio paging systems;
- the liberalisation of the laws on the use of very low-powered radio transmitters in many countries.

The fact is that silent, *i.e.* vibrating, devices have advantages for both hearing and for deaf and deafblind people; consequently, there is a larger market for such devices.

Pager systems generally have the further advantage of being able to transmit different types of alarm and alerting signal and to distinguish between at least some of the different types of signal by using obviously different patterns of vibration. Pager systems are available from a number of different manufacturers and suppliers, including Bellman, Connevans and Easylink UK.

The Connevans system PV2 (http://www.connevans.com/) consists of a vibrating pager and a number of transmitters, which Connevans calls trigger units. However, a system of one or more trigger units can be connected to more than one pager, for instance to allow everyone in a household to be alerted. The pager unit is portable and can fit into a pocket. It should be fairly close to the body, *e.g.* on a belt or in a shirt, trousers or skirt pocket, but not a coat pocket. There are three different vibration patterns, which indicate fire alarm, telephone and other alerts. In the case of alerts other than fire and telephone, the channel number (see Table 7.2) is displayed at the same time as the vibration. When more than one device signals at approximately the same time, the different alerts are indicated in the following order of priority: first a fire alarm, then the telephone, followed by other alerts.

There are three different types of fire alarm trigger unit: domestic, commercial and source powered, for all of which the channel is F. There are seven other types of trigger unit. Some of the properties of the different trigger units are given in Table 7.2.

The telephone, doorbell, alarm clock, PIR and domestic and commercial fire alarms have an external sound piezo option. There are standard and lower frequency piezo sound sensors. The lower frequency device is more suitable for commercial fire alarms and private telephone systems. The wiring of the piezo on the doorbell is a wired ring and sleeve, whereas on the piezos used with the other trigger units it is a wired tip and sleeve. Def Chan indicates the default channel. The trigger units can be fastened to a wall or a door.

The pager unit uses two AA size long-life or rechargeable batteries and the trigger units one alkaline-type PP3 size battery. The use of rechargeable batteries is not recommended in the trigger units, as the terminal voltage is slightly lower and they self-discharge too quickly. The low-battery indication is able to distinguish whether the low battery is in the pager or in one of the trigger units and, in the latter case, in which one.

Where there are two doors, a single trigger can be used, or each bell could be connected to a separate trigger unit to indicate to users which door the bell has rung at. The doorbell trigger unit can also be connected into door-entry systems. The connection should be made across the buzzer inside the handset or speaker box inside the user's home and not at the external door. Similar connections are used whether the doorbell uses mains electricity via a

Table 7.2 Properties of different types of trigger unit (courtesy of Connevans Ltd, UK).

Trigger unit name	Channels	Trigger sensitivity	Type of sensing	Standard accessories	Comments
Telephone	1	N/a	Sound or light opto-coupler	Ringer and adapters	Normal connection is to use standard telephone socket
Doorbell	2	110 dB	Voltage or sound	1 m connecting lead	Voltage triggering range 1–30 V DC and 1–20 V AC r.m.s., wired across bell
Baby alarm	3	85 dB	Sound	None	Unit is placed near to, but out of reach of, the child
External switch	4	N/a	Closing switch/short circuit	1 m connecting lead	Can be used with any closing contact switch or relay
Call alarm	5	N/a	Closing switch/short circuit	Nurse call switch	Either the integral or external button can be used
Alarm clock	6	95 dB	Sound	External piezo sound sensor	Use the external piezo or connect directly to a modified clock
PIR	7	110 dB	Sound	External piezo sound sensor	Same sensitivity as the fire PTU, but with different alert for general use
Domestic fire alarm	F	110 dB	Sound	External piezo sound sensor	The external piezo is placed on a domestic smoke alarm
Commercial fire alarm	F	110 dB	Sound or voltage	External piezo sound sensor	Direct connection is possible, voltage triggering range 1–30 V DC and 1–20 V AC r.m.s.
Source-powered fire alarm	F	N/a	N/a	None, the source voltage lead is ordered separately	Activated and powered from the alarm system at approximately 20 mA, source operating voltage range of 9–48 V with appropriate lead

transformer or a battery. As the trigger unit does not have a noticeable power drain, it can be used with most low-voltage buzzers or bells or any device with an external sounder.

The external switch trigger unit has an enclosed lead with a 3.5 mm jack plug at one end to allow direct connection to equipment. It is intended to respond to a closing contact switch, such as the external (relay) switch on a burglar alarm system. When the unit is connected to a system such as the relay on a burglar alarm, the contacts should be isolated from the actual alarm system so there are no mains or other power on either contact. Although it is very similar to the call switch unit, the external switch trigger unit is not recommended to be used as a substitute call trigger unit and would require the test button to be held down for a longer time. However, the switch can be used with a surface bell-push switch when there is no house doorbell or for installation on a sales counter to call for assistance. There is also an accessory kit, consisting of an actuator magnet and a magnetically operated proximity switch, which can be used to inform users when someone leaves a room. A surface switch is included so that the system can be isolated when not required.

7.7 Learning Highlights of the Chapter

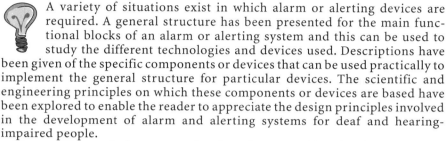

A variety of situations exist in which alarm or alerting devices are required. A general structure has been presented for the main functional blocks of an alarm or alerting system and this can be used to study the different technologies and devices used. Descriptions have been given of the specific components or devices that can be used practically to implement the general structure for particular devices. The scientific and engineering principles on which these components or devices are based have been explored to enable the reader to appreciate the design principles involved in the development of alarm and alerting systems for deaf and hearing-impaired people.

Three different design approaches have been considered. Of these, design for all, *i.e.* the design of alarm and alerting systems that can be used by everyone, independently of disability, age, race, size or other factors, has a number of advantages. However, it is unfortunately only rarely used in practice, and modification of systems designed for hearing people is more common.

Such systems are almost always unsatisfactory or completely unusable by people with hearing impairments unless the signals used are modified. Particular problems relate to the intensity level and frequency (range) of the signal. For many people who are deaf, the intensity level is too soft to be audible or the audibility level is not sufficiently loud for the sound to be effective as an alarm. For others, the frequency of the sound is in a range that is inaudible, although they may be able to hear at other frequencies. Alternatively, the signal may be audible when the listener is close to the device, but not from another part of the house or even across the room from where the device is situated, or audibility may prevented by closed doors or other obstacles. A systematic and fundamental presentation has been given in the chapter of the design of alarm and alerting devices that can be used by people who are deaf or hearing impaired. This includes a systematic presentation of the technologies required in the different design approaches.

Projects and Investigations

1. Evaluate a number of different alarm and alerting devices with regards to design for all principles. In particular, determine what features of the devices are consistent and inconsistent with this design approach and how the devices could best be modified to make them consistent with design for all principles.

2. Design and build an inexpensive portable alarm clock that can be used with different output transducers, including the following:
   - a vibrating pad
   - a flashing light
   - a buzzer with adjustable frequency and volume.
3. Design and build a multifunctional alarm and alerting system that can be used with different output transducers, including the following:
   - a vibrating pad
   - a flashing light
   - a buzzer with adjustable frequency and volume.
4. Design and build a system to carry out the following functions:
   - receive an auditory signal from an alarm or alerting device;
   - distinguish the type of signal using the fact that most alarm and alerting devices have a frequency spectrum consisting of one or two discrete frequency components;
   - output the signal to a vibrating pad with a distinct frequency or pattern of vibration that corresponds to the input signal.

References and Further Reading

References

Bannister, B.R., Whitehead, D.G., 1991. *Instrumentation Transducers and Interfacing.* Chapman and Hall.
Boyleslad, R.L., Nashelsky, L., 2002. *Electronic Devices and Circuit Theory*, 8th edition. Prentice Hall International.
Carson, R.S., 1990. *Radio Communications Concepts: Analog.* John Wiley and Sons.
Cooke, M.J., 1990. *Semiconductor Devices.* Prentice Hall.
Dally, J.W., Riley, W.F., McConnell, K.G., 1993. *Instrumentation for Engineering Measurements*, 2nd edition. John Wiley and Sons.
Decker, T.N., 1996. *Instrumentation. An Introduction for Students in the Speech and Hearing Sciences*, 2nd edition. Lawrence Erlbaum Associates.
Floyd, T.L., 2002. *Electronic Devices*, 6th edition. Prentice Hall International.
Gardner, J.W., 1994. *Microsensors Principles and Applications.* John Wiley and Sons.
Lathi, B.P., 1983. *Modern Digital and Analog Communication Systems.* Holt-Saunders.
Leven, A. 2000. *Telecommunication Circuits and Technology.* Butterworth Heinemann.
Morris, A.S., 1993. *Principles of Measurement and Instrumentation.* Prentice Hall International.
Noll, A.M., 1995. *Introduction to Telecommunication Electronics.* Artech House.
Ohba, R. (Ed.), 1992. *Intelligent Sensor Technology.* John Wiley and Sons.
Sedra, A.S., Smith, K.C., 1989. *Microelectronic Circuits.* Saunders College Publishing.
Smith, J., 1986. *Modern Communication Circuits.* McGraw-Hill Series in Electrical Engineering. McGraw-Hill.
Stremler, F.G., 1982. *Introduction to Communication Systems.* Addison-Wesley.
Usher, M.J., 1985. *Sensors and Transducers.* Macmillan.
Usher, M.J., Keating, D.A., 1996. *Sensors and Transducers Characteristics, Applications, Instrumentation, Interfacing*, 2nd edition. Macmillan.

Further Reading

Books

Beards, P.H., 1987. *Analog and Digital Electronics, a First Course*. Prentice Hall International.
Collin, R.E., 1985. *Antennas and Radiowave Propagation*. McGraw-Hill International Editions, Electrical Engineering Series. McGraw-Hill.
Freeman, R.L., 1975. *Telecommunication Transmission Handbook*. Wiley-Interscience
Johnson, C., 1993. *Process Control Instrumentaton Technology*, 4th edition. Regents/Prentice Hall.
O'Dell, T.H., 1991. *Circuits for Electronic Instrumentation*. Cambridge University Press.

Suppliers of Alerting Systems and Alarm Devices

The list of commercial distributors and manufacturers is not exhaustive; it is just a sample of the many devices available and some of the places from which they can be purchased. This information can be used to learn about what is available.

Ameriphone, 7231 Garden Grove Blvd, Suite E, Garden Grove, CA 92641-4219, USA. Tel.: +1 (714) 897-0808 (voice); +1 (714) 897-1111 (tty); +1 (714) 897-4703 (fax). Products include: Alertmaster AM-100, AM-300, and AM-6000 Wireless Notification System.

BT Guide for People who are Disabled – Hearing. Found only on-line, but provides distributors for every product shown. Internet: http://www.bt.com/world/community/aged_and_disabled/2general.htm. Products include: telephone ringers (adjustable, extension); visual telephone signallers; remote/wireless telephone ringer with adjustable volume and pitch (tone); remote/wireless visual telephone signaller.

Connevans Ltd, 54, Albert Road North, Reigate, Surrey, RH2 9YR, UK. Tel.: +44 (0)1737 247571; text: +44 (0)1737 243134; Internet: www.connevans.com. Products include a wide range of alerting and alarm devices.

Deafworks, PO Box 1265, Provo, UT 84603-1265, USA. USA voice relay: (800) 877-8973; TTY: (801) 465-1957; fax: (801) 465-1958 Internet: http://www.deafworks.com. E-mail: info@deafworks.com. Products include: light flashers (general purpose); alarm clocks; remote wireless signallers; baby cry alarms; doorbell flashers; telephone/tdd signallers; technical manuals.

EasyLink Electronics, Factory 7, Grange Road, Geddington, Northants, NN14 1AL, UK. Tel.: +44 (0)1536 744788; fax: +44 (0)1536 262217. Internet: http://nthost.nildram.co.uk:10075/index.html. E-mail: enquires@easylink.uk.com. Products include: door and telephone bells – visual and vibrating; baby cry alarms; bed vibrating alarm clocks; telephone signallers – visual and vibrating; carbon monoxide/fire alarms.

HARC Mercantile Ltd, Division of HARC of America, PO Box 3055, Kalamazoo, MI 49003, USA. Products include: Blinker-Buddy electronic turn-signal reminder.

Scottish Sensory Centre, University of Edinburgh, Holyrood Road, Edinburgh, EH8 8AQ, Scotland, UK. Tel.: +44 (0)131 651 6501. Internet: http://www.ssc.mhie.ac.uk/Vpages/F1/V170.htm. Products include: flashing and vibrating alarm clocks; flashing and vibrating baby alarms; flashing door bells; flashing door knockers; flashing and vibrating smoke alarms; flashing and vibrating telephone signallers; combined alerting remote and wireless systems; includes a comprehensive list of product suppliers.

Silent Call Corporation, PO Box 868, Clarkstown, MI 48347-0868, USA. Tel.: +1 (313) 673-0221 (voice); +1 (313) 673-6069 (tdd). Products include: Gentex 7000 series photoelectric smoke detectors, Gentex 710CS and 710 LS photoelectric smoke detectors and fire alarm; Shake-Up smoke detector and signal unit.

8 Dual Sensory Impairment: Devices for Deafblind People

8.1 Learning Objectives

The main aim of this chapter is to give readers an understanding of the role of assistive technology in supporting deafblind people and extending the options open to them. Specific aims include the following:

- obtaining an awareness of the demographics of the deafblind population;
- reviewing the range of assistive devices for deafblind people and understanding the engineering principles on which they are based;
- appreciating existing solutions and the need for new solutions to enable deafblind people to participate in the new information and communication systems emerging in today's society.

8.2 Definitions and Demographics of Deafblindness

The term deafblind refers to a person with a combined loss of hearing and sight. Deafblind or dual sensory-impaired people can be divided into four groups:

- Those who were born deaf and blind, for instance if the mother suffered rubella (German measles) during pregnancy.
- Those who were born deaf or hearing impaired and then lost their sight. One condition in which this occurs is Usher's syndrome; this is a form of retinitis pigmentosa.
- Those who were born blind and then lost their hearing. The term blinddeaf is occasionally used.
- Those who become deafblind, most commonly as a result of old age, or through an illness or accident.

Estimates of the number of deafblind people vary widely, depending on the definition used. According to Deafblind UK about 23,000 people in the UK are deafblind, excluding the large number of elderly people with some degree of sight and hearing. Deafblind UK believes that the total number of people with a combined sight and hearing loss could as high as 250,000. However, with regard to the development of assistive technology, the class of deafblind people who are not able to use devices developed either for deaf or for blind people is particularly important. This gives a smaller number of maybe 250 per million of the population in the industrialised countries, or about 14,500 in the UK. However, estimates of about 20,000 deafblind people in the USA (Ouellette) say more about the different definitions in use than the greater prevalence of deafblindness in the UK.

The numerically largest group of deafblind people are those over retirement age. This group may have a number of other age-related impairments, but generally have some usable sight and/or hearing. The next most common cause of deafblindness is Usher's syndrome. Another medical condition that leads to deafblindness is the Lawrence Moon Biedl syndrome of retinitis pigmentosa.

Some assistive devices for deaf or blind people can also be used by deafblind people. However, devices for blind people are increasingly using audio output, such as synthetic speech, so there are fewer inexpensive devices with tactual output. For instance, the number of electronic calculators with Braille output is falling, since the cost of synthetic speech output has dramatically reduced in recent years. These trends have benefited blind people but have significantly reduced the choice available to deafblind people.

This is particularly important, since the number of deafblind people is considerably smaller than the number of deaf or blind people, making the costs of developing and manufacturing assistive devices specifically for deafblind people relatively high. In the past, non-profit organisations often subsidised both development and manufacture, but these organisations are now under pressure to become more commercial and minimise their financially loss-making activities.

Thus, on the one hand, there has been a decline in lower price and often lower technology assistive devices and, on the other hand, advances in information and communications technologies have opened up a wide range of possibilities for increased independence and employment for deafblind people. However, the associated hardware and software is often much more expensive than information and communications technology for hearing and sighted people, and considerable training may be required to use the systems effectively. In addition, organisations serving deafblind people also need to develop training and support skills for these high-technology systems.

The role of state provision varies considerably from country to country. In the past, the Eastern Bloc countries provided relatively generous funds for assistance to deafblind individuals who had above-average intelligence; the change in the economic environment has resulted in cutbacks in these services. In Western countries, the lead is usually taken by voluntary organisations with some subsidy from the state.

8.3 Communication for Deafblind People

Communication by deafblind people, who have little useful hearing and vision, uses the sense of touch. Touch can be classified as passive and active. Passive touch involves skin sensitivity to pressure, temperature, pain and other sensations when objects make direct contact with the skin. Information obtained by passive touch is called *tactile*. Active touch involves *tactual* information obtained by a combination of the skin's cutaneous sensations (tactile) and the body's kinaesthetic sensitivity to spatial position and movement. Tactile information can be used to describe the type of contact with an object (such as static or vibrating) and properties of the object (such as its texture), whereas tactual information can be used to actively investigate objects and their properties and to interact with the environment (Fleischer and Durlach, 1993).

The two main approaches to communication for deafblind people are fingerspelling and Braille. Both of them can provide the basis of automated communication devices. Many deafblind people become blind later in life, whether they are born deaf or hearing impaired, as with Usher's syndrome, or lose both hearing and sight later in life. In addition, Braille is relatively difficult to learn later in life. Therefore, in practice, many deafblind people do not read Braille, and fingerspelling is more widely used. The deafblind manual alphabet (fingerspelling) is similar to the manual alphabet for deaf people, but the letters are formed on the listener's hand (see Figure 8.1(a) and (b)). A related approach, which is considerably slower than deafblind manual but which is generally easier for non-deafblind people to learn, is the block alphabet or Spartan. This involves tracing capital letters on the listener's palm. Hands-on signing is an adaptation of sign language for people with low vision.

Braille is a system of reading and writing for blind and deafblind people; see Figure 8.2. It is based on a rectangular six-dot cell with 64 different configurations. It is named after its inventor, Louis Braille, who developed it from a

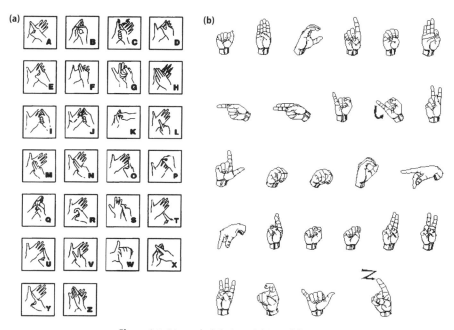

Figure 8.1 Manual alphabet: (a) UK; (b) USA.

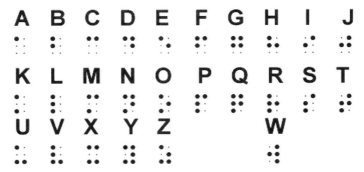

Figure 8.2 Letters in Braille.

system called night writing, which was developed for communicating with troops after dark. Each letter is represented by a particular arrangement of the six dots. Numbers are represented by a numeral symbol followed by the letters A–J to represent the numbers 1–10. There are also short forms for some common words and combinations of Braille dots in a cell for contractions of two or more letters.

Braille can be embossed by hand or by using a machine, called a Brailler, onto thick paper to give raised dots and is read by moving the fingers across on top of the dots. A Braille book is typically 20 times as bulky as the print edition. Therefore, a form of shorthand is employed which uses 189 abbreviations and contractions giving a space saving of about 25%. About 13,000 people in the UK regularly read Braille out of one million people who could be registered as blind or partially sighted. This low proportion is due to the difficulty of learning Braille by people who lose their vision later in life, the fact that some blind and partially sighted people are still able to read text and that some causes of vision impairment, such as diabetic retinopathy, also affect the sense of touch.

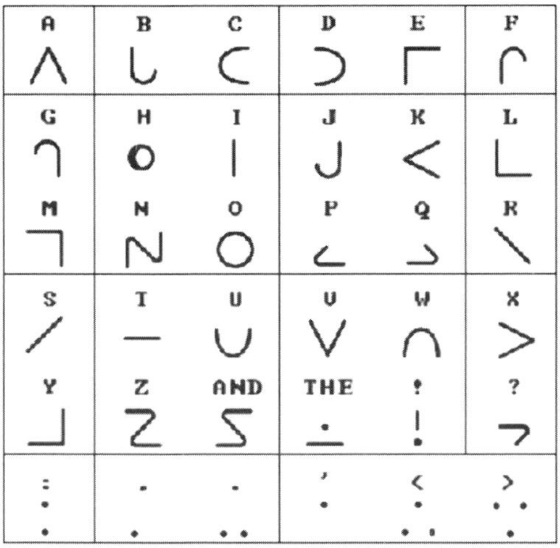

Figure 8.3 Moon alphabet.

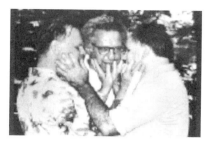

Figure 8.4 Communication by Tadoma (courtesy of Nathaniel and Hansi Durlach).

Moon (Figure 8.3) was developed by Dr William Moon in 1847. Since it has similarities to ordinary print characters, it is easier to learn for people who have previously read visually. However, it has the disadvantage of having about 80 times the volume of the print version and four times that of the Braille version. The high cost of production has meant that very few books are printed in this medium. The number of Moon readers has dwindled to about 400, most of who are in the UK. Until recently, Moon was produced boustrophedon, which has the advantage of not requiring backtracking from the end of one line to the beginning of the next and the disadvantage of requiring alternate lines to be read in different directions.

Tadoma (Figure 8.4) is a method of communication of oral speech through tactile contact (Alcorn, 1932; Vivian, 1966). It involves placing a hand on the speaker's face, with the thumb lightly over the lips and the fingers spread on the cheek and upper neck. This allows a deafblind person to feel lip and face movements and the vibration of the vocal cords as each sound is made. Even sounds that look alike on the lips, such as "F" and "V", feel different. Deafblind people with some vision can use it in conjunction with lip-reading.

It was developed at the Perkins School for the Blind, in the USA, as a method of teaching deafblind children to speak. Although only a very small number of deafblind adults use Tadoma, studies have shown that it can give good speech reception and high levels of communication efficiency without requiring exceptional tactual sensitivity from the user (Schultz *et al.*, 1984; Chomsky, 1986; Reed *et al.*, 1989).

8.3.1 Assistive Technology for Deafblind Communication

Assistive devices can have an important role in enabling deafblind people to communicate with a much wider range of people, leading to increased access to information and increasing independence. The simplest form of communication device is a magnetic board with raised metal letters (as used on notice boards). This has the advantage of simplicity, but it is very slow. A faster device has a keyboard connected to a single-cell Braille display, as shown in Figure 8.5.

However, this is more expensive and can only be used by deafblind people who can read Braille. There are a number of more sophisticated electronic

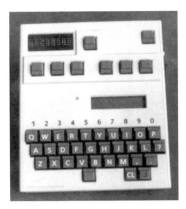

Figure 8.5 Screen Braille communicator.

devices that can be used over the telephone via a modem (a device that converts the digital signals into analogue signals for transmission along a telephone line, as discussed in Section 6.4.2).

8.4 Braille Devices

A number of different Braille devices are produced commercially. Electronic devices include:

- 40-, 65- and 80-cell refreshable Braille displays
- Braille notetakers, which are often multifunction
- text–Braille translation programs
- Braille embossers.

8.4.1 Braille Displays

A Braille display is a tactile device that is used to read text from a computer or Braille input from a Braille notetaker and to output Braille; see Figure 8.6. It consists of a row of "soft" cells, which have six or eight metal or nylon pins. The eight-dot configuration is becoming more common for computer use. These pins are controlled electronically so they move up and down and display characters on the display of the source system, which is either a computer or a Braille notetaker. In the eight-dot versions, dots seven and eight can be used to show the position of the cursor in the text, for European eight-dot Braille, or for advanced mathematics or computer coding.

Placing a number of cells next to each other gives a soft or refreshable Braille line, which can be read by touch. Refreshable Braille displays only read one line of text at a time. There are generally directional keys to facilitate navigating a document. Full-size Braille lines generally consist of 80 cells to facilitate access to computers and information technology, as this is the number of characters that fits across a typical computer monitor. These large displays also include a

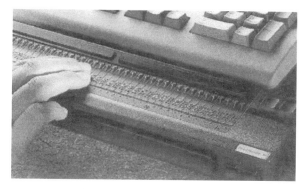

Figure 8.6 Using a Braille display.

cursor routing function, in which the cursor can be moved directly over a particularly letter using the cell router button or a touch sensor. Smaller Braille displays are cheaper and, therefore, are more affordable for many users, but they display a line of text in a number of stages, for instance in four stages for a 20-cell line. The display is connected to the computer by a serial cable.

Issues to consider when selecting a Braille display include the following:

- compatibility with the computer platform used
- the number of Braille cells active on the display
- whether the display has its own power source
- whether the display has extra keys that can be programmed with additional commands.

There are a number of different refreshable Braille displays, such as:

- PowerBraille 40, 65 and 80 from Freedom Scientific Blind/Low Vision Group, where the number indicates the number of Braille cells active.
- Braille Windows Display from Freedom of Speech Inc. There are 85-cell desktop and 45-cell portable versions for use with Windows 95 or Windows 3.x.
- Braille Voyager, ALVA Delphi Braille Terminals and the ALVA Satellite Series from Humanware Braille Solutions. The Voyager has its own power, can be used independently of a screen reader and uses logical Braille keys. The ALVA is available in 23- and 43-cell portable and 45- and 85-cell desktop versions.
- Braillex EL2D 80 and Braillex EL 80 from Papenmeier GmbH. The EL2D 80 has 80-cell Braille and 20-cell vertical display, whereas the EL 80 has 80 cells plus two status cells. Both can be used as screen readers for DOS and with Windows 95/98, NT and Linux.

8.4.2 Multifunction Braille Notetakers

Electronic Braille notetakers are generally multifunctional devices, somewhat analogous to palmtop computers or personal organisers for sighted people, but

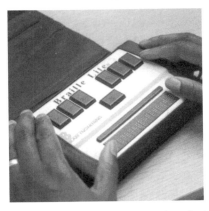

Figure 8.7 Portable Braille notetaker incorporating scientific calculator, stopwatch and diary functions, and that can transfer files to and from a computer.

rather larger in size and at a much higher price. In addition to word processing, address book and diary functions, some of them also give e-mail and/or Web access facilities. Popular examples include the Braille Lite produced by the Freedom Scientific Blind/Low Vision Group(Figure 8.7). It is available in 20- and 40-cell models with eight-dot input, allowing for a backspace, carriage return key and one-key commands. Both models are approximately 29.4 cm × 12.8 cm × 3.8 cm in size and 900 g in weight.

They have complete word-processing capabilities, including a built-in spell checker. There is grade 2 Braille translation in the Braille input mode and output to a Braille embosser. E-mail facilities can be obtained from the notetaker through most Internet service providers. Accessory software can be used to expand the functionality to include money management, spreadsheet, scientific graphic and mathematics. The 14 Mb of internal storage can be expanded by using removable SanDisk Storage cards in the Compact Flash™ port. WinDisk connectivity allows file sharing with a PC, and there is JAWS for Windows support.

8.4.3 Text–Braille Conversion and Braille Embossers

Since there is a shortage of skilled transcribers, computer systems are often used to translate text to contracted Braille, which is then output on a special embosser. The algorithms for this translation are not simple, since the rules governing the use of contractions depend on pronunciation and meaning. For example, there is a contraction for "mother" that can be used as part of a longer word as long as it does not bridge a syllable boundary as in "chemotherapy". The Duxbury Braille translator for MS windows (http://www.duxburysystems.com/) can translate between text and Braille in both directions, but creating a Braille document from text is its most common use. It has drivers for all the commercially available Braille embossers and can print black and white "simulated Braille" graphics on most printers supported by windows. It can format documents and can be used as a Braille editor. It is accessible via a mouse, speech, Braille or a keyboard. Although its code and style are built round WordPerfect versions 5.0–6.1, it can import from other word processors and earlier Braille editors.

Commercially available Braille embossers include the following (http://www.utoronto.ca/atrc/reference/tech/brailleemb.html):

- Tactile Image Enhancer from Repro-Tronics Inc.
- Index and Thiel Embossers from Sighted Electronics in the USA or Techno-Vision Systems Ltd in the UK
- Braille Blazer, and VersaPoint Duo from Freedom Scientific
- Braillo Comet, Braillo 2000 and Braillo 400S from Braillo, Norway AS
- Index Basic-D and Index Basic-S from Index Braille Printer Company
- Paragon Braille Embosser from Pulse Data HumanWare.

The Braille Blazer can emboss Braille paper and special plastics in a range of sizes varying from 2.5 to 21.3 cm wide, as well as index cards. It is compatible with any PC or Blazie notetaker. It prints 15 characters per second in six-dot or eight-dot Braille. The landscape emboss feature can create long-format spreadsheets or screen dumps. It is 33.8 cm × 20 cm × 12.5 cm with the lid closed and weighs 5.5 kg. There is an internal speech synthesiser. The Blazer is at the domestic end of the market, but there are other, more expensive, embossers with higher printing speeds and a greater range of facilities and options that are more suitable for commercial and professional use (Figure 8.8).

The increasing use of graphics in printed books raises both technical and perceptual problems. Although many diagrams can be converted to an embossed form, simply converting an existing visual diagram to tactual form without making any changes is unlikely to be satisfactory in conveying the information in the graphic or illustration. It may be necessary to replace each image by a series of tactual images of increasing complexity to allow readers to first obtain an overview and then build up the detail. Other approaches include modifying the image to make it easier to comprehend and appreciate tactilely and supplementing it with introductory and/or explanatory text.

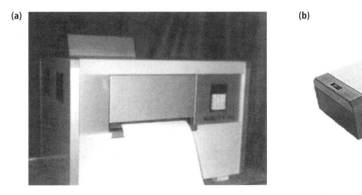

Figure 8.8 Braille embosser (600 pages per hour).

8.5 Automating Fingerspelling for Deafblind Communication

The manual alphabet is the main means of communication for many deafblind people. Therefore, development of automated approaches to deafblind manual or fingerspelling is particularly important, as most non-deafblind people are unable to communicate in this way. As well as its use in face-to-face communication, automated fingerspelling can form the basis of telephone and other long-distance communications for deafblind people. In this way, it can increase their independence and access to information and employment opportunities. Different deafblind manual languages have developed in a number of different countries, and the details of the different languages have had an effect on the appropriate technical solutions for automation. For instance, the deafblind manual languages in the USA and UK differ in two important ways:

- The use of different hand movements for each letter.
- Differences in the relative hand positions. In the USA, the listener's hand covers the speaker's hand, whereas in the UK the message is spelt into the listener's left hand, which remains fixed.

It is the second difference that has had a significant effect on the engineering solutions used to automate the USA and UK deafblind manual alphabets. The fingerspelling hands discussed in Sections 8.5.1–8.5.5 describe successive developments in automating US fingerspelling, whereas Section 8.5.6 describes a device for automating the UK deafblind manual alphabet. Section 8.5.7 looks at speaking-hand and talking-glove systems.

8.5.1 Developing Mechanical Fingerspelling Hands for Deafblind People

In this and the following three sections, the development of mechanical fingerspelling hands in the USA is discussed. This uses material that is largely drawn from Jaffe (1994a). The initial development of a mechanical hand demonstrated the feasibility of the concept of using a mechanical device to communicate the US fingerspelling language to the listener. It also showed that the device could produce each letter in the same way on a consistent basis, making comprehension easier. Subsequent developments refined and improved the original design in the following ways:

- making the fingerspelling movements more fluid and natural;
- increasing the speed of fingerspelling;
- eliminating pauses and neutral positions between the letters;
- improving the feel of the hand by changing the materials used and making the ends of the fingers rounded;
- improving the formation of some of the letters;
- making the hand smaller and lighter;
- incorporating a facility to allow adjustment of fingerspelling speed and the hand positions used to make the letters;

- improving the interfacing so that the mechanical hand could be controlled by any device producing R232 data.

These design improvements were achieved by modification of both the hardware and software in the original design, as discussed in this and the following sections.

The first mechanical fingerspelling hand was developed by the South-West Research Institute in San Antonio in 1977 (Laenger and Herbert, 1978). It demonstrated the feasibility of communicating information typed on the keyboard through electrical logic circuitry to a mechanical hand, which responded by forming the corresponding letters of the manual alphabet. The deafblind listener could receive the communication by placing a hand over the mechanical one to feel the finger positions. However, there were several technical problems, such as not forming all the letters properly, slow speed and lack of fluid motion, which made the letters more difficult to understand.

8.5.2 Dexter I

The next development came in the mid-1980s, when four graduate students at Stanford University devised the Dexter robotic fingerspelling hand (Danssaert et al., 1985; Gilden and Jaffe, 1986, 1988; Gilden, 1987a; Jaffe, 1987). Dexter I, as it is now termed, consisted of four machined aluminium fingers and a thumb joined together at the palm. It projected vertically from a box. The digits had a range of motion similar to human fingers and operated independently of each other. A pneumatic rotary activator pivoted the palm in a rotary fashion about a vertical steel rod. Pneumatic cylinders pulled the drive cables, which flexed the individual fingers and thumb, and spring-driven cables extended the fingers. Air pressure, controlled by electrically operated valves, activated the cylinders. A microcomputer system controlled the valves and both were housed in separate assemblies below the hand.

The original design consisted of an 8085 microcomputer, Forth programming language, memory and counter/timer support, which generated the signals that determined the rate of hand motion and the duration of each finger position. The hardware was subsequently revised to consist of a Z80 microprocessor card, two medium-power drive cards and a high-current DC power supply, all housed in an STD bus card cage. The CPU card contained counter timers, memory and serial interfaces. User messages were communicated over a serial link from an Epson HX-20 laptop to the self-contained target system.

The finger movements corresponding to each letter were determined by two to six valve operations, separated by a programmed pause. The states of the 22 valves were determined by the ASCII value of each letter of a message typed on the keyboard. The microcomputer controlled the opening and closing of the bank of valves. These valves determined the air pressure in the pneumatic cylinders, which pulled on the drive cables, which acted as the finger "tendons". Although Dexter had difficulties with the letters J and Z and, unlike human finger-spellers, had a neutral position between letters, the use of the same motions for a given letter made it easily intelligible.

8.5.3 Dexter II and III

Building on the development of Dexter I, three Stanford graduate engineering students designed a second prototype, Dexter II, in 1988 (Jaffe, 1989a,b). It used DC servomotors to pull the drive cables of a much smaller redesigned hand, thereby eliminating the need for a supply of compressed gas. As with its predecessor, incoming serial ASCII text was translated into the movements of a mechanical hand, which could be felt and interpreted as finger-spelt letters. The hand, a right hand, the size of a 10-year-old child's, was oriented vertically on top of an enclosure housing the servomotors. These motors were connected to a pulley and drove the motion of each hand. As with the original Dexter, Dexter II was constructed like a skeleton human hand. The fingers butted against a cylindrical knuckle, and a cord passing through the finger and the knuckle acted as a ligament to keep the finger in place and allow its articulation.

The hand was able to move in the following ways: each finger could flex independently, the first finger could move away from the other three fingers, the thumb could move across the fingers and the wrist could flex. The motion-control software allowed smooth operation of 676 different pathways and gave the hand sufficient flexibility to mimic the motion of the human hand in fingerspelling reasonably accurately.

The finger "tendons" were wire cables anchored at the fingertips and wound around pulleys, turned by powered motor shafts. The force to straighten the fingers when cable tension was released was provided by torsion springs. The STD-bus enclosure, Z80 microprocessor card and Epson HX-20 computer were still used, but the pulse-width-modulated waveforms to control the DC servomotors were now produced by two commercial counter timer cards. Dexter II's computer software used the ASCII value of each letter typed on the Epson HX-20 keyboard to access a memory array of stored control values and program the pulse-width-modulation chips to operate the eight servos and flex the fingers. This gave coordinated finger movements and hand positions, *i.e.* fingerspelt letters that could be interpreted as the letters of a message. Although neither Dexter system could exactly reproduce the hand movements of fingerspelling, their approximations were sufficiently close to be relatively easily learnt. Dexter II evolved into Dexter III (shown in Figure 8.9); this was considered for commercial production, but does not appear to have made the transition.

8.5.4 Fingerspelling Hand for Gallaudet

As in the Dexter II design, the Gallaudet hand (Figure 8.10) was moved by servo motors connected to a pulley (Jaffe, 1993a,b). The fingers were made of Delrin segments connected by a strip of carbon fibre, which provided the flexible hinge and restoring force to extend the fingers. Each finger could be flexed or extended by rotation of the motor shaft and pulley. The hand motion was controlled by a Z180 Smartblock eight-bit microcontroller that accepted R232 serial data and controlled eight DC servomotors. The controller was compact enough to fit into the hand enclosure.

The Forth programming language provided a simple user interface and enabled modifications to the finger positions or system parameters. The

Dual Sensory Impairment: Devices for Deafblind People

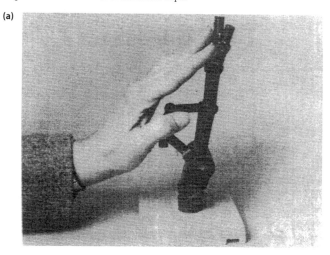

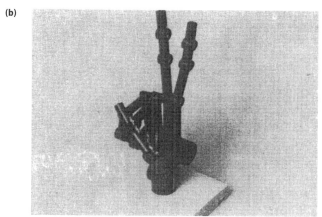

Figure 8.9 Dexter III fingerspelling hand: (a) reading the hand; (b) view of hand for Dexter III (courtesy of David Jaffe, Department of Veterans Affairs, Rehabilitation Research and Development Center, Palo Alto, CA).

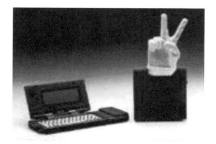

Figure 8.10 Fingerspelling hand for Gallaudet (courtesy of David Jaffe, Department of Veterans Affairs, Rehabilitation Research and Development Center, Palo Alto, CA).

elimination of the neutral position between letters gave more fluid fingerspelling movements. The software included a permanently installed and adjustable finger position table for each letter pair. This made it possible to change the hand positions to make the letters easier to read. The fingerspelling speed was adjusted by a six-position rotary switch. The first five positions selected increasing speeds by changing the length of the pauses between letters and the sixth position provided a programmable speed.

8.5.5 Ralph

The design of Ralph (robotic alphabet) is similar to that of the Gallaudet hand (Jaffe, 1994a,b; Jaffe *et al.*, 2001). However, a servomotor connected by a lever arm to a rod drives the hand motion and the fingers are rounded, making them feel more natural. Ralph is shown in Figure 8.11.

The eight servomotors are operated by control signals produced by the microcontroller software from the incoming serial ASCII data. The fingers are made in three segments, mechanically linked to each other. The rods move a system of linkages at the base of the fingers and these linkages flex the individual fingers and the wrist. The elimination of the pulleys has increased fingerspelling speed and made Ralph more compact.

Ralph uses the same computer hardware as its predecessor. The Forth software is organised in 17 modules. These modules enhance the Forth kernel, and provide an assembler, an ANSI display driver, serial port utilities, timer port and clock utilities, speed switch driver, timing control, fingerspelling algorithm and user interface, amongst other facilities. Like the Gallaudet hand,

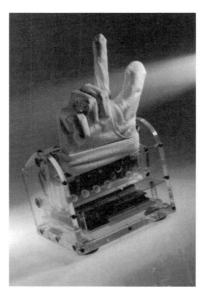

Figure 8.11 Ralph fingerspelling hand (courtesy of David Jaffe, Department of Veterans Affairs, Rehabilitation Research and Development Center, Palo Alto, CA).

Ralph also has a menu-driven user interface that allows the finger positions and system parameters to be changed.

Ralph can be controlled by any device that produces RS232 data, including terminals, modems, computers, optical character recognition (OCR) scanners, speech recognisers and modified closed-caption systems. The user interface is provided by a menu system, which gives easy access to unit functions, such as displaying and setting the microcontroller parameters, testing hand motions, editing hand position data and entering letters for fingerspelling. In the fingerspelling mode, key-presses are entered on the keyboard and translated by software into commands for the DC servomotors. Rotation of the motorshafts moves the rods connected to the fingers' mechanical linkage and transforms keyboard input into fingerspelling movements.

Ralph's ability to respond to computer input means that it can be connected to a telecommunications device for the deaf to provide deafblind people with telephone as well as face-to-face communications. It can also be connected to computers to provide improved access to information and employment potential.

The current prototype is compact: it weighs about 900 g without a battery and is 11.25 cm × 13.75 cm at the base and is 25 cm tall to the tip of the index finger; see Figure 8.11. It has suction cups to hold it to the table. It uses a 6 V power source, either battery or mains. The individual letters, transitions between letters and speed of presentation can be edited to suit individual preferences. The design is quite fast, with a capability of several characters per second. However, incorporation of wrist rotation would improve intelligibility and current limiting could be used to increase the motor life.

8.5.6 The Handtapper – a UK Development

The design of the Handtapper is significantly different from that of the US fingerspelling hands due to the different approaches to fingerspelling in the USA and UK. In the UK manual alphabet the communication is spelt out letter-by-letter onto the listener's left hand. The listener's hand remains fixed while the message is spelt out, and this fact was exploited in the development of a Handtapper device to automate the deafblind alphabet.

Twelve solenoids mounted below a hand-shaped base-plate produce a clear and localised vibration when activated by a 30 Hz chopped DC voltage. The individual locations and combinations of the solenoid locations can be correlated to the manual alphabet. Some fine-tuning with deafblind end-users was necessary to optimise the locations, which are shown in Figure 8.12.

A seven-key Braille keyboard allows the user to control the flow of material and to read, review and re-read a message. The keyboard operations are given in Table 8.1.

Handtapper applications include:

- reading electronic literature, such as books and correspondence via a computer interface;
- reading electronic mail via a modem connection;
- word processing and similar tasks via computer connection;
- access to telecommunications.

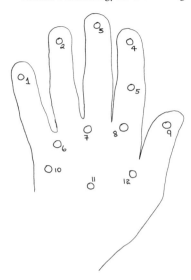

Figure 8.12 Handtapper solenoid positions.

Table 8.1 The keyboard operations table of the UK Handtapper.

Key	Alone	With repeat (RPT) key
DN	Forward one sentence	Forward a paragraph
UP	Go back one sentence	Go back a paragraph
RT	Move right one letter	Move right one word
LT	Move left one letter	Move left one word
RPT	Repeat one letter	–
START	Go to beginning of text	–
END	Go to end of text	–

8.5.7 Speaking Hands and Talking Gloves

Speaking Hands

The speaking hand was a UK project for a device based on a data-glove that enables deafblind people to send the UK manual alphabet to a computer. Future developments are envisaged to allow a computer to communicate with the user by inflating small balloons in the glove. This would put pressure on the fingertips analogous to communication from another person.

The Talking Glove System

The Talking Glove was developed as a Stanford University Project in 1988 (Kramer and Leifer, 1987, 1988, 1999, 1990; Kramer, 1991). Finger flexion associated with

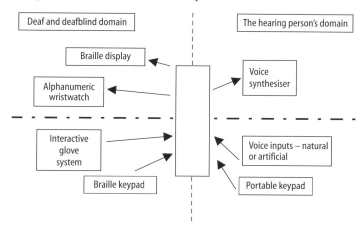

Figure 8.13 A complete Talking Glove system.

fingerspelling was measured by attaching sensors to a glove worn by a deafblind person. A microcontroller was able to use this information to deduce which letter was being formed and send the character to a display or a speech synthesiser. Thus, a Talking Glove system (Figure 8.13) allows deafblind people to communicate with hearing and sighted people and could be used in combination with Ralph to give two-way communication.

The system has acceptable fingerspelling performance, and the company Virtual Technologies was set up to market the system. A commercial fingerspelling recognition package called GesturePlus was released in 1995, but at the high price of $3500. The CyberGlove costs about $6000. In addition, a computer is required to run the system.

8.5.8 Comparison and Availability

All the mechanical hands described in Section 8.5 have been tested with small numbers of deafblind people, who have generally been very enthusiastic about them and eager for commercially available products. The resulting feedback has been used to improve letter formation. The learning rate for the Handtapper was found to be about 20 letters in 30 min for the small sample of five deafblind people. In an 8 hour evaluation of Ralph, over 2 days, a deafblind person familiar with the Gallaudet hand was able to identify 75% of short sentences the first time and identify them either completely or except for one word the second time (Jaffe, 1994a,b). Ralph and its predecessors are one-way communication systems that allow a hearing and sighted person to communicate with a deafblind person, the Talking Glove gives communication in the other direction between a deafblind and a hearing and sighted person. The Handtapper allows communication in one direction to the deafblind person.

A commercial fingerspelling package based on the Talking Glove has been produced in the USA, but it is very expensive, even without the associated Cyberglove and computer. Handtapper and Ralph have been developed to the prototype stage, but finance and/or an interested firm would be required to develop these further and to manufacture and distribute the devices.

8.6 Other Communication Aids

This section discusses a number of other communication aids. Other devices that use text Braille conversion will be presented in Sections 8.10 and 8.11 on information technology and telecommunications.

8.6.1 The Optacon and Optical Character Recognition (OCR)

The Optacon discussed here is interesting in that it illustrates the development of assistive technology for deafblind people as a spin-off from other projects, in this case an unsuccessful project by NASA to develop a tactual system for communication with astronauts during lift-off. It also illustrates the disadvantages that spin-off technologies may have in terms of performance, since they have not been developed specifically for deafblind people and deafblind people have not been involved in the design and development. In the case of the Optacon, it had a low reading speed. This is typically 100 words per minute (wpm) after training and compares to a good Braille reader at about 250 wpm and a sighted reader at more than 500–700 wpm.

The Optacon (Figure 8.14) is a reading aid for blind and deafblind people. The Optacon uses a hand-held camera connected to 144 piezoelectric elements and gives a vibratory image of the print characters under the fingertips. Character recognition was left to the user. Each vibrator operated at about 250 Hz, which is the most sensitive frequency for tactual reception at the fingertips for most people.

A number of systems to recognise printed characters have been developed for inputting text to computers. Such systems have immediate application for deafblind people since the information can be output in Braille. OCR is now

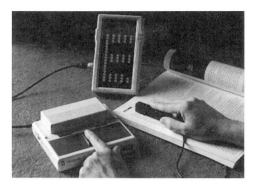

Figure 8.14 The Optacon.

Arial   Charles III III

Times Roman   Charles III Ill

Tiresias   Charles III Ill

Figure 8.15 Tiresias and some other typefaces.

very accurate for clearly printed texts, but some typefaces can give problems, and none of these systems is able to read handwriting satisfactorily.

The use of a standardised typeface has advantages with regards to character recognition. The Tiresias typeface (Figure 8.15) was originally developed for subtitling on digital terrestrial television, where legibility was considered to be of primary importance. It is now also used for teletext and interactive television, and has been adopted as the resident typeface for the European multimedia platform. It may also be easier for deafblind people with some vision to distinguish characters in Tiresias.

8.6.2 Tactile Sound-recognition Devices

The Tactaid II+ and Tactaid 7 convert sounds to vibrations on small pads attached to the body. More details can be found at the Web site, http://www.tactaid.com. There are only two pads and, therefore, two channels on the Tactaid II+, whereas there are seven channels and pads on the Tactaid 7. Each channel corresponds to a frequency band. Tactaid 7 also has an automatic noise-suppression circuit that reduces steady background sounds. It is able to provide information on speech characteristics, including voiced or voiceless, inflection, temporal cues and the first two formants that aid in vowel recognition. The units are battery operated and consist of a small box with wires to the pads. Attaching the pads to areas where the long bones are prominent, such as by a ring to the fingers or on a wristband, makes it easier to feel the vibrations.

Tactaid 2000 (Figure 8.16) is a six-channel modification of Tactaid 7. It is designed to present tactile cues that allow differentiation of the difficult to hear high frequency speech sounds. Five vibrators cover the speech spectrum from 2000 to 8000 Hz, allowing detection and discrimination of the sounds in this range, and a single detachable vibrator provides the output for sound

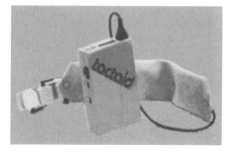

Figure 8.16 Tactaid (courtesy of Audiological Engineering Corporation).

frequencies less than 2000 Hz. The device can be used alone or together with hearing aids or cochlear implants.

8.7 Low-technology Devices and Domestic Appliances

Many of the devices discussed in this chapter, and the book as a whole, draw on state-of-the art high technology. However, there are also a number of useful devices that use much simpler and/or older technologies, some of which will be discussed in this section. Since most of these lower technology devices are used in the home, this section will also briefly discuss the marking of domestic appliances and groceries.

One relatively simple approach is device modification by the replacement of the output transducer to give a vibratory rather than a visual or audio output. This approach may have considerable potential in making devices accessible to deafblind people, but the number of devices currently available with vibratory output is small due to the high development and manufacturing costs for a small national market. Such devices include a liquid-level indicator (see Figure 8.17) and light probe (see Figure 8.18). In the liquid-level indicator the device vibrates when the conducting liquid connects the pair of probes. An intermittent tone and vibration indicate that the cup is nearly full, whereas a continuous tone and vibration indicate that it is full.

The vibratory light probe can detect the presence of light directly from the light source and can be used to tell if an electric light is on or check the status of indicator lights on domestic appliances, such as a washing machine. The amplitude of vibration is proportional to the intensity of light detected.

A vibrating room-thermometer operates by moving a pointer to a position where a tone is heard and vibrations can be felt. It is marked with tactile dots and large print. The unit can be wall mounted and measures temperatures between −5 and +35 °C.

Since (totally) deafblind people gain important information largely through the sense of touch, recognition of different products requires them to have a distinctive size, shape, texture or embossed or other tactile markings.

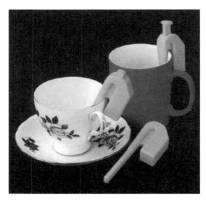

Figure 8.17 Liquid-level indicator with vibratory output.

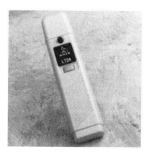

Figure 8.18 Light probe with vibratory output.

However, there has been an increasing standardisation of packaging, which has resulted in, for instance, aerosol containers of polish and hairspray feeling the same, thereby making recognition much more difficult. There is, therefore, a need for embossed or other tactile markings to enable deafblind (and blind) people to distinguish different products. An embossed triangle is now used on the packaging of dangerous substances. Although clearly essential, this is insufficient, and there is a need for at least the type of product and the price to be marked on all products either using Braille or a simplified tactile code, possibly using a small number of symbols to represent the most common household products. A few items have been specially designed to be easy to differentiate by touch to help blind people. For instance, in the UK, differently sized banknotes indicate different denominations (see Figure 8.19).

There have been a number of proposals for using barcodes to help blind and deafblind people sort their groceries at home. The barcode gives the product number, so a databank would be required to relate this number to the product name or label information. In theory, a barcode reader can be connected to a database of full product information via the telephone or Internet, and provide an output in Braille. In practice, the cost of establishing and running such a service has not made it attractive to potential operators. Therefore, any practical system might have to be automated, with only a limited number of options for querying the system, such as

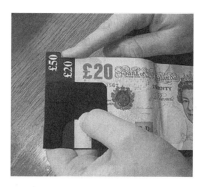

Figure 8.19 Banknote identifier.

- product type and name
- product type, name and quantity in appropriate units
- full product information, including all ingredients.

Manufacturers would probably consider it in their interests to submit full product information to the database and, therefore, would do so voluntarily without legislation being required. However, having to obtain product information in this way is considerably more complicated than obtaining it by reading the packaging. Therefore, the database should preferably supplement basic information in Braille or other tactile format.

In the past, embossed markings could be added to the controls on most domestic appliances, such as washing machines, cookers and central heating. However, an increasing number of appliances are now using dynamic visual displays rather than electro-mechanical controls. Braille or large visual displays could be connected, possibly using developments such as Bluetooth, but this is likely to increase the cost significantly and probably also increase the the difficulty of using the appliance. Therefore, persuading manufacturers to continue to produce at least some domestic appliances with electro-mechanical controls is probably a better option.

8.8 Bluetooth

Bluetooth is a short-range wireless networking technology that facilitates interconnection of mobile computers, mobile phones, headsets and computer peripherals without rewiring cables (McGarrity, 2001). Although it has some potential for supporting deafblind people through the provision of information, the limited range of less than 10 m is likely to prove a severe restriction on the facilities that can be provided. Bluetooth could probably be used through a system of primary and secondary links to provide product information from barcodes in a supermarket, but could not be used to provide connection to a centralised database of information.

There are also potential applications of using Bluetooth via a handheld unit with vibrating output to give information about the status of traffic lights and to request additional crossing time. However, the status information could be obtained with a portable sound monitor from traffic lights that give an auditory signal or from an adaptation of a light indicator to make it frequency sensitive. There may be advantages in using Bluetooth rather than current radio-frequency transmission systems in, for instance, home alarm and alerting systems. Another application could be the connection of different assistive devices to a wide range of appliances and equipment in the home and workplace. A low-cost system with a much greater range than Bluetooth could have a useful role in providing environmental information to deafblind and blind people.

Bluetooth is designed to be low cost and low form factor. It uses the unlicensed instrumentation, scientific and medical (ISM) band around 2.4 GHz. There is, therefore, a possibility of interference from other applications that use this band, such as cordless telephones, garage-door openers and outside-broadcasting equipment, as well as from microwave ovens, which emit

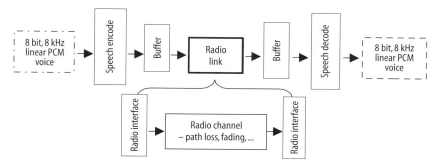

Figure 8.20 Communications link between transmitter and receiver.

radiation in this bandwidth. This frequency band is also used by two other wireless networking standards: 802.11b or "WiFi" and Home RF on 802.11b.

The Bluetooth specifications define voice and data communication requirements for transmission over a radio channel with a maximum capacity of 1 Mb s^{-1}. Bluetooth transmits at low power (1 mW) and, therefore, is intended for short distances of less than 10 m. It uses the Gaussian frequency shift keying (GFSK) modulation scheme. Frequency hopping is used to avoid interference from other devices transmitting in the band. Appropriate coding schemes can be used to recover Bluetooth transmissions when they collide with another device, though this is an occasional occurrence. A new hop frequency is used in each of the 625 µs slots into which transmission time is divided.

Bluetooth devices can be primary (master) or secondary (slave) in transmission, with the primary device initiating connection to one or more secondary devices. The communications links between the primary transmitter and secondary receiver for voice transmissions is illustrated in Figure 8.20.

8.9 Alerting Devices for Deafblind People

The basic structure of an alarm and alerting system was discussed in Chapter 7. It was seen that these systems consist of input and output transducers, signal-conditioning elements and signal transmission. However, when considering alarm and alerting systems for deafblind people, particular consideration has to be given to the implementation and the user controls in addition to the output transducer. The controls on alarm and alerting devices are generally tactile, in the form of buttons and/or switches, with visual indications of the settings. The use of visual markings on tactile user controls will pose problems for many deafblind people. To maximise accessibility, such markings should be made as clear as possible through the use of large symbols and good colour contrast; additionally, they should be supplemented by tactile markings, for instance in Braille or through the use of raised symbols.

Four different devices are discussed in this section: two of the devices have been developed in a university context, through student projects, and two are commercially available products, one of which has been developed specifically for deafblind people and the other for profoundly deaf people. One of the university devices is still in the prototype stage and was developed specifically for deafblind people, although it also applies design for all principles. The other was developed for a specific deafblind person using a modification of existing devices. Two devices include signal-transmission components. The design of three of the devices has resulted in both an output transducer and user controls that are fully accessible to deafblind people, whereas one of the commercial devices has user controls that allow deafblind users to access some, but not all, device functions.

8.9.1 Vibrating Alarm Clocks

This section discusses an alarm clock (Figure 8.21) specifically for deafblind people that is being developed at the University of Glasgow through student projects (Teo, 2000; Teo and Hersh, 2001; Rozario, 2002). It has reached the prototype stage. There are a number of alarm clocks currently available for either deaf or blind people, but none for deafblind people. However, most existing alarm clocks do not have user controls that are accessible to deafblind people and which allow them to set and check both the time and the alarm time using touch.

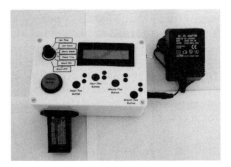

Figure 8.21 Vibrating alarm clock (courtesy of Garvin Rozario).

Tactile user control for setting and checking the time have been incorporated by using push buttons to set the time and the alarm time and small vibrators to check both the actual time and the alarm time. The original version was slightly larger and required the use of both hands for separate buttons and vibrators. The current prototype has been reduced in size through the use of relays that can function both as push buttons and as vibrators (see Figure 8.22).

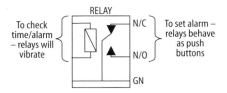

Figure 8.22 Relay used as push button and vibrator (courtesy of Garvin Rozario).

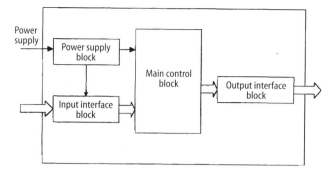

Figure 8.23 Hierarchical design concept, main blocks (courtesy of Joseph Teo Choon Kok).

This has advantages in increasing portability. The clock is a 24-hour type, and the first, second, third and little fingers are used to set the "tens" and digits of the hour and the "tens" and digits of the minutes respectively. The function-select buttons used to determine which operation was carried out in the original version have been replaced by a six-way rotating switch for selecting functions. A snooze feature with a large snooze button, which also doubles as an enter button, has also been added.

The design concept is based on a hierarchical design approach consisting of discrete single function blocks, with the major blocks (shown in Figure 8.23) as follows:

- power supply block
- user input interface block
- main control block
- output interface unit.

The power supply block, as seen in Figure 8.24, has the following components:

- a constant-current regulator circuit, which is designed to produce a constant current that trickle charges the battery so that it ceases charging when the battery is fully charged, but which supplies power as long as the battery is plugged in;

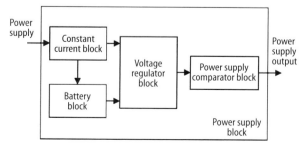

Figure 8.24 The power supply block (courtesy of Joseph Teo Choon Kok).

- an 8.4 V PP3 energiser rechargeable battery with capacity of 150 mA h. This is significantly less than the 550 mA h of a 9 V PP3 alkaline battery;
- a power indicator, which indicates when the battery is supplying less than 6 V;
- a 7805 voltage regulator to regulate the power supply from 9 V to 5 V.

The user-input interface consists of the following:

- a six-way switch to select the clock function to be implemented;
- a snooze/enter button, which functions as a snooze button to interrupt the buzzer or vibrating alarm for a brief period and as an enter button to confirm the operation selected on the six-way switch;
- four small buttons for entering the digits and tens of the minutes and hours of the actual time and the alarm time to be set.

The main control unit consists of a microcontroller, with a CPU, memory and input/output all on one IC chip. The microcontroller takes the signals from the different inputs, processes them and transmits the results to the appropriate outputs. It also runs the clock process through an integrated 16-bit free running counter powered by a clock derived from the 8 MHz crystal oscillator connected to the microcontroller.

The output interface includes both output actuators and user controls. It consists of the following:

- four small vibrators for checking the digits and tens of the minutes and hours of the actual time and the alarm time set
- a loud buzzer to wake deafblind users with some hearing
- a vibrating pad to act as an alert
- a liquid-crystal display panel for deafblind users with some vision to read the time.

8.9.2 A Multifunction Domestic Alert System

A multifunction domestic alert system was developed at the University of Southampton for a specific deafblind user and has been built and installed in his house (Damper, 1993; Damper and Evans, 1995). The system (Figure 8.25) is designed to alert the user to either of his two telephones ringing, the doorbell

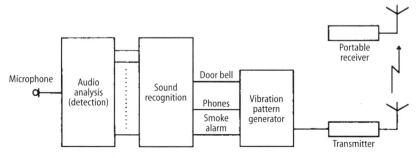

Figure 8.25 Block diagram of alerting system.

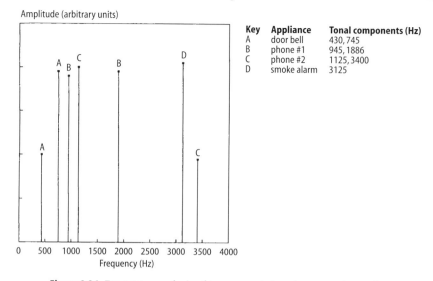

Figure 8.26 Frequency analysis of tape-recorded environmental sounds.

and a smoke alarm sounding and to distinguish between the different alerts. This system illustrates the modification of several single-function alarm and alerting devices for hearing people to give one multifunction device for a deafblind person.

The design modification is based on a sound detection and recognition unit in a fixed position in the hallway of the client's house, within 10–15 m of all relevant sound sources. This unit determines the source of the sound and transmits the information over a single remote channel to a portable unit worn by the user. The different alerting sounds have tonal components at different frequencies, as shown in Figure 8.26. These distinct tonal components form the basis of a discrimination system using simple analogue active filters. The uniform bandwidth of 100 Hz used for all the tone-detection filters gives a maximum sensitivity or Q value of 31.25. Additional noise filters centred on 1550 and 2550 Hz and of bandwidth 200 Hz are used to sample the spectrum in the regions in which the appliances do not have spectral components. Twelve filters, rather than the minimum of eight required, are included to facilitate adaptation of the system for other users. Potentiometer controls are included to allow adjustment of filter centre frequency and gain.

A programmable logic device (PAL 16L8), with 12 inputs and eight outputs, is used as the recognition module for the different alerting sounds. This allows the flexible allocation of the different filters to the recognition of different environmental sounds. A radio frequency transmission system based on a cordless door chime from Innovations is used to transmit the signal to the user, with vibration codes generated by switching the transmission on and off. Different vibration codes are used to distinguish the doorbell, telephone and smoke alarm. The vibrating output is produced by a 3 V DC motor, with a small brass disc at one end to provide an eccentric out-of-balance weight.

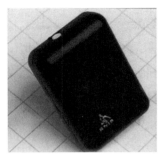

Figure 8.27 Tactiwatch (courtesy RNIB).

8.9.3 Tactiwatch

Tactiwatch (http://www.rnib.org.uk/wesupply/products/prodcat/catvibr.htm#tact) is a hand-held watch that has been designed specifically for deafblind people (Figure 8.27). Once set, the time can be read by pressing the recessed switch on the top of the unit. The output for telling the time consists of pulses of varying duration that vibrate the unit, *e.g.* giving short pulses for hours, long pulses for tens of minutes and short pulses for minutes. The main disadvantage is the inability of the deafblind person to set the alarm on the watch.

8.9.4 Tam

Tam, from Summit, is a lightweight sound monitor for profoundly deaf people. It is worn like a watch on the left wrist. A very thin wire connects the device to a small control box, which can be clipped to clothing or worn in an inside pocket. The watchband gives a clear firm vibration when triggered by a sound above the level set by the user. Some users are able to use it to distinguish between different everyday sounds such as a telephone ringing and a door slamming. It can alert deafblind people to someone entering the room or trying to communicate with them and can be helpful in crossing a moderately busy road. The main drawback is the long charging time of 10 hours.

8.10 Access to Information Technology

Developments in information technology are potentially very significant for deafblind people. On the positive side, these developments could open up a wide range of new opportunities for deafblind people and enable them to communicate on equal terms with hearing and sighted people, *e.g.* through e-mail. This requires the availability of appropriate interfaces, including text–Braille conversion and haptics, to allow deafblind users to access information technology. It also requires appropriate design of software and hardware to ensure compatibility and that deafblind people can access the full range of services provided by information technology.

On the negative side, deafblind people frequently have low incomes and adapted (information) technology is generally relatively expensive. In addition, deafblind people are likely to have more difficulty than hearing and sighted people in accessing the training they need to use information technology and gain the full benefits from this use. The inability to access information technology and to participate in the information society is likely to be even more detrimental for deafblind than hearing and sighted people. Therefore, it is very important that information technology is accessible to deafblind people. This section discusses the accessibility of information technology to deafblind people and presents a text browser for deafblind people.

The advent of the personal computer with Braille or magnified visual output has opened up opportunities for a significant increase in access to information for deafblind people. However, although software for producing large characters on the monitor is relatively inexpensive, Braille displays have remained expensive.

The text-based operating system DOS is easier to use for many deafblind people than systems that use a graphical user interface, such as Windows. However, keeping to DOS restricts the choice of software, as most new software is written for the Windows environment. The use of haptics in computer interfaces may allow blind and deafblind people to navigate spatially organised computer systems, such as Windows. Haptics is based on a dynamic combination of touch and proprioception or sensitivity to changes in body position. It should allow deafblind and blind computer users to access at least some of the graphical interface elements and, therefore, to benefit more from their computer systems.

E-mail systems are predominantly text-based and, therefore, are relatively easy to use with a Braille display. The World Wide Web is more problematic, in that many sites employ graphical representations without an adequate text alternative. The sites that are fully accessible tend to belong to government departments, and the most inaccessible sites are the popular home-shopping sites. Even with these restrictions, the Internet has the potential for significantly increasing access to information by deafblind people. What is needed is a range of affordable user-friendly terminals that provide access for deafblind people who need non-visual output but who do not read Braille.

The World Wide Web Consortium (W3C) was founded in October 1994 to help make the Web more accessible to everyone. It has set up the Web Accessibility Initiative (WAI) to make the Web fully accessible, including to disabled people (http://www.w3.org/WAI/). The WAI is considering the five key areas of technology, guidelines, tools, education and outreach, and research and development. W3C has developed a series of 14 guidelines on making Web sites accessible. These include the following:

- provide equivalent alternatives to auditory and visual content;
- provide context and orientation information and clear navigation mechanisms;
- ensure that tables and pages featuring new technologies transform gracefully.

A Web-page evaluation tool called Bobby (www.cast.org/bobby) was created by the Centre for Applied Special Technology (CAST) in 1996 to encourage

Web-page designers to follow the W3C guidelines. It has been upgraded continually and can be used to test Web pages and search engines against the W3C accessibility criteria. Sites that pass the test can display the Bobby logo. It is likely that, as a result of recent legislation on disability in many countries, an increasing number of Web sites will be legally required to make themselves fully accessible and could face legal action if they do not.

8.10.1 The Universal Communications Text Browser (Ucon)

Ucon was developed by S.W.H. Software (http://www.swhsoftware.demon.co.uk) to give deafblind and visually impaired people improved access to the World Wide Web, e-mail and telecommunications through Braille. It is also compatible with the Handtapper and can be used with speech on some systems. The software is fully functional under Windows, although it is currently DOS based. This gives full access to people with older computer systems.

Ucon uses e-mail to access Web pages and displays them in Braille in a text-only reading mode. Links to other Web pages, e-mail addresses and telephone numbers can be "clicked" as they appear in the Braille display for use or storage in the Ucon directory. Ucon can also read Web pages saved by other browsers and display them as text with the links available for use. HTML files can be accessed directly and displayed in Braille with the page links accessible.

The default is to supply all text without formatting information, such as blank lines, which are not relevant to deafblind readers. There is also the option to show the on-screen layout of the text, which can be helpful in reading tables. The text search feature can find any sequence of words, regardless of spaces and line breaks between them, and search Web pages and source files independently of link and format information. An automatic bookmark facility records the reader's place, to allow them to break off and resume reading easily.

E-mail communications are supported. The Microtext teletext adaptor card for the PC can be used to facilitate the Braille reading of teletext pages, including live subtitled television programmes. The automatic sequencing of pages allows users to read consecutive pages, such as news headlines, without having to wait for each one. The use of subtitles allows users to stop reading and come back to a programme where they left off. Ucon gives access to telecommunications with auto dialling of telephone numbers for both voice and text calls. There is full support for direct text calls and a text answerphone, as well as the facilities to store numbers or dial them without having to store them first, both directly from the text. This gives a similar service to the deafblind as to sighted readers, who are able to dial a number from a magazine without having to write it in their address book first.

8.11 Provision of Telecommunications Equipment and Services

Alongside information technology, access to telecommunications determines whether individuals can access information and participate fully in society.

Access to telecommunications is particularly important for deafblind people who may experience social isolation, since it allows more interactive communication than is possible, for instance with e-mail. Despite the importance of access to telecommunications, the needs of deafblind people for telecommunications equipment and services are in general poorly served in most countries. However, there are a number of systems available. This section describes some of these systems. The section is divided into two subsections, which discuss hardware, and software and access to services respectively.

8.11.1 Hardware

The American VersaBraille system is a computer with a built-in Braille display (Figure 8.28). It was first tested in the early 1980s, but is no longer being manufactured. It allows deafblind people to communicate by telephone with other deafblind people or deaf users of text telephones and with hearing people through relay services.

Another US product, the Braillephone from Audio Visual Mart Inc. (http://www.av-mart.com/Braillephone.htm), was developed to provide a good portable communications system for deafblind people (Figure 8.29). The system allows the user to communicate using either a text telephone or a relay service, such as Typetalk, over the telephone lines. Braillephone also supports face-to-face communication between deafblind people or between deafblind and sighted people. Braillephone can be used to access most MS-DOS, Windows 3.1, or Windows 95 computer systems when used with appropriate software. It has a 23-cell eight-dot refreshable Braille displays and a 25,000-character memory. The user can switch between Braille and QWERTY keyboards. There is a 20-character visual display and rechargeable battery system. Braillephone's™ plug-in palm-sized vibrating data detector provides hands-free continuous monitoring of the status of all information, including the telephone ringer. This allows the user to be fully informed of the status of the conversation while keeping their hands free to type and read the Braille display.

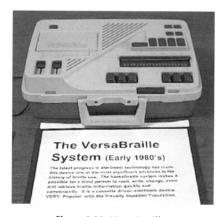

Figure 8.28 VersaBraille.

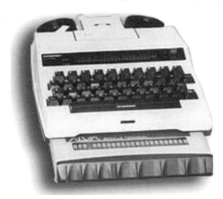

Figure 8.29 Braillephone (courtesy of Audio Visual Mart, Inc.).

Telebraille III from Telesensory (http://www.deafblind.com/telebrl.html) was designed as a telecommunications device for the deaf (TDD) to allow a deafblind person and a person using a TDD to communicate by telephone (Figure 8.30). It can also be used in face-to-face conversations between a deafblind and a sighted person. For telephone conversations, the modified UltraTec Supercom TDD can either be connected directly to the telephone line with a conventional telephone jack or the telephone receiver can be coupled to the Supercom TDD by placing the handset on the acoustic coupler. The modified 20-cell six-dot Braille display is then used for reading and either the Braille or the QWERTY keyboard for writing. In face-to-face conversation, the two components are separated. The sighted partner types on the QWERTY keyboard of the Supercom textphone and sees the information on the 20-character visual display. However, this display is standard size and not particularly useful for people with low vision. Vibration of the 20th Braille cell is used to indicate the Braillephone ringing, busy or a speech signal on the line. Up to ten messages of 255 characters each can be recorded on the automatic TDD answering machine. There is a connection port to a printer or Braille embosser to provide hard copies of messages. The addition of Gateway software allows

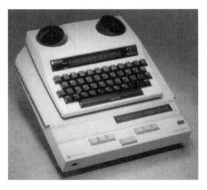

Figure 8.30 Telebraille (courtesy of Telesensory).

the Telebraille to be connected to a desktop or laptop computer and used in DOS applications.

The LiteTouch Telephone Communicator and Infotouch are both portable communication system for deafblind Braille readers, which consist of three small components that can be easily connected. In the case of LiteTouch, these components are a Braille Lite personal data assistant, an UltraTec SuperPrint E modified textphone and a tiny signal detector. Telephone access for LiteTouch is provided through a smart microprocessor that automatically scrolls characters sent or received by the textphone across the Braille Lite 18-cell refreshable Braille display. The signal detector gives a strong vibration when the telephone detects a ring, busy signal or audible indication that the other party is speaking.

In the case of Infotouch, the three components are a portable Romeo Braille printer, a Superprinter TDD and a vibrating data detector. The printer and Superprinter have carrying cases and the detector can be put in a pocket. Messages can be typed using either six-key Braille or a conventional keyboard and are displayed on the Romeo Braille printer. Text can be automatically embossed as it appears, without waiting for a full line. The messages can also be displayed on a 20-character LED display or transmitted by telephone through the Superprinter TDD. The TDD can answer incoming calls with a message that has been programmed in and the caller can leave a Braille message.

UltraTec (http://www.ultratec.com/) have produced a large visual display for TDD users that gives ten times magnification. The large visual display can be connected to an external port of the Superprint 4425A to obtain a permanent record of the conversation, with adjusted print style.

8.11.2 Software and Access to Telecommunications

The Swedish Deafblind Association (FSDB) has developed the conversation program Telo for people using Braille or magnifying displays. Telo has been modified to allow the use of bulletin board systems. It is available free of charge in both English and Swedish. FSDB has also successfully campaigned for equipment to be subsidised, and all deafblind people in Sweden are supplied with a computer, complete with modem, readers and software free of charge. The FSDB service group has been set up to provide training in the use of this equipment.

HASICOM (Hearing and Sight Impaired Communication) was set up in the UK in the early 1980s to support full participation of deafblind people in everyday life and is now operated by Deafblind UK. The HASICOM network currently has about 50 users of Braille or large-print screen facilities, with availability and take-up constrained by the limited funds of a voluntary organisation. Users can communicate with ordinary voice telephones over the UK national relay service, Typetalk, where an intermediary operator relays the conversation in both directions. At present, the HASICOM service mainly provides equipment for experienced Braille users and deafblind people with some residual vision.

In the USA, some states provide telephone access equipment to disabled people through a fund supported by all telephone subscribers. When an approved commercial version of Ralph, or other fingerspelling hand is developed, it could be provided free of charge to deafblind people under this programme.

The Telephoning with Deafblind People Project (http://www.tichnut.de/phone/) has developed software to enable computer telephone conversations between deafblind and hearing and sighted people over the computer. There is a choice of DOS or Windows and English or German versions. Calls can be indicated either by vibrator or through the PC speaker. In the Windows version, both communication partners communicate via a window divided into two parts, with the whole conversation shown in one part and the text to be sent in the other. This software can be used on any PC or notebook with a modem.

Software has been developed that can be used in conjunction with Braille telephone devices to give deafblind people access to closed captions of television information. For instance, the Braille TeleCaption System (http://www.ggtechservices.com/files/Tele.txt) provides news, weather, sports and educational TV programmes to deafblind people in the USA. Data is translated into grade 1 Braille and can be read with a Telebrailler or other Braille telephone devices. The Closed Caption Braille computer system allows deafblind people to read closed-captioned television programmes in Braille. The data input–output and translation are controlled by the computer software; the hardware consists of a videotape recorder, an IBM compatible computer and a closed-caption-to-Braille computer card. The system is connected to the Telebraille via a telephone handset and the closed captioning is displayed in either grade I or grade II Braille. However, not all technological developments have benefited deafblind people. For instance, analogue television is compatible with Braille teletext output, and gives basic access to the news. However, digital teletext is graphically based, so this is no longer possible.

Future developments could include radio-based systems for short-range interconnection of both domestic and public terminals. Systems such as Bluetooth have the potential to facilitate the connection of assistive devices to a whole range of equipment. If this technology performs successfully, then it could provide significant support to deafblind people in living and working independently.

8.12 Future Research Directions

Considerably more assistive technology devices have been developed for blind or deaf people than deafblind people. In some cases, assistive technology devices for deaf or blind people can be converted to devices for deafblind people by replacing audio or visual output by tactile or tactual output, whereas in others a total redesign will be required.

It is also significant that a number of positive developments in the area have been as the result of student projects. This has the advantages of applying creative and innovative solutions and facilitating developments that would probably not have occurred otherwise. The disadvantages are a considerably extended development period, as products often have to be worked on by several students in succession, and the difficulties in moving from a prototype to a marketable product, since there are generally no direct links between the development stage and a firm or other organisation that is able to produce and market the device.

Owing to the importance of tactile and tactual input in conveying information to deafblind people, there is a need for research on the sense of touch, including both perception and cognition. Related areas of research include different ways of representing and transmitting information in tactile or tactual form to maximise information content and understanding, as well as how residual vision and hearing can best be supplemented by tactile and tactual information.

Devices for automating communication based on the US and UK deafblind manual alphabets have been developed, but they have not gone beyond the prototype stage. Further developments in this area could include making the devices more portable, for instance by allowing them to be carried in a pocket and then opened out to an appropriate size for use, and making the fingerspelling movements more natural. There is also a need for the development of devices for the conversion of the deafblind manual alphabet to high-quality natural-sounding synthetic speech with a choice of voices and accents to provide further support for communication by deafblind people who do not have oral speech.

Deafblind people in non-English-speaking countries also require communications devices. There is a need for research effort into how these can best be provided, including the feasibility of a universal or multi-lingual translation device, which could carry out the following two operations:

- conversion of text (or speech) input in any language into any deafblind manual language output;
- conversion of any deafblind manual language input into text or synthetic speech output in any language.

The development of a universal or multi-lingual translation device would also have advantages in terms of allowing deafblind people to read (untranslated) materials in foreign languages and to travel abroad independently. One alternative would be the separate development of devices for each oral and deafblind manual language. However, owing to the small national markets for automated fingerspelling devices, it may prove to be easier to develop and market a multi-lingual translation device than separate devices for each oral and deafblind manual language. Another approach would require further research to investigate the details of the different deafblind manual languages world-wide to determine whether deafblind manual languages can be categorised into groups that use similar principles to facilitate the development of automated fingerspelling devices for each group of languages.

There are likely to be continuing developments in information and telecommunications technology for sighted and hearing people. Research will be required to keep up with these developments and to determine how best they can be used to increase the options open to deafblind people, as well as to ensure that all the new developments are accessible to them. Developments such as Bluetooth will require further investigation to determine their real potential and applications for supporting deafblind people. Bluetooth is currently limited by the short transmission distance. There is, therefore, a need for further research to develop an analogous low-cost system, either based on Bluetooth or using different principles, that could be used in transmitting information from centralised databases to deafblind people.

Another important area where research is still required is supporting independent travel by deafblind people. A number of mobility aids have been developed for blind people, but nothing specifically for deafblind people, though some of the mobility aids have vibration in addition to audio output. However, the most successful mobility aids are still the long cane and the guide dog. There has been less work on the development of orientation aids for determining current position and navigation aids, such as tactile or tactual maps.

To be successful, future research and development should involve deafblind people, so that the resulting technologies, products and devices are user friendly and serve a real purpose.

Projects and Investigations

1. Design and build an inexpensive battery-operated calculator with tactile output.
2. Consider a system for obtaining tactual output from teletext on digital television.
   (a) Investigate existing systems that perform related functions.
   (b) Draw up detailed design specifications in consultation with deafblind end-users.
   (c) Obtain a detailed design.
   (d) Build a prototype device.
   (e) Test the device with deafblind end-users.
3. The UMTS terminal is for use by a deafblind person.
   (a) Investigate existing systems that perform related functions.
   (b) Draw up detailed design specifications in consultation with deafblind end-users.
   (c) Obtain a detailed design.
   (d) Build a prototype device.
   (e) Test the device with deafblind end-users.
4. Compare and contrast the underlying technologies and principles used in the US and UK fingerspelling hands.
5. Consider an improved design of a fingerspelling hand.
   (a) Investigate existing fingerspelling hands.
   (b) Draw up a critique of existing fingerspelling hands and determine which features require modification.
   (c) Draw up detailed design specifications in consultation with deafblind end-users and using the critique of existing fingerspelling hands.
   (d) Obtain a detailed design.
   (e) Build a prototype device.

(f) Test the device with deafblind end-users.
6. Consider conversion from the deafblind manual alphabet to synthetic speech.
   (a) Investigate the literature on text speech conversion and other related topics.
   (b) Draw up detailed design specifications in consultation with deafblind end-users.
   (c) Obtain a detailed design.
   (d) Build a prototype device.
   (e) Test the device with deafblind end-users.
7. Investigate the deafblind manual languages used in different countries and the feasibility of developing a multi-lingual translation device for deafblind people.
8. Consider a device to aid deafblind people to cross the road.
   (a) Investigate currently available mobility and navigation aids for deafblind and blind people.
   (b) Make a critique of existing aids.
   (c) Determine what principles of existing aids could be adapted.
   (d) Draw up detailed design specifications in consultation with deafblind end-users and using knowledge obtained from existing aids.
   (e) Obtain a detailed design.
   (f) Build a prototype device.
   (g) Test the device with deafblind end-users.

References and Further Reading

References

Alcorn, S., 1932. The Tadoma method. *Volta Review* 34, 195–198.
Chomsky, C., 1986. Analytic study of the Tadoma method: language abilities of three deaf-blind subjects. *Journal of Speech and Hearing Research* 29, 332–347.
Damper, R.I., 1993. New alert system for deafblind people. *Talking Sense* 39 (3).
Damper, R.I., Evans, M.D., 1995. A multifunction domestic alert system for the deaf–blind. *IEEE Transactions on Rehabilitation Engineering* 3 (4), 354–359.
Danssaert, J., Greenstein, A., Lee, P., Meade, A., 1985. A fingerspelling hand for the deaf-blind. ME210 Final Report, Stanford University.
Fleischer, D.A., Durlach, N.I., 1993. Measuring the dimensions of sensory communication at RLE. *RLE Currents* 6 (2), http://rlweb.mit.edu/Publications/currents/6-2cover.htm.
Gilden, D., 1987a. A robotic hand as a communication aid for the deaf-blind. In: *Proceedings of the 20th Hawaii International Conference on Systems Science*, Hawaii.
Gilden, D., 1987b. Time and again, say in without feeling: two new devices for deaf–blind people. In: *Proceedings of the 10th RESNA Conference on Rehabilitation Technology*, San Jose, CA.
Gilden, D., Jaffe, D.L., 1986. Dexter, a helping hand for communicating with the deaf–blind. In: *Proceedings of the 9th Annual Conference of Rehabilitation Engineering (RENSA)*, Minneapolis.
Gilden, D., Jaffe, D.L., 1988. Dexter, a robotic hand communication aid for the deaf–blind: research news. *International Journal of Rehabilitation Research* 11 (2), 198–199.
Jaffe, D.L., 1987. Speaking in Hands. *SOMA: Engineering for the Human Body* 2 (3), 6–13.
Jaffe, D.L., 1989a. Dexter II – the next generation mechanical fingerspelling hand for deaf–blind persons. In: *Proceedings of the 12th Annual RESNA Conference*, New Orleans, USA.

Jaffe, D.L., 1989b. Dexter – a fingerspelling hand. *OnCenter – Technology Transfer News* 1 (1).
Jaffe, D.L., 1993a. Third generation fingerspelling hand. In: *Proceedings of the Technology and Persons with Disabilities Conference*, Los Angeles, USA.
Jaffe, D.L., 1993b. The development of a third generation fingerspelling hand. In: *16th RESNA Conference*, Las Vegas.
Jaffe, D.L., 1994a. Evolution of mechanical fingerspelling hands for people who are deaf–blind, clinical report. *Journal of Rehabilitation Research and Development* 31 (3), 236–244.
Jaffe, D.L., 1994b. RALPH: a fourth generation fingerspelling hand. 1994 Stanford University, Rehabilitation R&D Center Progress Report.
Jaffe, D.L., Schwandt, D.F., Anderson, J.H., 2001. Technology transfer of the Ralph fingerspelling hand. In: *Conference on Intellectual Property in the VA: Changes, Challenges, and Collaborations*, Arlington, VA.
Kramer, J., 1991. Communication system for deaf, deaf–blind and non-vocal individuals using instrumented gloves. US Patent 5,047,952, Virtual Technologies.
Kramer, J., Leifer, L., 1987. An expressive and receptive communication aid for the deaf, deaf–blind and nonvocal. In: *Proceedings of the Annual Conference IEEE Engineering in Medicine and Biology Society*, Boston, USA.
Kramer, J., Leifer, L., 1988. The talking glove: an expressive and receptive verbal communication aid for the deaf, deaf–blind and nonvocal. *SIGCAPH Newsletter* (39), 12–16.
Kramer, J., Leifer, L., 1989. The Talking Glove: a speaking aid for non-vocal deaf and deaf–blind individuals. In: *Proceedings of RESNA 12th Annual Conference*, pp. 471–472.
Kramer, J., Leifer, L., 1990. A talking glove for nonverbal deaf individuals. Technical Report CDR TR 1990 0312, Centre for Design Research, Stanford University.
Laenger Sr., C.J., Herbert, P.H., 1978. Further development and tests of an artificial hand for communication with deaf-blind people. Southwest Research Institute, March.
McGarrity, S., 2001. Bluetooth voice Simulink model. *MATLAB Digest*, Volume 9, Number 4 (November 2001), www.mathworks.com/digest.
Reed, C.M., Delhorne, L.A., Durlach, N.I., Fisher, S.D., 1989. Analytic study of the Tadoma method: effects of hand position on segmented speech perception. *Journal of Speech and Hearing Research* 32, 921–929.
Rozario, G., 2002. Vibrating alarm clock. University of Glasgow Department of Electronics and Electrical Engineering Final Year Project Report.
Schultz, M.C, Norton, S.J., Conway-Fithian, S., Reed, C.M., 1984. A survey of the use of the Tadoma method in the United States and Canada. *Volta Review* 86, 733–737.
Teo, J., 2000. Improved design vibrating alarm clock. University of Glasgow Department of Electronics and Electrical Engineering Final Year Project Report.
Teo, J., Hersh, M.A., 2001. An improved design vibrating alarm clock for deafblind people. Preprints CVHI 2001, Castlevecchio Pascoli, Italy.
Vivian, R., 1966. The Tadoma method: a tactual approach to speech and speech reading. *Volta Review* 86, 282–292.

Further Reading

Books

Bliss J.C., 1978. Reading machines for the blind. In: Gordon, G. (Ed.), *Active Touch*. Pergamon Press, Oxford, pp. 243–248.
Gill, J.M., 1982. Production of tangible graphic displays. In: Schiff, W., Foulke, E. (Eds), *Tactual Perception: A Sourcebook*. Cambridge University Press, pp. 405-416 (ISBN 0-521-24095-6).
Gill, J.M., 1983. New aids for the blind and deaf–blind. In: Perkins, W.J. (Ed.), *High Technology Aids for the Disabled*. Butterworth, pp. 56–63 (ISBN 0-407-00256-1).
Gill, J.M., 1985. *International Guide to Aids and Services for the Deaf–Blind*. Research Unit for the Blind (ISBN 0-902215-63-9).
Gill, J.M., Silver, J., Sharville, C., Slater, J., Martin, M., 1998. Design of a typeface for digital television. In: Placencia Porrero, I., Ballabio, E. (Eds), *Improving the Quality of Life for the European Citizen*. IOS Press, pp. 248–252. (ISBN 90-5199-406-0. Also at http://www.stakes.fi/tidecong/632gill.html.)

Gill, J.M., 2000. *Which Button? Designing User Interfaces for People with Visual Impairments.* Royal National Institute for the Blind. ISBN 1-86048-023-3. Also at http://www.tiresias.org/controls.

Kates, L., Schein, J.D., 1980. *A Complete Guide to Communication with Deaf–Blind Persons.* National Association of the Deaf, Silver Spring, MD.

Michael, M.M., 1990. Making the difference for deaf–blind travelers in mass transit. In: Uslan, M.M. (Ed.), *Access to mass transit for Blind and Visually Impaired Travelers.* American Foundation for the Blind, New York, pp. 136–151.

Ouellete, S. (undated). Deaf–blind population estimates. In: Watson, D., et al. (Eds.), *A Model Service Delivery System for Deaf–Blind Persons.* University of Arkansas Rehabilitation Research and Training Centre on Deafness/Hearing Impairment.

Reed C.M., Durlach, N.I., Braida, L.D., 1982. *Research on Tactile Communication of Speech: A Review.* American Speech and Hearing Association Monograph, No. 29.

Schein, J.D., Schiff, W., 1973. A field evaluation of devices for maintaining contact with mobile deaf and deaf–blind children: electronic communication with deaf and deaf–blind persons. Deafness Research and Training Center, New York University School of Education, New York.

Shipley, A.D.C., Gill, J.M., 2000. *Call Barred? Inclusive Design of Wireless Systems.* PhoneAbility. (ISBN 1-86048-024-1. Also at http://www.tiresias.org/phoneability/wireless.htm.)

Technical Papers

Bliss, J.C., Moore, M.W., 1974. The Optacon reading system. *Education of the Visually Handicapped* 6 (4), 98–102.

Bliss, J.C., Moore, M.W., 1975. The Optacon reading system. *Education of the Visually Handicapped* 7 (1), 15–21.

Franklin, B., 1988. Effects of tactile aids on communication skills of deaf–blind children. *International Newsletter for the Deaf–Blind* 5 (2), 21–24.

Fukishima, S., 1993. View ahead: the technology for deaf–blind individuals. In: *Proceedings 10th TRON Project International Symposium,* Tokyo, Japan, pp. 169–172.

Gill, J.M., 1975. Auditory and tactual displays for sensory aids for the visually impaired. *Research Bulletin of the American Foundation for the Blind* (29), 187–196.

Gill, J.M., 1982. Telephone-linked communication aids for the deaf–blind. *Inter-Regional Review* (71), 4–8.

Goldstein, D., 1993. Technology for deaf–blind people. *Technology Update* (August), 1–10.

Grigson, P., Lofmark, N., Giblin, R., 1991. Hand-tapper III: a prototype communication device using fingerspelling. *British Journal of Visual Impairment* 9 (1), 13–15.

Harkins, J.E., Korres, E. Jensema, C.J., 1993. Final report – a robotic fingerspelling for communication and access to text for deaf–blind people, Gallaudet University.

Hinton, D.E., 1989. Research and technological aids for people who are deaf–blind. *American Rehabilitation* 15, 7–10.

Jaffe, D.L., Schwandt, D.F., Anderson, J.H., 1996. Ralph fingerspelling hand. 1996 University of Stanford Rehabilitation R&D Center Progress Report.

Kruger, F.M., 1976. Technology and the deaf–blind: electronic devices expand the horizons of the deaf–blind. *Computer Decisions* 8 (10), 46–48.

Moore, M.W., Bliss, J.C., 1975. The Optacon reading system. *Education of the Visually Handicapped* 7 (2), 33–39.

Reed, C.M., ca 1982. The implications of the Tadoma method of speechreading for spoken language processing. American Speech and Hearing Association. www.asel.udel.edu/icslp/cdrom/vol3/1002/a1002.pdf.

Reed C.M., Delhorne, L.A., Durlach, N.I., Fisher, S.D., 1990. A study of the tactual and visual reception of fingerspelling. *Journal of Speech and Hearing Research* 33, 786–787.

Smithdas, R.J., 1994. Technology and deaf–blind populations. *See Hear!* 12, 12–16.

Szeto, A.Y.J., Christiansen, K.M., 1988. Technological devices for deaf–blind children: needs and potential impact. *IEEE Engineering Medicine and Biology* 7 (3), 25–29.

Zuckerman, D., 1984. Use of personal computing technology by deaf–blind individuals. In: *Proceedings of the 17th Hawaii International Conference on Systems Science,* Honolulu, HI, pp. 420–423.

Zumalt, L.E., Silver, S., Kramer, L.C., 1972. Evaluation of a communication device for deaf–blind persons. *New Outlook for the Blind* 66 (1), 20–25.

Web Sites

Information and Devices for Braille and Moon
http://www.rnib.org.uk/braille/welcome.htm
http://www.rnib.org.uk/wesupply/fctsheet/moon.htm
http://www.utoronto.ca/atrc/reference/tech/refbraille.html
http://www.freedomscientific.com/

Both Braille and Moon TrueType fonts can be downloaded from the RNIB Web site at http://www.rnib.org.uk/wesupply/archive/welcome.htm. These fonts can be used on any PC with any version of Windows, but there is no version for Macintosh.

Information about Deafblindness
http://www.deafblind.co.uk
http://www.deafblindscotland.org.uk
http://www.deafblinduk.org.uk
http://www.deafblind.com
http://www.sense.org.uk/

Equipment and Software for Deafblind People
http://www.deafblind.com/dbequipm.html
http://www.swhsoftware.demon.co.uk/
http://www.tiresias.org/equipment/eb21.htm
http://www.freedomscientific.com/
http://www.blazie.co.uk
http://www.deafblind.co.uk/equipment.html
http://www.duxburysystems.com/resources/

9 The Final Product: Issues in the Design and Distribution of Assistive Technology Devices

9.1 Development and Distribution of Devices

Developing assistive technologies and devices is, in itself, insufficient. To be of benefit, devices have to be produced in sufficient numbers and to reach end users. In some cases, the end users will also require training in the use of the devices to get the most benefit from them. In order to move from the prototype stage to a device in the hands of end users the following are required:

- sufficient funding to cover the costs of further developments of the prototype, end-user tests and initial marketing or distribution;
- a distribution network;
- a support system for users, including training, information, advice and repair facilities.

However, these three aspects are, in many ways, interrelated. The distribution network and support system (if any) may be provided at a common location or by the same organisation and the type of distribution, including the costs (if any) to the users are at least partly determined by financial questions. The focus in this section is on assistive technology devices for deaf and deafblind people, but much of the discussion is also valid for other groups of end users of assistive technology.

The initial research and development of assistive technology products may take place in industry or in research institutes and universities, sometimes in the context of student projects. The nature of the final product and the relatively small markets mean that developments initiated through student projects are more important than is generally the case. This has both advantages and disadvantages. The advantages include the following:

- the development of ideas and products, such as many assistive technology devices, that are not immediately or obviously commercial;
- the ability to draw on a wide range of talent and investigate unorthodox or unproven ideas;
- making students more aware of the issues involved in designing assistive technology.

However, there are disadvantages. In particular, there is no direct link to industry or an organisation that is able to produce and distribute the product. Consequently, although a very large number of potentially useful assistive technology devices are developed in universities, only a very small proportion of them actually reach end users. Industry and universities operate in very different ways. Although many universities and research institutes are becoming more commercial, there is still a culture, or at least an ideal, of sharing knowledge and ideas. This runs counter to industrial practice, which is largely governed by the needs of commercial confidentiality. Many firms will only agree to develop a product that can be patented or protected, and this usually precludes publishing the results. Even if results have not been published in journals or at conferences, there may still be problems when devices have been developed by a succession of students. It will generally be assumed that they have discussed their work with other students and colleagues, even when this is not in fact the case. This particular problem can be avoided by students signing non-disclosure agreements before they start work on a particular project, but this runs contrary to much of academic practice and may not be considered favourably by either academic supervisors or the students themselves.

However, the development of devices in industry also has disadvantages. The market is relatively small, and many deaf people have low incomes. Therefore, research and development of assistive technology devices may not seem a commercially viable proposition. There are, therefore, only a relatively small number of firms that produce assistive technology devices for deaf and hearing-impaired people. Some of these firms specialise in assistive devices, whereas for others it is only one component, and possibly even a relatively minor one, of their wider operations. For instance, infrared assistive listening devices are generally manufactured by firms that specialise in the production of infrared conference equipment.

There are particular problems in developing and marketing assistive devices and products for deafblind people. The number of deafblind people is considerably less than the number of either deaf or blind people. In addition, the way in which the field has developed has led to a focus on issues and technology for people with single rather than multiple impairments. Thus, assistive devices for deafblind people form a small, highly specialised niche market to an even greater extent than devices for deaf and blind people. However, assistive technology is one area where the development of global and Internet markets could have social benefits, since the numbers of people requiring particular assistive devices world-wide are much larger than the numbers in any given country, making the production of assistive devices on a commercial basis more viable.

Manufacturers of assistive technology devices do not necessarily act as their distributors, and assistive devices will frequently be available only, or mainly, from specialised outlets for products for deaf and hearing-impaired people. For instance, in the UK many products are supplied on commercial terms by the RNID shop, and it is also possible to obtain products free of charge from centres run by social work departments. A smaller number of products, such as telephones with amplification and large buttons, are available from standard outlets. However, these products are generally better categorised as design for all rather than assistive devices.

Currently, assistive devices are produced and distributed by charities, non-governmental organisations, private firms, hospitals, social work departments and private and public clinics. The charge levied on the user varies according to the source. In some cases the users are required to pay the full market price, whereas in other cases the devices are cost free to some or all users or the devices may be supplied with a partial subsidy. The balance between different sources of assistive devices varies in different countries. Thus, access to assistive devices, and whether and how much individuals are required to pay for them, may depend largely on where they live, with some countries and areas of particular countries having considerably better provision than others. Access to assistive devices is generally poorer in rural than in urban areas.

There could be a number of advantages in taking up a US suggestion, which has not (yet) been implemented, of setting up local or regional assistive technology resource centres. Such centres should preferably be funded by taxation and provide services and devices free of charge to users. They would be staffed by personnel across the full range of disciplines of relevance to the development of assistive technology, including engineers, social workers and medical personnel.

In their function of distributors of assistive technology products and devices, these centres would be able to support users in evaluating their assistive technology needs and to provide information and advice on the currently available devices that best meet their needs. The engineering and other technical personnel would be able to tailor devices developed for the general user to meet the needs of specific users or user groups. Training in the use of the device, advice and support would be available to ensure that all users gained the maximum benefit.

Centres of this type would also be able to host assistive device user-support or self-help groups, so that end users would be able to exchange information and learn from each other. In some cases it might be the end-user groups that brought the availability of new devices to the attention of centre staff and other (potential) end users. The centres could also provide resources and other support for consultative fora to investigate where there are gaps in existing provision, so that new devices are required, or where modifications of existing devices would be better able to meet users' needs. Mobile facilities linked to the centres would be required to support, for instance, deaf and hearing-impaired people living in rural areas and deaf people with other disabilities who might find public transport inaccessible or who experience fatigue or other difficulties when travelling.

Although there would probably be considerable up-front costs in setting up centres of this type, they would be offset many times by both the social and economic benefits with regards to improving quality of life and the ability to live and work independently. Even in purely financial terms there is likely to be a net gain, as the increased availability of assistive technology that is suited to the specific user, as well as training in its use, would enable more deaf and deafblind people to obtain better paid and more satisfying employment.

9.2 Working with End Users

Much of assistive technology *research* is about the design of new products, processes and devices for disabled people. Carrying out the design process effectively requires the involvement of end users. In particular, only (potential) users of a particular product, process, device or service:

- know their particular requirements.
- can test what does and does not work in practice.
- can accept or reject devices, products, processes and services.
- determine whether a product, process, device or service is acceptable from all points of view, as users may reject them on grounds other than functionality.

To be most effective, user involvement should occur from the start of the research, design or development process, as this is when decisions are made. Changes introduced at a later stage may be both considerably less effective and more expensive. However, many scientists and engineers find it difficult to work with end users and, therefore, either do not involve them at all or only do so at the final stage of testing a finished product. Though better than nothing, this is often much too late.

There are three main possibilities for bringing end users into the research, design and development process:

- Participation in which end users (generally representing particular organisations) are involved in the decision-making processes and are considered part of (one of) the research team(s).
- Consultation in which advice is sought from end users at different stages, including testing prototypes and finished devices.
- Involvement of end users as research "subjects".

The same or different (groups of) end users may be involved in all three roles.

9.2.1 Methods for Involving End Users

A range of different methods has been developed for consultation and involving end users and others in decision making. In principle, most of these methods are equally applicable to deaf, hearing or hearing-impaired people. It is relatively easy to adapt techniques such as brainstorming (which is a method for generating ideas by people shouting them out) to groups of deaf people who sign. However, particular care is required when a group consists of people who communicate in different ways (for instance by using sign language, deafblind manual language, oral speech and oral speech with lip-reading) to ensure that everyone is able to participate equally and that all contributions are taken note of and equally valued.

9.2.2 FORTUNE Concept of User Participation in Projects

End-user participation in research and development projects has itself been the subject of research. For instance, the FORTUNE (www.fortune-net.org) research project has developed a concept of user participation based on the following seven principles:

1. Partnership as a basis.
2. Users as members and/or representatives of organisations.
3. Users should receive payment on the same basis as other participants.
4. Guaranteed accessibility of all relevant materials and premises.
5. All partners guarantee confidentiality, respect and expertise.
6. Detailed project plan, including time and resource planning for user participation.
7. Partnership is implemented from the start of the project.

Involving users as partners gives them a role in decision making and can help to ensure they are treated with respect. It is also a way of recognising the importance of end-user involvement. The involvement of end users as members and representatives of organisations means that they can obtain support and feedback from the organisation and present a wider range of perspectives. It also needs to be recognised that individuals with a particular disability are not identical. They have a wide range of different characteristics and needs and may be affected by the same disability in different ways.

Providing payment on an equal basis is another way to ensure equality with other participants. It also provides recognition of the importance of end-user involvement and the fact that it is more than a volunteering activity. Planning for user involvement is necessary to ensure it is effective and that resources are available. As discussed already, end-user involvement from the start of the project is likely to be more effective than bringing it in at a later stage.

9.3 Communication Issues

The participation or other involvement of (lay) deaf and hearing-impaired people in research projects involves two types of communication issue:

- the use of jargon, scientific and engineering terms;
- different ways or styles of communicating or the use of different languages.

The first issue is relevant to the cooperation of all mixed groups, involving engineering and scientific "experts" and the lay population, whether or not they include deaf people. Training and resource materials may be required on both sides. For instance, a glossary of technical terms, explained using non-technical language, could be useful. The scientific and engineering participants also need to be careful not to use technical language where non-technical terms could be used. They should also learn to communicate in appropriate ways with people without a technical education.

The second issue is specific to the participation of people with disabilities. For instance, the group may involve:

- deaf people who use sign language;
- people with unclear speech;
- people with hearing impairments who lip-read;
- deafblind people who use the deafblind manual language and require text materials to be provided in Braille.

These issues are part of the wider context of accessibility. It will often be necessary to:

- provide interpreters – this will include sign language interpreters, deafblind manual language interpreters and interpreters for people with unclear speech;
- provide text materials in differing formats;
- provide infrared listening devices or an induction loop;
- provide highly skilled typists to input a text version of oral communications to allow access through Braille or projection onto a screen;
- ensure all participants are seated appropriately and there is adequate lighting, to allow them to lip-read or see interpreters;
- provide note-takers for deaf participants who use sign language or lip-read.

It should be the responsibility of all participants, particularly the hearing participants, to ensure that the communication needs of deaf and hearing-impaired participants are met. To ensure this, communication needs should be discussed in advance of any meetings.

Sufficient time should be allowed for interpretation. Therefore, a longer time period may be required for meetings and interviews, and this should be allowed for in planning. It is also important to clarify the way in which technical and other special terms are being communicated by interpreters or translated into Braille, to prevent misunderstandings or differing interpretations.

9.4 Other Important Issues

9.4.1 Deaf Culture and Deaf Awareness

In the context of assistive technology for deaf and hearing-impaired people, end users include:

- older people, who have age-related hearing loss;
- people born deaf or with a hearing loss;
- people who have acquired a hearing loss through accident or illness.

All these groups can include people with other disabilities in addition to a hearing loss.

Many people born deaf identify as part of the Deaf Community. They use sign language (British sign language or BSL in the UK) rather than oral speech, and they have a vibrant culture based on sign language. One of their main concerns is for the recognition of sign language and Deaf culture. They require alarm devices that alert them by visual and tactile signals and telephony devices that allow them to communicate through sign language or text.

The situation for people who are hearing impaired (not totally deaf) or experience hearing loss later in life is often different. They generally do not know sign language and require devices that will enhance any residual hearing, or assist them to behave as though they have no hearing loss. They frequently want these devices either to be inconspicuous or to have an application to hearing people, so that it is not obvious they have a hearing loss. However, this distinction between the attitudes of people who were born deaf and those who are hearing impaired cannot automatically be assumed.

9.4.2 Ethical Issues

Like other types of technological research, research and development in the area of assistive technology raises ethical issues; these can be divided into two categories:

- research aims and applications;
- conduct of research and presentation of results.

Unlike in many other areas of research, in the development of assistive technology devices, the second category generally presents more problems than the first one. Therefore, the discussion here will focus on the second category. The development of assistive technology may involve work with human "subjects" and will require awareness of the following:

- ethical research policies of the university or organisation at which the research is based;
- national and international legislation and regulations;
- national and international standards.

Working with human subjects raises the following issues (amongst others):

- honest communication
- confidentiality
- safety and risk.

Honest communication includes information on:

- The main aims of the research or other activity.
- The desired involvement of the individual or group of deaf or hearing-impaired people and how long this is likely to take.
- The availability of payment or expenses for participation. There are also issues as to the ethics of organising user participation without payment.
- What training, if any, will be provided.
- Expected outcomes and how likely they are to occur, *e.g.* whether they are fairly definite or only probable and whether a percentage can be given to the probability. Information on outcomes should include likely benefits and whether these are general, *e.g.* advancement of knowledge or more specific, *e.g.* for a particular group of deaf people. There should also be an indication of the time span over which benefits are likely to occur and whether they are likely to occur in time to affect the specific individual or group of people with disabilities participating in the research.
- The status of any information supplied and, in particular, whether it is confidential and/or anonymous.

As generally interpreted, confidentiality and anonymity of information do not prevent the resulting statistical data being openly published; as long as informants are informed of this when data are collected. Therefore, if confidential and anonymous data are collected on, for instance, the usage of assistive listening devices by deaf people, the percentages of deaf people using particular devices or types of device can be openly published.

Ethical considerations about risk imply that:

- One group of individuals should not be exposed to risk and another group to which they do not belong receive the benefits.
- Individuals or groups of people should not be exposed to risk without their informed consent. This informed consent must involve a full understanding of the situation, the extent of the risk and the likely benefits to themselves and/or others.
- There should be some correlation between the nature and extent of risk and benefit, *e.g.* people should not be exposed to serious risk for minimal benefits.
- Alternative approaches that avoid risks should be used wherever possible. Saving money by using less expensive techniques is not a valid reason for exposing people to risks.

9.4.3 Data Protection Legislation

Many countries have legislation about data collected from individuals, and this is likely to affect assistive technology researchers. As a typical example, the UK Data Protection Act 1998 (http://www.dataprotection.gov.uk/) requires anyone processing personal data to comply with the following eight principles of good practice, which state that data must be:

- fairly and lawfully processed
- processed for limited purposes
- adequate, relevant and not excessive
- accurate
- not kept longer than necessary
- processed in accordance with the data subject's rights
- secure
- not transferred to countries without adequate protection.

Assistive technology researchers are required to register under this Act if, for instance:

- they collect and record data on living individuals;
- data collection is for research purposes;
- the individuals can be identified from the data or the data and other information in the possession of the researcher(s).

Acknowledgements

The editors would like to thank Roddy Sutherland (Stowe College, Glasgow) for some of the information on commercialisation of products and devices.

References and Further Reading

 Further Reading

Books

Bowling, A., 1997. *Research Methods in Health*. Open University Press (ISBN 0-355-19885-6).
Bryman A. 2001. *Social Research Methods*. Oxford University Press (ISBN 0-19-874204-5).
Bühler, Ch., 2000. *FORTUNE Guide – Empowered Participation of Users with Disabilities in Projects*. Evangelische Stiftung Volmarstein, FTB.
Cook, A.M., Hussey, S.M., 1995. *Assistive Technologies: Principles and Practice*. Mosby Inc. (ISBN 0-8016-1038-9).
Martin, M.W., Schinzinger, R., 1996. *Ethics in Engineering*, 3rd edition. McGraw-Hill International Editions (ISBN 0-07-114195-2).

Web Sites

The online ethics centre for science and engineering research design explained can be found at http://onlineethics.org/.

Biographies of the Contributors (in Alphabetical Order of Family Name)

Conny Andersson

Conny Arrhenius Andersson was born in Sweden. After an education in electronic design in Sweden, he was responsible for the Research and Development department at the Swedish County Council company from 1975 to 1992. One of the largest projects, apart from electronic designs of audio-related products, was an automatic quality production test system for hearing aids, where every single hearing aid was automatically tested (55,000 units yearly) regarding vital basic acoustic parameters and statistical evaluation. This gave totally new knowledge of the quality variation for different hearing-aid brands and valuable statistical information.

During a 10 year period, he was also active as an expert at the Karolinska Institutet in Sweden on determining what hearing aids should be represented in the Swedish market. From 1990 to 1994 he was active as a teacher for hearing aids and assistive devices (technology and algorithms) at the University of Stockholm, Karolinska Institutet.

In 1993 he joined the company Bo Edin AB as a manager of the R&D department, where his main interest was in constant-current amplifiers for wireless audio information to hearing aids and algorithms for constant levels of speech in microphones. This is now called Dual Action AGC with variable attack and decay times. Bo Edin specialises in the development and manufacture of audio induction-loop systems technology. They have a wide international market and sell approximately 11,000 loop systems yearly. His work as the Convener for the new IEC standard for inductive loops began in 2000 and has already involved a change of the standard by including a measurement procedure using artificial speech.

During the period from 1977 he has given many talks and lectures in Europe. For example, in the UK, presentations were given at Heathrow (1977), London (1980) and Bristol University (1999) and three talks were given in 2002. He gave a Tutorial Workshop on induction-loop technology at the European Union sponsored Conference on Vision and Hearing Impaired Assistive Technology (CVHI, 2001) in Pisa, Italy.

When he is not travelling, Conny Andersson enjoys his family activities and is interested in world cinema, but, wherever he is, he finds time to enjoy distance running to relax and find inspiration.

Douglas Campbell, BSc, PhD, CEng, FIEE, CPhys, FInstP, FRSA, MILT

Douglas R Campbell was born in Glasgow, Scotland, in October 1947. He was educated at Lenzie Academy and while working as a technician with Barr and Stroud Limited, ICL and The University of Strathclyde he obtained an ONC and HNC by part-time study. He entered the University of Strathclyde as a student in 1969 and was awarded a BSc Hons (1st Class) in Electrical and Electronic Engineering in 1972, and a PhD in 1976 for research work in the field of identification techniques applied to distributed parameter systems. He was a lecturer at Paisley College of Technology (now The University of Paisley) during 1976. From 1977 to 1980 he worked on motion simulation aspects of aircraft flight simulation, leaving from the position of Principal Research Engineer with Rediffusion Simulation Ltd to join the Department of Electrical and Electronic Engineering at the University of Paisley as a lecturer. He was promoted to Senior Lecturer in 1984, designated Reader in 1991, and appointed to a Personal Chair in 1996. Professor Campbell is a Fellow of the Institution of Electrical Engineers, a Fellow of the Institute of Physics, a Fellow of the Royal Society for the encouragement of Arts, Manufacture and Commerce, and a Member of the Institute for Learning and Teaching in Higher Education.

His current research interests are in the field of speech signal-processing algorithms, systems and devices and are conducted within the Applied Computational Intelligence Research Unit in the School of Information and Communication Technologies at the University of Paisley. Recent awards to support research into speech enhancement and digital signal processing for hearing aids have come from the UK EPSRC, The Scottish Office Department of Health, Motorola Ltd, Defeating Deafness (The Hearing Research Trust) and The Leverhulme Trust.

His leisure interests include hill-walking, windsurfing, swimming, badminton, music and the visual arts.

Alistair Farquharson, MSc

Alistair Farquharson joined BT in 1984 after graduating from Edinburgh University. He has many years of experience working with communication protocols and analogue modems, particularly those related to Group 3 fax machines. Over the past few years he has been developing the International Telecommunications Union V.18 recommendation for text telephones and was editor of the recommendation. He is now working with broadband technologies and has a keen interest in bringing textphones into the multimedia age.

Stephen Furner, BA, IEng, MIIE, CPsychol

As a consultant in Human Factors for BT, Stephen Furner has applied advanced usability engineering techniques to the research, design and development of BT products and services. He has led multinational teams of technical experts researching convergent technologies, and has managed national and international R&D projects for BT. Stephen regularly reports the results of the research he carries out for BT at professional conferences, in technical journals and through the technical press and public media. His current research interests include computer haptics, social uses of computing and communications, and self-positioning mobile data services. Stephen is both a Chartered Psychologist and an Incorporated Engineer. He originally joined BT as a trainee telecommunications technician in London, working on the development of the UK Telex network. After qualifying in engineering, Stephen went on to study social science and moved into the area of human interaction with advanced communications and computing technology at the BT Laboratories.

John Gill, OBE, PhD, CEng, FIEE

John Gill is Chief Scientist at the Royal National Institute of the Blind; he was previously a senior research fellow at Warwick and Brunel universities. He is a chartered engineer and a Fellow of the Institution of Electrical Engineers. He has published over 200 papers on technology and disability, and he has visited 40 countries in connection with this work. His current research interests are coding of user preferences on smart cards, design of fonts, and accessibility of information and communication technology systems.

Marion Hersh, BA, MSc, PhD, MIMA, CMath, MIEE, CEng, MIEEE

Dr Hersh is currently a Lecturer in the Department of Electronics and Electrical Engineering, University of Glasgow. She previously held an appointment as a Post-doctoral Research Fellow (1982–1985) at University of Sussex.

Her current research interests fall into three main areas:

- assistive technology for deaf, blind and deafblind people;
- the application of fuzzy and soft computing techniques to sustainable design and decision making;
- ethics and social responsibility issues in science and engineering.

She has run the successful conference series entitled "Vision and Hearing Impairment: Rehabilitation Engineering and Support Technologies for Independent Living" with funding from the EC High-Level Scientific Conferences Programme jointly with Professor M. Johnson of the University of Strathclyde. Current research projects in the area of assistive technology include the development of principles of sustainable and accessible design, open and distance learning for people with mobility impairments with colleagues from Germany, Hungary and Romania and intelligent audiometry with her research student Roddy Sutherland.

As well as research, Dr Hersh also has well-developed teaching activities in the area of assistive technology, including an undergraduate module written together with Professor M.A. Johnson. She also regularly supervises undergraduate projects in assistive technology and is looking to market or otherwise distribute an alarm clock for deafblind people developed through these projects.

Other recent research projects have included the Application of Fuzzy Methods and Other Soft Computing Techniques to Sustainable Design and Decision Making in collaboration with Dr I. Hamburg, Institut Arbeit und Technik, Wissenschaftszentrum Nordrhein Westfalen, Germany, and Mr L. Padeanau of the University of Craiova, Romania. Dr Hersh is currently finalising a book on Computational Mathematics for Sustainable Development, co-authored with Dr Hamburg and also to be published by Springer Verlag. Dr Hersh is a Member of the Institute of Mathematics and its Applications, the Institution of Electrical Engineers (UK) and the Institute of Electronic and Electrical Engineers (USA).

Alan Jackson, BSc, MIEE

Alan Jackson graduated from UMIST in 1983 with a BSc (Hons) in Electronics. Alan joined BT Laboratories in October 1983 working on advanced telephone terminals involving analogue transmission design and microcomputer control for the residential market. The work evolved into specialist terminal design for users with disabilities, *e.g.* Claudivs II (talking keypad), ADC home-phone to suit visual and dexterity needs, ADC payphone, text terminal and customised standard products.

Alan is currently an Internet Designer with BTexact Technologies (formerly BT Labs) working on solution design for business applications.

Michael A. Johnson, BSc, DIC, MSc, PhD, FIMA, CMath, MIEEE

Professor Johnson's academic career has concentrated on control engineering, theory and applications. He has significant industrial control applications and research experience. He is the author and co-author of books and papers on power generation, wastewater control, power transmission, and control benchmarking. Previous European Union project experience includes the ESPRIT Projects MARIE and IMPROVE. Currently, he is team leader for Strathclyde in a THERMIE Project to implement the results of the IMPROVE project in real Italian and Spanish national applications. He has had a number of student projects in the area of assistive technology and has successfully trained over 35 engineers to PhD level in last 15 years. He is Series Editor to Springer-Verlag-London monograph series Advances in Industrial Control and to the new Springer-Verlag-London Advanced Textbooks in Control and Signal Processing. AUTOMATICA Associate Editor (1985–2002).

His interest in assistive technology came through teaching commitments, which included student group study dissertations at second-year level and assorted project supervision at Masters and undergraduate levels. These were used to explore some electrical and electronic engineering aspects of assistive devices for the hearing impaired. Subsequent collaboration with Dr Hersh at the University of Glasgow has led to a set of targeted activities in this area. These include a new course module, a new conference series and some research projects in the area.

Professor Johnson is a member of Deafblind UK, and the British Retinitis Pigmentosa Society.

Jay Lucker, BA, MA, EdD, CCC-A/SLP, FAAA

Jay R. Lucker is an audiologist and speech–language pathologist who has had a varied professional career. Living his entire life in the USA, he was educated at the City University of New York: Hunter/Lehman College for his undergraduate degree and Hunter College for his graduate work. He completed his postgraduate work at Columbia University in New York, where he earned a Doctorate of Education in audiology and auditory perception focusing his work on how children with auditory difficulties perceive speech and make sense out of what they hear.

Jay has had a varied career, working in school systems, hospital and clinic settings, private practice, and higher education. He was an Associate Professor in the Department of Speech, Communication Sciences, and Theatre at St John's University, in Jamaica, NY, Professional Associate/Professor in the Department of Communication Disorders at Mercy College, Dobbs Ferry, NY, and Associate Professor in the Department of Audiology and Speech–Language Pathology at Gallaudet University, Washington, DC. He is currently in private practice, again, specialising in auditory processing.

His research and clinical work have focused upon how we perceive speech and understand what we perceive. His work has also focused on counselling families who have members with auditory disorders. Although his work in both auditory perception and counselling has been with all age groups, most of his focus has been with children. He has lectured internationally and continues to make presentations on a variety of topics related to auditory processing and counselling. His publications are varied, but focus on aspects of processing and counselling primarily with children.

Jay holds dual certification and licenses in three states (in the USA) as an audiologist and speech–language pathologist. He also holds certification as a special education teacher of the speech and hearing handicapped. He is a Fellow of the American Academy of Audiology. Jay is active in many professional associations, holding positions as Vice-President, Co-Founder and Member of the Board of the National Coalition on Auditory Processing (NCAPD), Washington/Baltimore area coordinator of the Children's Mentoring Program of the Alexander Graham Bell Association of the Deaf, Program Chair for the District of Columbia Speech–Language–Hearing Association, and member of the American Speech–Language–Hearing Association and American Academy of Audiology as well as the Speech–Language–Hearing Associations of the states of Maryland and Virginia.

Keith Nolde

Keith Nolde joined BT in 1977 working in the Circuit Laboratory in London. In 1980 he was sponsored by BT to study for a Mathematics with Electronics degree at Southampton University. After graduating, he joined Regulatory

Standards and was responsible for equipment approvals. In 1984 he transferred to BT's laboratories at Adastral Park to join the telephone design team. Several years later he became involved with open software standards for communications (OSI) and this is where his interest in UNIX (and later LINUX) began. More recently, he returned to terminals development and lately has been involved in ADSL modem evaluation and customer support for BTopenworld.

Erhard Werner, MSc, PhD

Dr Werner has concentrated most of his engineering activities on electroacoustic devices, including the wireless transmission of audio signals. In a career spanning over 24 years in responsible R&D positions with a leading German manufacturer, he began a very early involvement with assistive technologies dating from the 1970s. This involvement started with cabled devices using fixed microphone installations and individual hearing aids in schools for disabled children. He went on to be involved in the evolution of radio frequency use for wireless hearing aids and the development of several other solutions using infrared light as the information carrier. This work included cooperation with academic institutions and links to international societies for wider applications other than those of just audio applications. During his industrial career, Dr Werner contributed to many projects in national and international standards organisations, *e.g.* IEC, ETSI, CENELEC and DKE.

Although he is now retired, he is still involved in several projects of these national and international standards organisations. His membership in societies like ASA, AES, VDE and DEGA also continues to lead to further work in his field of interest, leading to many contributions in technical journals, and books and presentations at conferences and conventions.

Mike Whybray, BSc, MSc, CEng, MIEE

Mike Whybray received an Honours degree (1st Class) in Electrical and Electronic Engineering from the University of Birmingham in 1977, joining BT Research Laboratories to work on reliability physics – studying water vapour contamination in semiconductor packages, failure modes of magnetic bubble memories, and CMOS latchup problems. In 1983 he gained an MSc in Telecommunications Systems at the University of Essex, and moved to the Visual Telecommunications Division of BTRL, where he led a group whose activities included developing videophones for deaf people, writing software for DSP-based videophones, and building demonstrators of advanced image-processing applications, such as intelligent surveillance and synthetic "talking head" displays. He currently leads the Advanced Video Services team at BTexact Technologies, developing systems for control of videoconferences, and new mobile and IP audio/video streaming systems. In his spare time he enjoys learning to play the cello, astronomy, reading and skiing.

Index

The starting page numbers for a **major section** for a keyword entry are shown in **bold numerals**.

A

accessibility design, telephones   192
acoustic feedback *see* electronic aids
acoustic immittance devices, calibration of   **65**
acoustic reflex threshold *see* immittance audiometry
acoustics of hearing   4, **73**
  amplitude   5, **6**, 8, 9, 10
  complex sounds   9, **10**, 12, 150
  decibel scale   **8**, 43
  filtering   4
  frequency   5, **8**, 9
  period   **8**
  phase   5, **7**
  simple sounds   **9**
  sound intensity   **8**, 38
  spectral analysis   4, **10**
actuators
  bells   **246**
  buzzers   **246**
  comparison, trigger units   252
  electro-tactile devices   **250**
  light emitting diodes (LEDs)   **248**
  lights   **247**
  television   **248**
  vibro-tactile devices   **249**
adaptive noise cancellation *see* electronic aids
aid-on-body considerations   **88**
alarm systems
  fire alarm   221, 251
  intruder detector   **225**
  smoke alarm   221
  suppliers   **255**
  see also actuators; alerting systems; amplifiers; sensors; transmission systems
alerting systems
  applications   **215**
  design issues   **216**
  design-for-all   217, 218
  design-modification approach   217, 218
  design-specialised   217, 218
  general components   **216**
  paging systems   **250**
  signal conditioning   **229**
  suppliers   **255**
  trigger units   252
  see also actuators; alarm systems; amplifiers; deafblind AT; sensors; transmission systems
amplifiers
  power   44, **230**
    Class AB   **237**
    Class C   **235**
  transistors   **231**
  tuned   **234**
  voltage   44, 230, **233**
amplitude   5, **6**, 8, 9, 10
  see also transmission systems
amplitude compression *see* electronic aids
amplitude modulation
  general concept   241
  infrared systems   155
analogue aid *see* electronic aids
anatomy
  central auditory nervous system   3, **27**
  of inner ear   **23**
  of middle ear structures   **18**, 27
  of outer ear structures   **15**
  see also ear anatomy

anti-phase loops *see* induction loop systems
artificial ears *see* audiometry
assistive technology devices
  design issues   297
  distribution issues   297
audio frequency systems *see* induction loop systems
audiograms *see* pure tone audiometry
audiology   41, 46
  see also audiometry
audiometry   45
  artificial ears   65
  audiometric equipment calibration   62
  audiometric equipment design   62
  bone vibrators, calibration of   65
  coupler
    2cc   66
    calibration of   64
    zwislocki   67
  earphone calibration   63
  kemar   67
  sound level meters, calibration of   64
  standards   61
  test decision process   46
  see also brain stem response audiometry; electric response audiometry; electrocochleography; immittance audiometry; measurement systems; pure tone audiometry
auditory (eighth) nerve problems   30, 33
auditory brainstem implant *see* hearing aid
auditory system   2, 3, 10, 14, 29, 33, 36, 41, 47, 56, 59, 79
  treatment of problems in   36
automated fingerspelling
  comparison of systems   273
  Dexter devices   267, 268
  Gallaudet device   268
  general issues   266
  glove systems   272
  handtapper device   271
  RALPH device   270
  talking hands   272
automatic gain control (AGC) *see* induction loop systems

B
behind the ear (BTE) aid *see* electronic aids
bells   246

blinddeaf *see* deafblindness
block alphabet   259
Bluetooth *see* deafblind AT
BOBBY (web) guidelines *see* deafblind AT
body worn (BW) aid *see* electronic aids
body-on-aid considerations   90
bone conduction aid *see* electronic aids
bone vibrators see audiometry
Braille   259, 260
Braille devices
  braillephone   287
  displays   262
  embossers   264
  notetakers   263
  optacon   274
  optical character recognition   274
  text converters   264
  versabraille   287
brain stem response audiometry   61
buzzers   246

C
carbon monoxide sensor   223
cavity, middle ear   20, 25, 33
central auditory nervous system   3, 27
central auditory pathways problems   30, 33
cochlea   24
  hearing loss due to problems in   30, 32
  sound processing in   27
cochlear implant *see* hearing aid
communication issues for projects   301
completely in canal (CIC) aid *see* electronic aids
complex sounds   10
coupler
  2cc *see* audiometry
  calibration of *see* audiometry
  zwislocki *see* audiometry
culture, deaf community   302

D
data protection legislation   304
deaf awareness   302
deaf culture   302
deafblind AT   261
  alerting devices   279
  Bluetooth   278
  BOBBY (web) guidelines   285
  domestic alerting system   282
  IT access   284
    computers   287
  light probe   276

Index

liquid level indicator   276
optical character recognition   274
room thermometer   277
suppliers   **296**
Taciwatch   284
tactaid devices   275
tactile marking   277
tactile sound recognition   275
TAM alerting device   284
telecommunications access   289
universal communications text browser (ucon)   286
vibrating alarm clock   **280**
web guidelines   285
see also automated fingerspelling; Braille devices
deafblindness   **257**
   block alphabet   259
   categories   257
   communication   258
   demographics   257
   manual alphabet (USA, UK)   259
   Moon   260
   retinitis pigmentosa   257
   SPARTAN   259
   Tadoma   260
   Usher's syndrome   257
   websites on   296
   see also Braille
decibel scale   **8**, 43
demodulator *see* transmission systems
design for hearing impairment, telephones   **178**
design issues, alerting systems   **216**
design, final AT product issues   297
design-for-all, alerting systems   217, 218
design-modification approach, alerting systems   217, 218
design-specialised, alerting systems   217, 218
Dexter devices *see* automated fingerspelling
differential temperature sensor   222
digital aid *see* electronic aids
digital telecommunications *see* telephony
diode characteristics, infrared systems, 160, 164
directional microphones *see* electronic aids
domestic alerting system *see* deafblind AT

E

ear
   anatomical structures   14
   anatomy   14, 15, 18, 23, 76

central auditory nervous system   3, 27
cochlea   2, 3, 15, 23, **24**
   as an engineering environment   **88**
   external auditory meatus   3, **16**
   functions   **15**, **17**, **22**, 27, 76
   hearing loss due to problems in middle ear   29, **32**
   hearing loss due to problems in the outer ear   **31**
   inner ear   2, 10, 21, 22, **23**
      anatomy   **23**
      auditory (eighth) nerve problems   30, **33**
      central auditory pathways problems   30, **33**
      cochlea
         functions of   **27**
         sound processing in the cochlea   27
      vestibule   **24**
   middle ear
      anatomy   **18**
      cavity   **20**, 25, 33
      functions of   **22**, 27
      ossicles   3, 18, **19**, 33, 38, 76
   outer ear
      anatomy   **15**
      functions of   **15, 17**
   physiology   **15**, **18**, **23**, 76
   pinna   2, 15, **16**
   treatments   **36**
   tympanic membrane   3, 18, 19, 22, 29, 33, 38
   vestibule   **24**
electric response audiometry   **59**
electrocochleography   **60**
electromagnetic principles *see* induction loop systems
electromagnetic radiation *see* infrared systems
electronic aids
   acoustic feedback   **101**
   adaptive noise cancellation   **104**
   aid-on-body considerations   **88**
   amplitude compression   **92,** 111
   analogue   **80, 87, 106**
   behind the ear (BTE)   80, **81**
   body worn (BW)   80, **81**
   body-on-aid considerations   **88**
   bone conduction   **84**
   categories   **80**
   completely in canal (CIC)   80, **83**
   digital   80, 87, 94, **106**, 112
   directional microphones   **97**

equalisation 91
frequency transposition 102, 111
history 87
in the ear (ITE) 80, 83
microphone arrays 102
radio based concepts 110, 112
signal processing strategies 91
sinusoidal modelling 98, 111
spectacles aid 80, 83
spectral contrast enhancement 95
spectral subtraction 98
unwanted signal reduction 96
voice activity detection 99
electro-tactile devices 250
embossers *see* braille devices
end-users
  communication issues 301
  data protection legislation 304
  ethics 303
  FORTUNE concept 300
  methods for inclusion 300
  working with 299
equalisation *see* electronic aids
errors
  environmental sources of 45
  physiological sources of 45
  types of 44
ethics 303
external auditory meatus 3, 16

F
filter
  band pass 10, 14, 60, 63, 111, 167
  high pass 14, 18, 111
  low pass 14, 55, 80, 111, 244
fire alarm sensors 221
fire alarm *see* alarm systems
fixed temperature sensor 221
FORTUNE concept 300
frequency 5, 8, 9
frequency response curves 10, 11, 43
  loop systems 148
frequency *see* transmission systems

G
gain
  in decibels 12, 43, 73
  system 11, 43, 73
Gallaudet device *see* automated fingerspelling
glove systems *see* automated fingerspelling

H
handtapper device *see* automated fingerspelling

hearing aid
  amplitude compression 92
  analogue 80, 87, 91, **106**
  auditory brainstem implant 86
  categories 80
  cochlear implant 85
  compatibility with telephones 192
  digital 79, 80, 87, 94, **106**
  history 87
  use with infrared systems, 169
  middle ear implant 85
  prescription 77
  principles 78
  receiver *see* induction loop systems
  schematic 72
  technical terms 73
  technology 72
  telecoil *see* induction loop systems
  see also electronic aids
hearing loss
  classification of 29
  degree of 30, 31
  due to problems in cochlea 30, 32
  due to problems in middle ear 29, 32
  due to problems in neural pathways 30, 33
  due to problems in outer ear 31
hearing
  acoustics of 4, 73
  in engineering terms 3, 73, 75, 92, 102
  see also audiometry
  see also ear, anatomy; ear, physiology

I
immittance audiometry
  acoustic reflex threshold 57, 59
  definitions 56
  measurements 57
  static acoustic immittance 57, 58
  tympanometry 57, 58
impedance *see* induction loop systems
in the ear aid (ITE) *see* electronic aids
inductance *see* induction loop systems
induction loop systems
  anti-phase loop 130
  audio frequency systems 117
  automatic gain control (AGC) 143
  calibration 135
  dynamic range of a loop system 146
  effect of different loop shapes 122
  effect of different materials 122
  electrical equivalent 136
  electromagnetic principles 118
  field strength meters 135, 148

hearing aid receiver or telecoil   120, 121
listening plane   122, 123
loop impedance   137
loop inductance   137
loop installation   132
loop plane   121, 123
loop resistance   137
loop system measurements   146
magnetic field
  direction   124
  distribution   124
  strength   123, 146, 147
    function of frequency   147
    function of level   147
measurement of the loop amplifier   147
multi-combination loop system   136
overspill   122, 124, **128**, 133
reverberation time   118
speech in noise   118
standards   124, 128, **149**
two-turn loop   141
worked examples   138, 141
infrared communications systems *see* infrared systems
infrared radiation *see* infrared systems
infrared systems
  advantages   172
  application requirements   155, 157, 169
  audio sources   159
  basic principles   153
  circuits   168
  design issues   169
  diode characteristics   160, 164
  disadvantages   172
  dynamic efficiency   159
  electromagnetic radiation   153
  ergonomic issues   170
  for audio applications   154, 169
  infrared radiation   153
  interference issues   170
  light emitting diodes   160
  light, visible   153
  operational issues   156
  photodiodes   164
  PIN diodes   164
  radiators   160
  receivers   164
  regulations   172
  standards   156, **172**
  system components   157, **158**
  system placement   170
  technical features   157, 169

transmitter signal processing   159
use with hearing aids   169
intruder detector *see* alarm systems
ionisation smoke detector sensor   222
IT access, computers *see* deafblind AT
IT access *see* deafblind AT

K
Kemar *see* audiometry
keyboard, text telephone   199

L
light as actuator *see* deafblind AT
light emitting diodes (LEDs)
  as actuators   248
  infrared systems   160
light probe *see* deafblind AT
lipreading with a videophone   205
liquid level indicator *see* deafblind AT
listening plane *see* induction loop systems
loop plane *see* induction loop systems

M
magnetic field
  direction *see* induction loop systems
  distribution *see* induction loop systems
  overspill *see* induction loop systems
  strength meters *see* induction loop systems
  strength *see* induction loop systems
manual alphabet (USA, UK)   259
masking *see* pure tone audiometry   51
measurement systems
  amplifiers in   42, **44**
  biological variables   44
  decibels   43
  frequency response curves   43
  gain   43
  sources of error   44
  types of errors   44
  see also audiometry
medical ear treatments   36
microphone arrays *see* electronic aids
microphone, as a sensor   228
middle ear
  cavity   20, 25, 33
  implant *see* hearing aid
  ossicles   3, 18, **19**, 33, 38, 76
  tympanic membrane   3, **18**, 19, 22, 29, 33, 38
modem, in text telephone   199
modulation *see* transmission systems

modulator *see* transmission systems
Moon   260

N
non-medical ear treatments   36

O
optacon *see* braille devices
optical character recognition *see* braille devices
optical character recognition *see* deafblind AT
ossicles   3, 18, **19**, 33, 38, 76
overspill *see* induction loop systems

P
paging systems *see* alerting systems
period   **8**
phase   5, 7, 241
photodiodes, infrared systems   164
photoelectric smoke detector sensor   222
physiological sources of errors *see* errors
physiology *see* ear physiology
piezoelectric sensor   226
PIN diodes, infrared systems   164
pinna   2, 15, **16**
portable speech processors   108
power amplifiers   44, 230
    Class AB   237
    Class C   235
pressure sensor   226
pure tone audiometer   52
    calibration of   64
    commercial designs   52
    standards   55
    technical description of   53
    technical specification of   55
pure tone audiometry   47, 48
    audiograms   47, 49
    masking   51
    noise   48
    test procedure   48

R
radiation *see* infrared systems
radio based concepts *see* electronic aids
radio based transmission systems   237
RALPH device *see* automated fingerspelling
resistance *see* induction loop systems
retinitis pigmentosa   257
reverberation time *see* induction loop systems

ringer pitch control *see* telephony
room thermometer *see* deafblind AT

S
sensors
    carbon monoxide sensor   223
    differential temperature sensor   222
    fire alarms   **221**
    fixed temperature sensor   221
    ionisation smoke detector   222
    microphone   228
    photoelectric smoke detector   222
    piezoelectric sensor   226
    pressure sensor   226
    sound sensor   **228**
sidetone control *see* telephony
signal processing
    see alerting systems; electronic aids; infrared systems
signing with videophone   207
simple sounds   **9**
smoke alarm *see* alarm systems
sound intensity   8, 38, 118
sound level meters *see* audiometry
SPARTAN   259
spectacles aid *see* electronic aids
spectral analysis   **10**, 75
    filtering   **10**, 12
speech in noise *see* induction loop systems
speech processors, portable   108
speech, sound intensity   118
standards
    audiometry   **61**
    induction loop systems   124, 128, **149**
    infrared systems   156, **172**
    pure tone audiometer   55
    text telephone   **201**
    V.18 in text telephone,   **201**
    videophone   208
        H.320   **209**
        H.323   **209**
        H.324   **209**
static acoustic immittance *see* immittance audiometry
superheterodyne receiver   239
suppliers
    alarm systems   255
    alerting systems   255
    deafblind AT   **296**

T
Taciwatch *see* deafblind AT
tactaid devices *see* deafblind AT
tactile marking *see* deafblind AT

Index

tactile sound recognition *see* deafblind AT
Tadoma   260
talking hands *see* automated fingerspelling
TAM alerting device *see* deafblind AT
telecommunications *see* deafblind AT; telephony
telephone technology *see* telephony
telephony
   accessibility design   192
   additional receiver   193
   amplification   193
   benchmarking   179
   call arrival indication (ringing)   190
   conceptual design   178
   design for hearing impairment   178
   digital technology   181
   hearing aid compatibility   192
   introduction   177
   iterative improvement   179
   the modern telephone   180, 182
   other accessibility features   195
   ringer pitch and volume control   193
   sidetone control   189
   starting the call   184
   transmission circuit design   187
   transmission of signalling information   184
   user centred telephone design   177, 178, 180
   visual display   194
   Wheatstone bridge circuit   189
   see also text telephone; videophone
television *see* actuators
text converters *see* braille devices
text telephone
   application aspects   196
   basic principles   196
   display   199
   in-call indicator   200
   keyboard   199
   line interface   198
   line status   200
   microcontroller   198
   modem   199
   standards   201
   talk-through procedure   201
   transmission circuit   198
   V.18 standard   201
transistors in amplifiers   231
transmission systems
   amplitude   241
   demodulator   244
   frequency   241
   modulation   241
   modulator   242
   phase   241
   radio frequency   237
   superheterodyne receiver   239
   transmitter   238
trigger units, comparison   252
   see also alerting systems
tuned amplifiers   234
two-turn loops *see* induction loop systems
tympanic membrane   3, **18**, 19, 22, 29, 33, 38
tympanometry *see* immittance audiometry

U

universal communications text browser (ucon) *see* deafblind AT
user centred telephone design *see* telephony
Usher's syndrome   257

V

versabraille *see* braille devices
vestibule   24
vibrating alarm clock *see* deafblind AT
vibro-tactile devices   249
video signal compression *see* videophone
videophone   203
videophone
   applications aspects   206
   basic principles   203
   frame rate   205
   future systems   210
   use with lipreading   205
   use with signing   207
   spatial resolution   205
   standards   208
     H.320   209
     H.323   209
     H.324   209
   video signal compression   203
   visual distortion   205
visible light *see* infrared systems
voice activity detection *see* electronic aids
voltage amplifiers   44, 230, **233**
volume control *see* telephony

W

web guidelines *see* deafblind AT
Wheatstone bridge circuit *see* telephony

Z

zwislocki coupler *see* audiometry